PSYCHEDELIC NEW YORK

INTOXICATING HISTORIES
Series Editors: Virginia Berridge and Erika Dyck

Whether on the street, off the shelf, or over the pharmacy counter, interactions with drugs and alcohol are shaped by contested ideas about addiction, healing, pleasure, and vice and their social dimensions. Books in this series explore how people around the world have consumed, created, traded, and regulated psychoactive substances throughout history. The series connects research on legal and illegal drugs and alcohol with diverse areas of historical inquiry, including the histories of medicine, pharmacy, consumption, trade, law, social policy, and popular culture. Its reach is global and includes scholarship on all periods. Intoxicating Histories aims to link these different pasts as well as to inform the present by providing a firmer grasp on contemporary debates and policy issues. We welcome books, whether scholarly monographs or shorter texts for a broad audience focusing on a particular phenomenon or substance, that alter the state of knowledge.

1 Taming Cannabis
Drugs and Empire in Nineteenth-Century France
David A. Guba, Jr

2 Cigarette Nation
Business, Health, and Canadian Smokers, 1930–1975
Daniel J. Robinson

3 Remedicalising Cannabis
Science, Industry, and Drug Policy
Suzanne Taylor

4 Mixing Medicines
The Global Drug Trade and Early Modern Russia
Clare Griffin

5 Drugging France
Mind-Altering Medicine in the Long Nineteenth Century
Sara E. Black

6 Psychedelic New York
A History of LSD in the City
Chris Elcock

PSYCHEDELIC NEW YORK

A HISTORY OF LSD IN THE CITY

CHRIS ELCOCK

McGill-Queen's University Press

Montreal & Kingston · London · Chicago

© McGill-Queen's University Press 2023

ISBN 978-0-2280-1671-7 (cloth)
ISBN 978-0-2280-1672-4 (paper)
ISBN 978-0-2280-1803-2 (ePDF)
ISBN 978-0-2280-1804-9 (ePUB)

Legal deposit second quarter 2023
Bibliothèque nationale du Québec

Printed in Canada on acid-free paper that is 100% ancient forest free
(100% post-consumer recycled), processed chlorine free

Library and Archives Canada Cataloguing in Publication
Title: Psychedelic New York : a history of LSD in the city / Chris Elcock.
Names: Elcock, Chris, author.
Series: Intoxicating histories ; 6.
Description: Series statement: Intoxicating histories ; 6 | Includes bibliographical
references and index.
Identifiers: Canadiana (print) 20220491623 | Canadiana (ebook) 2022049164X |
ISBN 9780228016717 (cloth) | ISBN 9780228016724 (paper) | ISBN 9780228018032
(ePDF) | ISBN 9780228018049 (ePUB)
Subjects: LCSH: LSD (Drug)—New York (State)—New York—History. | LCSH:
Hallucinogenic drugs—New York (State)—New York—History. | LCSH:
Recreational drug use—New York (State)—New York—History.
Classification: LCC HV5822.L9 E43 2023 | DDC 362.29/4097471—dc23

Contents

Figures   vii

If You're Going to New York City   5

1 Psychoactive Licence: Drugs and Urban Bohemia in a World Capital   18

2 Leary before LSD: Psilocybin, High Society, and the Birth of a Psychedelic Movement   42

3 Chemical Archetypes: From Experimental Science to Psychedelic Therapy   63

4 New York on Acid   86

5 Building Utopia: Nina Graboi, the East Village, and the Psychedelic Counterculture   107

6 Kaleidoscope Eyes: Isaac Abrams, Psychedelic Art, and Multimedia Light Shows   132

7 Changing Scenes: Prohibition and the Demise of Psychedelic Idealism   155

8 The Sixties Happened in the Seventies   180

A Wave That Never Rolled Back   198

Acknowledgments   205

Notes   207

Index   255

Figures

4.1 From left: Dan Rattiner, Walter Bowart, and brothers Allen and Don Katzman. 14 January 1966. Reproduced from nyujournalismprojects.org. *98*

5.1 Inside the Psychedelicatessen circa 1967–68. Reproduced courtesy of Susun Weed. *126*

6.1 An invitation to the Abrams' psychedelic art exhibition. Reproduced courtesy of Isaac Abrams. *140*

9.1 White Light Fungal Delight. 2022. Reproduced courtesy of Isaac Abrams. *202*

PSYCHEDELIC NEW YORK

To all those who helped along the way

If You're Going to New York City

"Turn on, tune in, and drop out." Timothy Leary solemnly paused between each verb to allow the message to sink in. He wore an immaculate white robe, and flowers crowned his head. The occasion was the first "Human Be-In" of 14 January 1967. At the San Francisco Golden Gate Park, more than 20,000 people heard Leary's infamous catch-phrase inviting psychedelic experimentation and withdrawal from society. The cream of the city's rock bands took part, as did some of the seminal countercultural figures of the time like Allen Ginsberg and Jerry Rubin.

The Be-In, however, was a false dawn for psychedelic enthusiasts. By October 1966, the state of California had prohibited LSD following reports of widespread recreational use. The following year, the so-called "Summer of Love" caused scores of teenagers from all over the country to flock to San Francisco's Haight-Ashbury district. Many of them had been awe-struck by television footage of the Be-in, and they were eager to make the scene. But what was meant to signal the heyday of psychedelia was marked by indiscriminate drug use and sexual violence.

Outside San Francisco, things got worse. In 1968, Leary was arrested for marijuana possession for a third time in Orange County, and two years later he was sent to prison. The next year, sociopath Charles

Manson ordered the followers of his LSD cult to murder five people in Los Angeles, and a few months later a group of acid-crazed Hell's Angels beat Meredith Hunter to death at the Altamont Rock Festival.

Over the past decades, these stories have been told endlessly in popular books and documentaries about the psychedelic Sixties. By feeding on those events and the vivid images they conjure, we are left with the impression that the psychedelic culture of the 1960s started with good intentions but followed an all-too-familiar path of disintegration[1] at a time when the civil rights and anti-war movements were also splitting as a result of internal radicalization.

Another consequence of this uneven coverage is that California remains the focal point of psychedelia. Notwithstanding Leary's communal experiments at Millbrook and the legendary Woodstock festival in upstate New York, the East Coast is hardly ever mentioned – never mind other parts of the country.[2] This book moves away from California by telling the story of psychedelic New York, which is just as historically important if not more so.

Lysergic Acid Diethylamide-25 was discovered in 1938 by Swiss chemist Albert Hofmann, who self-experimented with the drug five years later.[3] LSD was colourless, tasteless, odourless, and dosed in micrograms (by contrast, mescaline, the other major psychedelic investigated at the time, was dosed in milligrams). The experience could vary quite dramatically depending on a set of variables such as the environment in which it was taken, the user's personality, the intention, the purity of the dose, and the dosage itself. As a result, the effects of LSD remained somewhat unpredictable, but a 100-microgram dose was usually enough to induce a full-blown psychedelic experience full of colourful and swirling visions, moments of deep introspection, as well as more disquieting moments. Stronger dosage could lead to users describing a disintegration of the ego or a mystical experience, depending on the interpretation. Most of the acute effects wore off after ten or twelve hours, but they often reported feeling milder effects for a few days.

After the war, psychiatrists in Europe and the Americas began conducting research into LSD. Initially, they were interested in the drug's ability to induce a temporary psychosis that might help them to better understand this disease of the mind. But they soon realized that it could also be used as an adjunct to treat mental illness and alcoholism.[4]

Meanwhile, the CIA was quietly experimenting with LSD and other mind-altering substances, hoping to find the ultimate truth serum or a weapon that could temporarily incapacitate large populations.[5]

In the 1960s, and particularly in the second part of the decade, a small but increasingly visible segment of Americans experimented with acid and other psychedelic drugs like the mescaline-containing peyote cactus, psilocybin (the main alkaloid in "magic mushrooms"), and DMT (dimethyltryptamine), creating a distinctive psychedelic culture. At its heart were certain influential figures, including Harvard professors Leary and Richard Alpert (later known as Baba Ram Dass), who formed a psychedelic movement.[6] This movement sought to radically transform American culture by presenting acid as a magic bullet that could trigger a life-changing experience in users and give them new ontological insights. With so many turned-on individuals, the logic went, the world would become a better place.

The alleged revelatory power of the psychedelic experience soon formed a counterculture that sought alternative ways of life in which acid use played an important part,[7] while others interpreted the powerful psychedelic experience as a reconnection with the Divine.[8] British intellectual Aldous Huxley, along with other influential writers, produced important psychedelic literature.[9] Different artists were fascinated by the visionary states of the drug experience and drew on them to produce ground-breaking art.[10]

In 1968, US authorities banned LSD and psychedelics, citing public health concerns, and they later discredited their main advocates.[11] Acid continued to be used recreationally (and illegally),[12] but the new legislation, combined with changes in the scientific culture of the time,[13] virtually ended psychedelic research and, in some instances, drove therapists underground.[14] Since the 1990s, however, psychedelic science has come back to the fore of psychopharmacology and the neurosciences.[15] Other voices are calling for an end to the prohibition of psychedelic substances by arguing that it is a form of religious persecution.[16]

This very brief overview suggests that the history of psychedelics[17] is complex. As this book documents, nowhere was this more apparent than in New York City, a global metropolis that has occupied a unique place in the world's imagination.

From its beginning as a trading post, New York has become one of the most culturally diverse cities in the world and the main gateway to the US: "One third of all the people and goods that ever entered the United States came through the mile-wide Narrows, now spanned by the Verrazano Bridge."[18] As a major entry port, it became attractive for business from its colonial days, and although recent decades have seen the wealth gap widen, postwar New York was in fact ruled by generous welfare policies.

But in this booming metropolis, which welcomed returning servicemen and mobilized women, as well as waves of migrants, successive mayoral administrations struggled to strike a balance between welfare, public utilities, economic growth, and deficit. In the early 1970s, the city was on the brink of collapse as a result of poor book-keeping, a declining manufacturing base, and nationwide suburbanization (a.k.a. "white flight") that began after the war.[19]

This social and economic crisis coincided with the growing use of addictive drugs, which was especially visible among working-class and minority communities in poorer neighbourhoods.[20] But while some New Yorkers were shooting up heroin and taking amphetamines, others had discovered the far more intriguing category of psychedelic drugs and its star pupil, LSD.

The story of New York psychedelia has yet to be told,[21] in large part because the San Francisco Bay Area is still perceived as *the* psychedelic hotspot of the 1960s. In particular, the city's Haight-Ashbury district attracted countless numbers of young Americans throughout the decade, and the hip quarter certainly harboured a colourful psychedelic culture. In most histories set in that area, acid rock band the Grateful Dead, Ken Kesey's psychedelic parties, and LSD manufacturer cum psychedelic philanthropist Augustus Owsley Stanley give it an aura of egalitarianism and illustrate the city's long-lasting spirit of tolerance.[22]

But psychedelic Bohemianism was just as present in New York City's Greenwich Village, which has long been considered the Bohemian capital of the United States.[23] In the second part of the decade, the neighbouring East Village became the East Coast counterpoint to Haight-Ashbury by harbouring a local counterculture. Psychedelic happenings like Kesey's were not an isolated phenomenon in the west but rather were rivalled by New York's sophisticated art scene, which also included seminal painters and multimedia artists.[24] In fact, the "Acid Tests" Kesey organized on the West Coast in the mid-Sixties may have been remembered as uniquely influential because of Tom Wolfe's hyperbolic chronicles of his swashbuckling acid adventures,[25] which "probably turned on far more people to psychedelic culture than the Acid Tests."[26] But Kesey, who freely admitted that he was "far more conservative than Barry Goldwater can imagine,"[27] never saw himself as a psychedelic prophet or a countercultural hero – "mostly just a talented writer who liked to get high and have fun with his friends."[28]

A closer look at New York not only reveals that the city cultivated its own psychedelic culture but points to a much deeper history of drugs that can be traced right back to Greenwich Village and Mabel Dodge Luhan's landmark peyote party in the early twentieth century. When the cactus came back to the Village in the mid-1950s, scientific investigations into LSD and mescaline were well underway in the city. The doctors studying the effects of these drugs on the human mind and the therapists using them as adjuncts did not have to look far for provisions. Indeed, chemical companies based in the city were making mescaline available for research,[29] and the Swiss firm Sandoz that owned the patent to manufacture LSD had a local branch there, which research teams from all over the country acknowledged beginning in 1950.[30]

Subsequently, Sandoz started a plant in Hanover, New Jersey – a stone's throw away from Manhattan. As early as 1957, LSD was crossing the Hudson River and reaching New York's Bohemian enclaves long before it was circulating in California.[31] A year later, Hofmann synthesized psilocybin, and by 1961 the drug was circulating around high society and the cultural vanguard, courtesy of Leary and Ginsberg.[32] And beginning in 1963, DMT was trickling out of a makeshift laboratory in Brooklyn, probably the first of its kind.[33] Hence, ordinary New Yorkers could easily access psychedelics in or outside therapeutic settings, and the circulation of these drugs had a major impact on the city.

As an international hub for immigration, finance, media, business, advertising, pharmaceutical development, psychoanalysis, jazz, the arts, and the avant-garde, postwar New York gave birth to a sophisticated psychedelic culture. Leary's time in California is well documented, but he was just as influential on the East Coast, where his psychedelic campaign would not have been the same without the help of the local wealthy and the jazz scene. Psychedelics also found keen supporters in the New York City media, including *Time* and *Life* magazines, along with newspapers like the *East Village Other* and the *Village Voice*. Business people saw a lucrative potential in psychedelia and set up psychedelic stores and nightclubs to tap into the growing market. Some psychedelic artists went into advertising when companies realized that the visual codes of psychedelia could lend an aura of hipness to various commodities.

This deep history of drugs points to another striking feature of New York psychedelia. In the Californian narrative, the psychedelic culture faded toward the end of the 1960s, freezing its geography and timeline in the process.[34] To be sure, the end of the decade and the early 1970s saw the passing of new federal legislation that deemed psychedelics highly dangerous and without medical potential; the arrests of Leary, Kesey, and several underground chemists; and declining LSD quality as a result of the prohibition.

On the surface, it would seem that New York City had followed a similar downward trajectory. In the second part of the decade, young users often lacked an experienced mentor[35] to guide them through the sometimes challenging acid trip. Many drug dealers were prepared to sell any product vaguely resembling LSD, such as the highly potent but dangerous STP (2,5-Dimethoxy-4-methylamphetamine). What's more, heroin, amphetamine, and cocaine dealers began pushing their products in a much more aggressive way to oust psychedelics, for it made more economic sense to sell habit-forming drugs than non-addictive substances that might be used once or twice in a lifetime.

Exaggerated warnings about psychedelics did not help. In 1966, the president of the New York State Council on Drug Addiction infamously claimed that "Gram for gram, ingestion for ingestion, LSD is far more dangerous than heroin"[36] – a highly misleading contention, given that acid is non-addictive and dosed in micrograms. Those who paid attention to these warnings might have reasoned that heroin was milder than acid. But for the better-informed drug users, this was nothing less than propaganda, and if authorities had lied about psychedelics, then perhaps they had also lied about heroin. In certain neighbourhoods where psychedelics had been plentiful, smack consumption increased accordingly when some drug users realized that they had yet to try the "king of drugs."[37] This occurred at a time when the baby boomers were more likely to experiment with drugs, and their significant numbers were enough to create an atmosphere of a drug epidemic.[38]

That New York's narcotic use peaked at the same time that the city seemed to be in a state of decay would be enough to conclude that psychedelia was following a similar decline. But that was not the case.

Such a reductive interpretation is premised on an indelible association of LSD with the Sixties even though many New Yorkers continued to experiment with psychedelics in the subsequent decades. It also assumes that radical psychedelia *was* psychedelia. But while New York's psychedelic counterculture did not survive the Sixties, it is just one part of the story.[39]

Indeed, the acid culture was still alive thanks to its art scene and the local graffiti artists who were painting under the influence around the city. Psychedelia also made inroads into the nascent disco scene through the historic parties organized by disc jockey David Mancuso. New York City continued to host psychedelic research well into the 1970s when the overwhelming majority of scientific investigations had come to a halt with the changing regulations of clinical trials in 1962 and after Sandoz recalled most of its LSD stock in 1966. In the meantime, Howard Lotsof had discovered the anti-addictive properties of the mysterious ibogaine, and in the following decades he built a broad coalition with the radical left and Black Power to investigate its pharmacology.

A close examination of this history thus challenges three widespread narratives: first, it counters the idea that psychedelia disappeared with the Sixties[40]; second, it disrupts the image of a dying city in the 1970s; and, via Lotsof's ibogaine movement and the other remaining clinical investigations, it points to greater historical continuity in psychedelic science, which was believed to have died in the mid-1970s,[41] only to be resurrected in the early 1990s and thereafter.[42]

In an attempt to do justice to what is an important but neglected aspect of postwar life, this history of psychedelic New York is based on a multi-dimensional interpretation of the drug experience and of the city's psychedelic culture. LSD had the power to alter consciousness, create incredible sensory experiences, and lead to moments of profound self-examination. But actual experiences remained somewhat unpredictable, and the insights that came about as a result of psychedelic experimentation could vary quite dramatically from one person to another.[43]

Some LSD users reported a feeling of transcendence that they understood as spiritual, regardless of their religious upbringing. Others concluded that the society they lived in was deeply flawed and desperately needed to be transformed. Still others saw the drug as an important tool to probe the mind and facilitate psychotherapy. And some interpreted the swirling visions as a deep aesthetic experience and claimed to have found a new artistic sensibility through their experimentation.

In turn, many of these users reported life-changing experiences that gave new directions to their lives. Some artists claimed that LSD was responsible for starting their careers. Others created syncretic psychedelic churches or turned to Eastern spirituality as a result of their experiences. Still others decided that psychedelics should be freely distributed to naturally bring about social change to American society. And psychiatrists, analysts, and lay people alike used LSD to treat mental illness and to deepen self-understanding.

Because the psychedelic experience could take users in so many different directions, these multiple meanings often overlapped. Some artists incorporated spirituality into their paintings while others created installations to disorient the senses in an attempt to replicate or amplify the psychedelic experience. Others embarked on a psychedelic campaign to change the world in a way that blended politics and religion. Some patients who underwent psychedelic therapy resented, under the influence, some of the social norms of the time and developed countercultural sensibilities. This is testimony to the unique nature of the psychedelic drug experience, in contrast to the effects of habit-forming drugs like heroin that remained far more predictable.

By analyzing LSD and psychedelics in this multi-dimensional fashion, the chapters ahead give a clearer voice to New York City's acid users. For instance, this book will not use the word "hippie."[44] While some hippies presented themselves as such, some New Yorkers are quite uncomfortable with the term. Psychedelic experimenter Brad considers it a "silly word,"[45] and former activist Chuck Gould is just as suspicious: "I never considered myself to be a 'hippie.' I don't think any of us did. The whole concept was kind of weird. 'Hippie': What is that?"[46]

Even in the Sixties, critics were blaming the media for the popularization of the word.[47] Radical leftist Abbie Hoffman was one of the first to openly dismiss hippies as "a myth created by media and as such they are forced to play certain media-oriented roles."[48] Art Kleps, who ran a psychedelic church in upstate New York and who was a prominent figure in the psychedelic movement, concurred: "The media and media mongers like Tim [Leary] used the term constantly but the Psychedelians [sic] I knew in the 60s almost never used it to refer to themselves."[49] A reader of the Village Voice likewise took issue with the word popularized by the "establishment press" and voiced his concern in much stronger terms by equating it with a form of bigotry.[50]

Non–drug users were just as critical because being hip implied that the rest of the population were un-hip "squares." In a letter to the editor of the *East Village Other*, one woman presented herself in satirical terms: "I am an Establishment Square. That is to say, I live in the Outer Reaches of Darkest Trenton, in a split-level house with my husband and two children. I have never taken (used?) pot, grass, or acid, and I don't intend to. My hair is short; I wear lipstick and high heels. I am faithful to my husband. I enjoy cooking and gardening."[51] This book avoids such reductions by presenting New York psychedelia as a complex cultural phenomenon that resists easy categorization.

Furthermore, the chapters ahead challenge the notion that acid users were predominantly teenagers or in their early twenties, which is part of another reductive understanding of the 1960s as the setting for a "generational quarrel."[52] At the turn of the century, others had likewise championed the Manhattan young as the guardians of modernity and the purveyors of radicalism. "In reality, however, bohemian circles in the 1910s were as mixed by generation as they were by sex and social origins, with middle-aged people … freely speaking with fresh-faced college graduates."[53] Regardless of the media coverage of drug use among the young, the experimentations of high school and college students is only one part of the picture.

On one hand, the increase in LSD consumption in the second part of the 1960s was indeed the result of a greater number of young Americans experimenting, and there are two likely explanations for this. First, the surge probably happened as a result of Leary's far more aggressive promotion of these drugs that explicitly pitted the young against adults. Second, the measures designed to curb non-medical acid use had the effect of shifting the source of supplies away from legal channels and the grey market. Whereas New Yorkers of all ages might have accessed LSD through their physician, their therapist, or a friend working at Sandoz, the gradual crackdown on the drug spelled the end of licit sources. Prospective users now had to turn to the streets, and younger people were more likely to risk contact with the drug underworld and substandard materials.

On the other hand, the increased media coverage that accompanied this trend created a distorted impression of a youth-driven LSD movement. The short-lived *World Journal Tribune* expressed this in a series of articles describing a "drug cult" in New York City and lamented the youthful nature of its population: "They are, in frighteningly increasing numbers, high school students, and a great proportion of them think they have found, in drugs, the answer to all their problems."[54] In another article, the paper allegedly interviewed "one of the leaders of the young drug cult" and underscored the supposed prevalence of LSD on college campuses.[55]

Yet there were no stereotypical LSD users, even though they were mostly white and educated.[56] In the late 1950s and in the first half of the Sixties, Leary's psychedelic research and Huxley's experimentations with mescaline and LSD drew a broad range of Americans regardless of age, gender, sexual orientation, religious background, political affiliation, and occupation.[57] New York media magnate Henry Luce, owner of *Time* and *Life* magazines, and his wife Clare Boothe are striking examples of this pluralism: both were mature adults who identified as Protestant conservatives, but they were quite open about their experimentation with LSD under medical supervision.[58] More broadly, these drugs were used by a wide pool of New Yorkers like stockbrokers and real estate agents, which makes it impossible to reduce the average acid user to a unique profile.

Consequently, there was never one but myriad experiences with and attitudes toward psychedelics. Lay users, members of the psychedelic movement, scientists, and religious figures frequently engaged in heated debates to decide what qualified as legitimate drug use. Just as the civil rights and anti-war movements were riddled with internal conflicts, psychedelia also had its fair share of tensions within.[59] On the surface, then, New York's complex psychedelic culture might be understood as the product of a turbulent decade marred by disagreement.[60] But discord can also be understood as a more positive form of pluralism,[61] and this book reveals that there were important moments of cooperation and mutual understanding in New York psychedelia.[62]

To better understand how a psychedelic experience could be influenced by environmental variables, this book pays close attention to New York City's geographical spaces. Several locations became key for psychedelic drug users because they offered the supportive environment necessary for the experience to unfold with minimal risk. The notion of "set and setting" is key to understanding the mechanisms behind the psychedelic experience.[63] It refers to a user's psychological circumstances (both immediate and long-term) and to the environmental variables surrounding the user. Set and setting are critical to the way a psychedelic experience may unfold. For instance, a person who has repressed trauma (long-term set) or who has just heard some bad news (short-term set) is likely to be affected by these factors during the course of the experience. Likewise, taking LSD in a stressful environment, rather than in a calm atmosphere, is likely to amplify those negative elements. The experience was also dependent on the purity of the drug as well as its dosage.

Before offering a quick overview of the chapters ahead, a few caveats are in order. First, although this book is set in postwar New York City, it will occasionally take the reader beyond the city limits because some of its central figures had important experiences outside the metropolis. Among those locations, Leary's Massachusetts home, his Harvard office, and his acid commune in upstate New York allowed several New Yorkers to discover psilocybin and LSD and in turn to influence local psychedelia.

Second, some readers may be dismayed to see Timothy Leary feature so prominently. When I began my research, I wanted to give a clearer voice to "ordinary" acid users, but I soon realized that Leary had exerted a unique influence on New York. In my portrayal, Leary comes across as a deeply flawed individual but one who nonetheless introduced many influential New Yorkers to psychedelics and left a visible imprint on New York psychedelia. In the process, this book puts to bed the myth that his chemical revolution was bottom-up and democratic rather than top-down and elitist, an argument that he advanced in his influential but unreliable memoirs. In fact, Leary's nationwide promotion of LSD only occurred *after* his arrest in December 1965, which led him to look for support while revelling in the media limelight.

Third, some of the sources that have been used for this book, such as memoirs and interviews, point to the challenges of memory on a topic that is highly subjective and sensitive. I have supplemented these valuable autobiographies and oral histories with a broad range of archival sources as well as secondary sources. I am of course indebted to the scholars whose work has informed and shaped this book, but to avoid overwhelming non-specialist readers, I have confined my mention of prior scholarly works to the book's endnotes where they are fully referenced.

Finally, any piece of social history focusing on a global metropolis must inevitably leave some topics and people out of the picture or super-ficially discussed. To be sure, the history of psychedelic rock[64] in New York City is underdeveloped, though I hope that greater attention to the local jazz scene will partially make up for this shortcoming. As well, in-depth perspectives on the psychedelic experiences of Black and Hispanic New

Yorkers are also lacking in the sources; however, the evidence gathered here suggests that these communities stayed clear of these drugs. And the tale of Howard Lotsof's research into the anti-addictive properties of ibogaine is only partially covered and deserves a full treatment.

The story of psychedelic New York will be told in the following chapters. Chapter 1 offers an overview of the city's romance with psychoactive drugs from the late nineteenth century to the early 1960s. It introduces Greenwich Village and its distinctive brand of Bohemianism, which attracted Beat writers and poets in the postwar era, and describes the city's jazz scene. This cultural vanguard gradually reframed illicit drug use along the lines of experimentation and transgression. By the end of the Fifties, New York drug users had rediscovered peyote in Manhattan, decades after Luhan had sampled the cactus. They also encountered less-known plants such as morning glory seeds, and the positive meaning ascribed to early psychedelic experimentation was largely the product of changing media coverage following the publication of Aldous Huxley's voyages into inner space.

Chapter 2 describes Leary's early psychedelic movement before he discovered LSD and reveals how the Harvard psychologist disseminated psilocybin among the New York wealthy and the avant-garde. Chapter 3 offers perhaps the most explicit illustration of LSD during the "long Sixties" by exploring nearly three decades of psychedelic science in New York. In doing so, it focuses on early experimental research groups and then discusses how the city's psychoanalytic circles became interested in psychedelic-based therapy. Chapter 4 shows how LSD began to trickle out of the laboratories to reach the streets. While Leary played a part in the process, many New Yorkers were discovering LSD by their own means and connections. By the mid-1960s, there were growing psychedelic scenes all around the city, which allowed users to develop their own understandings of the drug.

The next two chapters exemplify the different paths psychedelics could take their users on. Chapter 5 focuses on Nina Graboi, a woman who had life-changing experiences with marijuana and psychedelics and who soon made inroads into the Greenwich Village scenes. Born Jewish in Vienna, Graboi was a Holocaust survivor and spiritual seeker who resented the climate of conformity of postwar America. She eventually became the director of the Center for the League for Spiritual Discovery, which served as a beacon for the local counterculture and for anxious parents worrying about their children's drug use. The final part of this chapter also illustrates how radical psychedelia moved away from the Village by carving out spaces in the East Village.

Chapter 6 likewise examines the transformations of psychedelic artist Isaac Abrams, one of the most underappreciated figures of the American history of psychedelia. Together with his then-wife Rachel, who also had meaningful psychedelic experiences, they organized a psychedelic exhibition that was very much the get-together moment for many of the New Yorkers who had been quietly experimenting up until that landmark event. This chapter also discusses Leary's own artistic collaborations with multimedia light-show artists and the influence of psychedelia on cinema.

Chapter 7 begins by discussing the backlash that occurred as a result of increased psychedelic drug consumption, particularly among the young New Yorkers who had been drawn to the thrills of communal living in the East Village. They were met by hostile locals who longed for better living in an area where illicit drug use was responsible for a great deal of damage to people and property. It was also around that time that several gurus arrived from India and advised acid users to shun drugs and get high on their alternative spirituality. Yet LSD use continued in midtown among well-heeled New Yorkers and on Madison Avenue when advertisers realized they could recycle the codes of psychedelia for commercial purposes.

The final chapter begins in Central Park in the early 1970s where a new generation of acid heads were experimenting in a more supportive setting than on the city streets. While heroin, cocaine, and crack dominated the downtown drug scenes during that decade and the 1980s, psychedelics did not disappear. Howard Lotsof's ibogaine movement gained traction, and LSD and psilocybin were joined by MDMA and new psychoactive compounds that were unknown to authorities. Meanwhile, psychedelic art had become a viable feature of New York's art scene, embodied by the work of Alex Grey and a 2007 psychedelic art exhibition at the Whitney Museum of American Art.

1

Psychoactive Licence
Drugs and Urban Bohemia in a World Capital

In the second half of the nineteenth century, the rise of the advertising sector and the growing influence of the pharmaceutical industry allowed New Yorkers to discover a number of household pills, syrups, and tonics containing psychoactive substances.[1] Thus began the city's involvement with mind-altering drugs. Addiction and the social problems that came with it did not leave the city in the following century, and gradually drug use made its way to the cultural avant-garde, which reappraised it along the lines of exploration and transgression.

In fact, meaningful drug use found an early audience in Greenwich Village, which likely witnessed the first ever peyote session run by a group of white Bohemians. The Villagers, who saw themselves as a breed apart, were always on the lookout for new ways of pushing the boundaries of experimentation and respectability, and it is no surprise that drugs gradually became part of their lifestyle. After World War II, narcotics and psychedelics alike became an important feature of life in the Village.

The transformation of drug use into a catalyst for cultural subversion received an important boost from some of New York's jazz players, who enabled the transition from swing to bebop during the 1940s. This new style, which had faster and more complex improvised lines, dissonant chord structures, and very few arrangements, was born on the fringes of the jazz world. Bop players rejected the commercialism of swing, and they longed to take jazz to unprecedented artistic heights so that white America would stop viewing their music as mere entertainment. These dissenting Black musicians became "an underclass within an underclass,"[2] and this distinctively subcultural edge was just as manifest in their drug use. Charlie "Bird" Parker, Miles Davis, Sonny Rollins, and John Coltrane were notorious for their heroin habits, which soon became an important feature of their subculture.[3] But the bop scene also nurtured the use of marijuana and amphetamines, which helped musicians to articulate their vision and listeners to appreciate their fast-paced sound.

Among the white New Yorkers to discover the local bop scene was a young aspiring writer by the name of Jack Kerouac, who was ambitiously looking for a ground-breaking form of literary expression that would transcend social conventions. Kerouac's apartment near Columbia University attracted more literary-inclined folks like poet Allen Ginsberg and an older writer named William Burroughs. The three of them drew tremendous inspiration from bebop musicians, their drug use, and their second-class citizenry. By the mid-1950s, they had successfully incorporated bop into a form of Beat literature that introduced Americans to drugs and Black culture. But in keeping with a longer tradition of Bohemian ambivalence toward Blackness,[4] the Beats became attracted to Blacks as a form of romantic primitivism and because they liked to think that they were just as alienated.[5]

Concurrently, peyote reappeared in the Village, along with other psychedelic plants like ibogaine and morning glory seeds. But this time around, they were here to stay. New York's influential publishing and media sectors effectively challenged the conventional ways of depicting psychoactive experiences, and this had important consequences for the local readership. Many New Yorkers were awe-struck by Aldous Huxley's elegant description of the mescaline experience, and soon news of a ground-breaking Beat style of poetry and literature simultaneously attracted cohorts of the nation's fledging Bohemians to the Village.

Drugs in the City

In the final decades of the nineteenth century, city-dwellers became acquainted with opium smoking, which had arrived in the United States with Chinese immigration. At first, American authorities did not mind opium because it was confined to the West Coast Chinatowns, but its reputation gradually changed as smoking trickled out of these areas and reached young men, prostitutes, gamblers, and criminals.[6]

In New York, news of clandestine opium dens in several Chinatown basements began to circulate during the 1880s[7] after San Francisco had become the first municipality to prohibit opium in 1875. Other drug users could be found congregating in a lavishly decorated house close to 42nd Street where they smoked a mixture of hashish, henbane, crushed datura seeds, and tobacco while drinking a coca-infused brew.[8] By 1909, federal legislation had prohibited the importation of opium for non-medical purposes, and in New York it became an eccentric luxury in the following decades, with "playboys, impresarios, show girls, high-class prostitutes, successful hustlers, and big-time gangsters" reported as indulging.[9]

In the meantime, opiate consumption was boosted by the commercialization of a highly effective pain reliever. Morphine, the main alkaloid of opium, was isolated in the early nineteenth century and promised a therapeutic consistency that crude opium lacked. In the second part of the century, the spread of the hypodermic needle gradually helped morphine to supplant medical opium. The Civil War, in particular, was decisive in the transition.[10]

The other major psychoactive drug that rapidly moved out of the medical realm was cocaine, which seemed to embody the miracles of modern science. It was used as a local anaesthetic (particularly for eye surgery) and a powerful stimulant that could also elevate the mood.[11] Non-medical use first appeared in southern cities like New Orleans among working-class Blacks looking for ways to sustain hard, often uninterrupted labour.[12] Coke soon reached northern cities, and in New York the police commissioner singled out the "prostitutes of the lowest order" and the "parasites" making a living off them.[13]

In the early twentieth century, oral opiate consumption began to wane, as a partial result of new pharmaceutical developments. In 1898, Bayer marketed the highly potent heroin as an effective cough syrup, and a year later the firm released aspirin, which soon replaced opium for many common afflictions. As non-medical cocaine became stigmatized and subjected to restrictions, many users grew frustrated by its subsequent scarcity and rising prices, and they started sniffing the cheaper heroin.

As the public and medical doctors became more aware of the dangers of opiate abuse, the federal government passed the Pure Food and Drug Act in 1906, which mandated drug manufacturers to list the ingredients of their products. A few years later, America began its century-long war on drugs with the 1914 Harrison Narcotics Tax Act. This landmark piece of legislation was devised to control non-medical drug use and was to have significant impacts both at home and abroad.[14]

But while authorities were targeting cocaine and opiate abuse, New York's cultural avant-garde was already looking elsewhere for more rewarding psychoactive experiences. That same year, New York became almost certainly the first city to host a psychedelic session with the peyote cactus. As Congress was about to approve the Harrison Act, anthropologist Raymond Harrington,[15] who had been fascinated by Native Americans since his childhood, introduced a group of Bohemian socialites to the mysterious plant in a Greenwich Village apartment.

The hostess was the influential patron of the arts, Mabel Dodge Luhan, who was known locally for her salons that brought together the cream of urban Bohemia. Luhan's get-togethers were in many respects the embodiment of the spirit of tolerance, subversion, and experimentation that reigned in the Village. Unhindered by puritanism, her guests could freely discuss topics like eugenics, women's rights, and capitalism while smoking cigarettes and sipping liqueurs.

A fitting illustration of their interest in the latest intellectual trends was psychoanalysis, which "promised not only hedonistic self-fulfillment but creative self-expression."[16] This new form of therapy arrived in the US thanks to intellectuals from Austria and Central Europe and owed part of its success to the new perspectives these immigrants brought on American culture by virtue of their outsider status.[17] Thanks to Luhan's gatherings, many of the country's leading radicals learned about a new development in psychology and soon used it to further their political crusade by condemning the "unhealthy" Protestant work ethic and the "repressiveness of genteel, middle-class 'civilization.'"

Among those who attended such evenings was Abraham Brill, the American translator of Freud, a founding member of the New York Psychoanalytic Society, and Luhan's subsequent psychiatrist.[18] As part of her quest to understand and revisit the self, Luhan also tried astrology and spiritualism, which "seemed to hold out as much healing potential as the rather implausible 'talking cure' recently introduced from Vienna." What really made them attractive, however, was that they seemed to embody the notion that "the mind could triumph over matter."[19] So when Harrington mentioned that he had brought to the salon a cactus that had the power "to pass beyond ordinary consciousness and see things as they are in Reality," Luhan was thrilled.

After Harrington warned the group that the peyote cactus was not to be trifled with and that Indians used it in carefully structured rituals, Luhan proposed that they all try it. Around 9:00 pm, a historic peyote ceremony was underway in a West 9th Street apartment, with everyone chewing away at the bitter cactus. Among the guests were actor and feminist activist Ida Rauh, her husband and socialist Max Eastman, and theatre designer Robert Edmond Jones, as well as a skin-and-bones anarchist who had vowed never to get a job.

As her body processed the peyote, Luhan noticed a numbness take hold of her mouth and limbs, and she had an irrepressible desire to laugh. Gradually, the group felt its self-consciousness dissolve under the influence and experienced changing colours and morphing environments. One of them reported a "death of the flesh" and claimed to have found a shortcut to the soul, while another guest "saw the walls of this house fall away and ... was following a lovely river for miles through the most wonderful virginal forest [he] had ever known." The anarchist just smiled as he gazed into the void.

Later on, Luhan retired to her bedroom, but as she lay there, she became restless and realized that she was stuck with the effects of the peyote, while the session carried on in her living room. Eventually, she went back to the group and discovered that one of the guests had disappeared. Fears of having to deal with the police took hold of her, but she then received a reassuring phone call from a friend who was taking care of the distraught guest.[20]

Luhan's worries were understandable. As a well-known public figure, she could not afford to have the press latch onto the sordid details of a drug party. The relatively unknown cactus might have been obscured by the rising rates of addiction, but as medical doctors and the police attempted to curb narcotic use, others were greatly concerned by peyote consumption in Native American settings. Just as opium's regulation was racially tainted by equating the drug with Chinese immigrants, the cactus was described "as a foreign menace, a Mexican drug damaging Indian bodies." Even some Native American Indians began to complain about licentious peyote orgies "run by good-looking males who were using the drug to enrich themselves and secure their own sexual conquests at the expense of their neighbors."[21] By 1918, several states had banned peyote, although federal prohibition remained narrowly elusive.

It is worth wondering why Luhan's combined interests in peyote, psychoanalysis, and unusual states of consciousness were not enough to start an informal group of like-minded people engrossed by psycho-active experimentation, particularly given that some local scientists were already examining the effects of mescaline on the human brain.[22] Unfortunately, nothing suggests that Luhan knew about this research, and New York City would have to wait another four decades for the cactus and mescaline to resurface in a far more favourable context.

After the passing of the Harrison Act, cocaine and heroin dominated New York's illicit drug market to a point where it most likely became the first American city to see those drugs supplant morphine in the early 1920s.[23] Because the effects of heroin were far more powerful, opiate users had a greater chance of developing a habit they might have otherwise avoided with opium, and dealers could easily mix it with other powders to maximize profits. During this transition, young working-class men became the main category of users, such as a young lad born to Italian-American parents in Greenwich Village, who began snorting heroin while working in a chandelier factory.[24]

The Harrison Act immediately created a black market in the Village's Italian area south of Washington Square Park. Back then, dealing was far more straightforward than in the following decades, defined by large-scale trafficking. "The Italian street dealers I was buying from got it from big drug dealers, maybe drug companies where they had somebody working," one former user recalled. "There was a drug company up on Thirteen Street, a big drug company, and people worked there and they were in a position to steal."[25]

As this story reveals, working-class areas in New York naturally allowed junk to flourish, but this only partly explains why it became the nation's heroin capital in the twentieth century. Back then, New York was home to the country's major pharmaceutical companies, and those firms made far more than was necessary for the legal market. Greater international cooperation led to more control over its legal production, but clandestine factories in Europe and China quickly began exporting junk to New York. By 1924, heroin had been prohibited,[26] and the United States entered a period of strict narcotic prohibition known as the classic era of drug control. In doing so, New York City became a transnational nucleus for trafficking while simultaneously providing its own residents with an endless flow of narcotics.

Other New Yorkers preferred alcoholic beverages, and they did not need to look far for supplies either. In the first decades of the twentieth century, New York was the nation's beer hub, with more breweries that Chicago, St Louis, and Milwaukee combined.[27] In Greenwich Village, writers like Ernest Hemingway, Scott Fitzgerald, and Dorothy Parker overindulged in booze, and as Luhan recalled, drinking hard was "was a very superior kind of excess that stimulated the kindliness of hearts and brought out all the pleasure." That men and women could drink together with little gender prejudice further illustrated the Village's ambition to become the country's shining light of modernity.[28]

The Prohibition of the 1920s turned the Village into an even more attractive proposition. There, New Yorkers could buy booze and home-made Italian wine in various stores and restaurants, and the illegality of the transactions was in keeping with the neighbourhood's spirit of transgression.[29] Bars like the White Horse Tavern and the San Remo Café served bootlegged alcohol throughout the era,[30] and although the state of New York ended Prohibition before the national repeal of the Volstead Act, many weekenders continued to patronize the speakeasies and clubs of the area.

If anything, the modern war on drugs, which ran parallel to and often overlapped with the "noble experiment" of alcohol interdiction, was a boon for criminal organizations. Locally, Jewish and Italian traffickers imported junk from overseas with the financial assistance of Arnold Rothstein, and other infamous mob figures like Waxy Gordon carried on using the existing bootlegging channels to trade heroin after Prohibition.[31] Soon, some extreme prohibitionists suggested using firing squads to permanently solve the problem.[32] Media mogul William Randolph Hearst was a bit more measured, but he immediately saw the narcotic issue as a fitting topic for his brand of yellow reporting, and he pushed an editorial agenda of strict prohibition in his widely read papers.[33]

By the end of Prohibition, illegal narcotics had reached New York women. In 1930, an author known by her "O.W." alias published a landmark drug memoir that offered an intimate account of her coke use. On one occasion, she ingested enormous quantities of the drug in a Manhattan hotel. All that powder gave her paranoid hallucinations, and she had to seek treatment in a local hospital. As she lay in bed, she could not help but notice nurse Gray's severely damaged nostril. "She made no bones about being a doper," O.W. wrote. "In the office was a big bottle marked 'Gray, Morphine Solution.' That was hers, and she took shots at times."[34]

In the 1930s, New York was particularly hard-hit by the economic recession, and the completion of the Chrysler and Empire State buildings were a minor source of rejoicing.[35] Amid these titanic projects that added to the metropolis' impressive skyline, the 1931 incorporations of the Buddhist Society and the New York Psychoanalytic Institute were probably unimportant to most New Yorkers. Yet they further cemented the city's position as an avant-garde capital, and they would significantly influence New York psychedelia during the postwar era.

The Buddhist Society became a flagship for those who had been studying Zen under Sokei-an Sasaki. In 1916, Sokei-an landed in Greenwich Village, where he lived in a Washington Square rooming house and wrote poems and stories. A few years later, he had a profound Zen experience that changed his life: "I saw a dead horse lying on the pavement in Sixth Avenue. Saw the physical details. Something happened. In that moment, nothing was left in my mind." He travelled back to Japan to complete his training, and by the late 1920s he was a Zen master. Initially, he gave talks in Central Park and in a bookstore, and subsequently he and his students incorporated as a religion and settled on West 70th Street.[36]

The New York Psychoanalytic Society, meanwhile, had been growing steadily thanks to many American analysts training in Europe, and the incorporation of the Psychoanalytic Institute drew many European migrants fleeing Hitler.[37] Around the same time, Abraham Brill realized that psychoanalysis needed to join forces with psychiatry to become more legitimate, and by 1934 psychoanalysis was part of that discipline thanks to his efforts.[38] A decade later, however, the Society began to split over whether psychoanalysis should have stricter training standards, leading to purges of non-conforming analysts.[39] Among those who walked away was Clara Thompson, who co-founded the William Alanson

White Psychoanalytical Institute in 1943. The Institute trained analysts at 20 West 74th Street by Central Park, and it offered an alternative to orthodox Freudianism by supplementing it with community service and with an interdisciplinary approach based on the social sciences. By the end of the 1950s, psychoanalysis was so firmly rooted among the city's Bohemians that "There were times when you felt like an outsider by the mere fact of not being in psychoanalysis."[40]

Buddhism and psychoanalysis significantly influenced the Greenwich Village Bohemians, but the cultural trend that seemed to best encapsulate their appetite for transgression was jazz. In 1934, they witnessed the opening of the Village Vanguard, and this jazz club cum literary salon became known for its racially integrated audiences at a time when even the famous 52nd Street clubs were known to enforce segregation. Unsurprisingly, the Vanguard welcomed the new sound of bop during the war,[41] just as the city's entire jazz scene was moving away from Harlem. and settling in Manhattan.[42] This allowed many patrons to discover two influential drugs that helped the local transition from narcotics to psychedelics: cannabis and amphetamines.

By then, the use of marijuana, which had arrived in the US with Mexican immigration in the early twentieth century, was increasing steadily. A combination of yellow reporting and an openly racist campaign spearheaded by the Federal Bureau of Narcotics' first commissioner, Harry Anslinger, transformed grass into a gateway drug leading to crime and insanity by tying its use to ethnic minorities and the underworld. Apart from a handful of dissenters, the medical profession backed up those sensational reports,[43] and this was more than enough to justify prohibiting weed. New York State banned it in 1934, and the federal government made legal transactions virtually impossible with the Marihuana Tax Act of 1937.

Around 1940, Charlie Parker was known in jazz circles as a grass dealer rather than as an exceptional saxophone player.[44] Other users could find the herb in Times Square, where many of the Prohibition-era speakeasies had been turned into jazz clubs, and in Harlem's after-hours clubs that became known as "tea pads." To find a tea pad, smokers could count on porters at railway terminals, and once they were inside, they usually asked the bartender or a waitress.[45] Eventually, New York Mayor Fiorello LaGuardia ordered an investigation into the problem, but the reports, which concluded that most users were unemployed and aged between twenty and thirty, could not corroborate suggestions that the drug made them aggressive and antisocial.[46]

As politicians and medical doctors debated the dangers of marijuana, some of them heard the first reports of amphetamine abuse among college students in the midwest.[47] In 1934, Smith, Kline & French released Benzedrine, which was initially marketed as an inhaler that could ease nasal congestion but soon became a thrilling chemical that promised to elevate the mood and improve efficiency. Benzedrine soon appeared in the jazz world and in a smash hit by Harry "Hipster" Gibson and Slim Gaillard, "Who Put the Benzedrine in Mrs. Murphy's Ovaltine?" which was banned by a Los Angeles radio station at the end of the war.

Before turning to heroin, Parker discovered speed in Kansas City, and other New York musicians likewise developed a habit with inhalers. Some of them simply emptied their contents and mixed them in their drinks before performing in Harlem and 52nd Street jazz clubs in the early 1940s.[48] Outside the jazz scene, Florrie Fisher, a regular heroin user who supported her habit by becoming a prostitute, encountered Benzedrine while serving time in jail. Fisher and the other female inmates simply asked the prison guards, who would sell them inhalers for $2.50 apiece.[49]

As the war was coming to an end, speed was strongly connected with a Black bebop subculture that was forever pushing the limits of the genre while simultaneously experimenting with pot, heroin, and cocaine. The combination of all the above made a tremendous impression on a group of Bohemians whose lives revolved around literary, sexual, and psychoactive experimentation in New York City. The Beats were about to sow the seeds of the psychedelic Sixties in Greenwich Village.

The Birth of Psychedelic Bohemianism

As the war was coming to an end, Jack Kerouac, Allen Ginsberg, and William Burroughs and his wife Joan Vollmer moved into a South Bronx apartment. Burroughs was mostly into heroin, but his friends soon introduced the Beats to Benzedrine, which immediately appealed to Kerouac.[50] Around the same time, the Beats explored the Times Square area and enjoyed the company of prostitutes, jazz musicians, and opiate users as they hung out in jazz clubs and all-night bars.[51] As they discovered New York's criminal and artistic underbelly, they found the perfect guide in Herbert Huncke, a native Chicagoan, con artist, and addict who had introduced Burroughs to heroin.

To describe Huncke as a veteran of drug use would be an understatement. Aged twelve, he had his first toke of marijuana and read about opium dens and smugglers, which made a lifetime impression on him. After cruising around the country, Huncke arrived in New York and settled on 42nd Street in 1939. He survived by becoming a prostitute, and in the 52nd Street jazz clubs he met Charlie Parker and Billie Holiday. He even did a few burglaries with Dexter Gordon. Huncke, who led a life on the margins of society, was so fascinating to the Beats that he became a character in their subsequent literary publications. The real Herbert, however, spent the next two decades going through the revolving doors of various prisons and addiction centres and could only read about their achievements in the papers.[52]

Gradually, Kerouac and Ginsberg attracted other Beats. Among those who joined their circles was Neal Cassady. In 1949, Cassady, Ginsberg, and Kerouac set off on a cross-country trip that formed the basis of Kerouac's masterpiece *On the Road*, which he wrote in April 1951 during an uninterrupted three-week Benzedrine binge.[53] In the meantime, Cassady had introduced speed to his lover Carolyn Robinson (whom he subsequently married). One day, Ginsberg, Cassady, and Robinson were having coffee close to Columbia, and the two men took apart an inhaler and soaked the saturated paper into their cups.[54]

To them, Benzedrine was an exciting drug, but around the same time Ginsberg began his love affair with cannabis. He discovered pot through the less-known Beat poet Gerd Stern, a Jewish refugee and college dropout who had landed in the same psychiatric institution as he had.[55] Like Ginsberg, Stern was attracted to Bohemian New York and soon discovered its illicit drug subcultures. He had his first smoke from a downtown hustler known as Jimmy the Greek, who could be found dealing grass in a cafeteria. These were "toothpicks of pot, which had precious little dope in them," jokes Stern, "but we managed to enjoy them."[56]

By then, the Beats had made Greenwich Village their home. In particular, Ginsberg and Kerouac were likely to be at the San Remo at 93 MacDougal Street. "A typically dark and smoky New York bar with a loud jukebox and crowded tables, the San Remo stayed open until 4:00 A.M.," to the delight of poets, writers, painters, actors, and intellectuals. It was at the San Remo that Ginsberg met W.H. Auden,[57] an older homosexual poet who eased his concerns about coming out by sharing his own stories[58] and who would most likely have told him that he started the day on amphetamines and ended it with alcohol and barbiturates.[59] There, Miles Davis could sometimes be found nodding in a corner after his latest heroin fix, and the Beats might also bump into one of Davis's main suppliers, a bisexual woman.[60] Davis had discovered heroin in 1949 during a spell of depression, which was not helped by the racial injustice of the time, but he managed to shake off his habit in 1954.[61]

For the Beats, Greenwich Village and postwar New York were also important sites to develop their interest in Zen Buddhism – a central dimension of their quest for a New Vision. By then, Sokei-an had passed away, but months before his death the Buddhist Society was renamed the First Zen Institute of America[62] and soon relocated to Waverly Place, close to Washington Square Park. Ginsberg discovered Buddhism at the New York Public Library in 1953 and particularly enjoyed the way Columbia lecturer D.T. Suzuki described satori. That same year, Kerouac also encountered Zen in a library, and thereafter the topic became a regular feature in their conversations and literary publications.[63] Their interest in Buddhism subsequently reached their readers and further enhanced the popularization that Zen scholar Alan Watts had initiated around the same period. Watts, who very briefly studied with Sokei-an, authored the first bestseller on the topic.[64]

Watts had also attended the institute, which attracted more seekers throughout the 1950s. But for its secretary, the popularization of Zen was more like a cultural fad rather than an authentic religious awakening: "Generally the crowd – the beats and hips and others who've just found out about Zen – can't take the tremendous discipline Zen imposes. They turn around and run."[65] Certainly, the Beats and most Americans were selective in what they borrowed from Zen and other forms of spirituality, but they were nevertheless sincere about their quest.

Meanwhile, New York City's interest in unusual states of consciousness was further stimulated by the 1951 inception of the Parapsychology Foundation at 11 East 44th Street. The foundation was created by Frances

Bolton and Eileen Garrett in an attempt to study paranormal occurrences like extra-sensory perception, out-of-body experiences, and psychic phenomena. Garrett had reached international prominence in the 1930s after reportedly collecting top secret information from the captain of a crashed dirigible during several mediumistic sessions. Bolton was a philanthropist and a member of Congress who came from an affluent family with connections to Standard Oil, and her wealth enabled Garrett to fulfill her long-lasting dream of creating such an institution.[66] By the end of the 1950s, the foundation had its own academic journal, which was created to act "as a two-way bridge between the field of parapsychological studies and the scientific community as a whole,"[67] while Garrett simultaneously edited the magazine *Tomorrow*.

The combination of spiritual pluralism, illicit drugs, sexual freedom, and a unique nightlife epitomized by its jazz scene soon made Greenwich Village the centre of gravity for young Americans fleeing the bigotry of the postwar era. Chester Anderson, who subsequently experimented with mind-altering drugs and became involved in radical politics, was relieved to find sanctuary in the Village. Anderson had been raised in Memphis, Tennessee, where he had experienced strict racial segregation. But growing up, he and his friends had come to realize that Jim Crow was wrong, and they saw the situation with their Black counterparts as "a source of endless embarrassment to thinking kids." This changed quite dramatically when he moved to the Village in 1952 and began having sex and taking drugs with Black New Yorkers.[68]

Poet Diane di Prima was just as disillusioned with postwar America, and her life story reveals that she was living the Beat way of life without knowing it. It was only after encountering Ginsberg's ground-breaking poem "Howl" in the latter part of the 1950s that she realized that like-minded souls were also pushing artistic, psychoactive, and sexual boundaries. In this way, her story goes against the idea that the Beat generation was a strictly male affair and suggests that women were already dismissing the cultural norms of the time without the help of men.[69]

In the early 1950s, di Prima moved to Greenwich Village with the ambition of becoming a poet. Like Ginsberg, she felt free of puritanical America and indulged in alcohol, pot, and bisexual sex free of judgment, and she enjoyed the jazz scenes and the climate of avant-garde, risk, and transgression of the Village. One of those places was the Swing

Rendezvous, a gay and lesbian bar run by the Mafia where she felt more at home than at her parents'. There she drank beer and did the dances that came with the new sounds of rock 'n roll and rhythm 'n blues with gay and straight men alike. She also befriended a thirty-year-old Italian racketeer and did not mind his heroin habit.[70]

Around 1952, she moved to the Lower East Side, which was then going through important demographic changes. The 1948 Displaced Persons Act enabled Russian, Austrian, Romanian, and Ukrainian refugees to move in, and in the 1950s some artists, writers, and poets could also be found there, even though they remained inconspicuous.[71] Di Prima found an apartment that belonged to a former rabbi who had anticipated the influx of the Sixties by acquiring a few tenements, cutting down the apartments to smaller sizes, and renting them to impoverished New Yorkers. For the Ukrainians, Poles, and Hungarians living in the area, it was mystifying that a young white middle-class woman would want to live in this rundown ghetto, but she could not have cared less.[72]

The large-scale housing development of the postwar years mostly occurred outside city centres, and the dilapidated Lower East Side fell under the category of "slum land" that could be rehabilitated by private funds and the partial aid of federal, state, and/or city subsidies. But the area was highly unappealing to investors because it was subject to rent-control policies, which took away rehabilitation incentives that might have attracted better-off tenants. Moreover, few of the brownstone buildings that typified the area could claim to carry architectural value that might have drawn interested buyers. Finally, by virtue of its central location, the prices there remained high. As a result, the Lower East Side's population did not diversify much in the postwar years, with the exception of semi-skilled Puerto Rican workers.[73]

As far as di Prima was concerned, the rent was cheap, and she was close enough to the action of the neighbouring Greenwich Village. Gradually, young runaways and Bohemians began to move into her apartment, and she routinely found herself in bed with several people. Among them was a mathematician who had dropped out of the Electronics Research Lab at Columbia and spent most of his time reading Indian philosophy and snorting cocaine.[74] Di Prima was not interested in coke, but a few months later she made some new friends who took her to the country where she had her first experience with marijuana.[75] Subsequently, she got a temporary job at the Quixote Bookstore on MacDougal Street, where she could read the latest avant-garde literature like the Beat poetry of Gregory Corso. There she fell in love with a young man who spent his days at the Quixote playing his guitar and shooting up smack.[76]

Authorities soon became concerned by the amount of illicit drugs available in the Village. In 1952, Sheridan Square was an important place for buyers, and five years later official reports found that this hotspot had moved south to the intersection of Carmine and Bedford Streets.[77] As di Prima remembered, "There were more and more drugs available: cocaine and opium, as well as the ubiquitous heroin, but the hallucinogens hadn't hit the scene as yet."[78] Throughout the decade, heroin and cannabis remained prominent in New York's drug marketplace. A mid-fifties study on New York jazz musicians and drugs revealed that they were more likely to have tried and used marijuana, rather than heroin, and that only a handful of them were taking cocaine because of the high cost.[79]

It was around that time that the Villagers first read about mysterious psychoactive substances that promised far more worthwhile experiences than the numbing high of the opiates or the amphetamine rush. Few Bohemians would have heard about the research into hallucinogenic drugs of the time, and the likeliest reason that these intrepid New Yorkers turned to vision-inducing plants and chemicals was an important shift in the media coverage of psychoactive substances.

The War on Drugs, combined with the McCarthyist politics of suspicion of non-conformity, had led to an extreme form of censorship that prohibited the depiction of the effects of mind-altering drugs like heroin, cannabis, and cocaine. But when the highly regarded Aldous Huxley described his experimentations with mescaline in such eloquent terms, even the most rabid opponent of drugs had to sit up and listen. In 1954, New York–based *Harper's* published his "Doors of Perception," and this landmark essay created an opening for journalists eager to cover astonishing psychoactive stories after decades of restriction and at a time when the obscenity laws were waning.[80]

Huxley's essay was also important because it explicitly linked these drugs and non-Western spirituality by borrowing freely from Hindu and Buddhist traditions. Long before his chemical encounters, he had written a book that synthesized the mystical literature of many religious traditions and speculated that there might exist a universal mystical reality.[81] To him, psychedelics had confirmed his intuition in spectacular fashion.

Two years later, another seminal piece of writing reached the awe-struck Village Bohemians and brought peyote, Eastern spirituality, and Beat culture to the cultural avant-garde. Di Prima was still a burgeoning poet when she was given a copy of Ginsberg's epic masterpiece "Howl" during a house party she had organized. As she read the opening lines, she had to leave the party to fully immerse herself in the revolutionary prose away from her guests. She sat down by the Hudson River and read the poem, sensing a historic moment: "The phrase 'breaking ground' kept coming into my head. I know that this Allen Ginsberg, whoever he was, had broken ground for all of us – all few hundreds of us – simply by getting this published." Beyond the obvious poetic quality, she immediately realized that there had to be a lot more people attempting to move poetry and literature toward a more natural language.[82]

Di Prima began corresponding with Ginsberg and his friends, and eventually the Beats agreed to meet her in the Prince Street loft of one of her gay friends.[83] The Beats showed up with a lot of cheap wine, pot, and hashish, and under the influence they began to "rap" uninterrupted prose. Kerouac then grabbed one of di Prima's notebooks and "uncorrected" the poems she had written – to him, writing was about spontaneity and should not be altered or corrected. The night was capped off with a memorable session of group sex and more pot.[84]

Black poet LeRoi Jones (subsequently Amiri Baraka) followed in di Prima's footsteps. Jones was enamoured by bop, and he had befriended a recent Zen Buddhist convert who worked at an eastern bookstore called Orientalia. Like di Prima, he moved to the Lower East Side in 1957 because the rent was cheap and it was the closest he could get to the Village. There, he hung out with other fledgling poets in the quarter's coffeehouses, but contrary to Chester Anderson he slowly began to see through the cracks of its much-vaunted spirit of tolerance. In particular, one of his friends cautioned him against the Italians who looked down on Blacks – particularly Black men dating white women.[85]

It was around that time that Jones got his first experiences with drugs. While most poets, artists, and Village-goers were smoking marijuana, he sometimes snorted junk. On one occasion, he was introduced to a "speedball" combining cocaine and heroin in a Hudson Street apartment, and the effect was overwhelming. "I'd never really been that high before," Jones recalled. "The heavy drugs almost dropped me to my knees, but somehow I made it out and down the stairs. And I staggered all the way cross town to East 3rd Street, throwing up any number of times as the world whizzed in circles around me."[86]

Then Jones discovered "Howl" and immediately realized it was something special: "It was a breakthrough for me. I now knew poetry would be about some things I was familiar with. That it did not have to be about suburban birdbaths and Greek mythology."[87] He began corresponding with Ginsberg, and in 1958 he decided to start a magazine, *Zazen*, which published Beat poetry. Eventually, Jones and his wife moved to the Village on West 20th Street, but the rent was high and he had to get a job as a copyeditor to pay the bills.[88]

In 1957, the publication of Kerouac's speed-filled *On the Road* along with "Howl"'s trial for obscenity gave even more publicity to the Beat phenomenon, which was covered in *Time*, *Life*, and *Newsweek*. Unsurprisingly, moralizing reporting in the tabloid press had the reverse effect and "helped to legitimize and authenticate the Beat subculture to adherents."[89] One of them was Janis Joplin, who had grown up in Port Arthur, Texas, with a strong feeling of alienation and a longing to meet people with an artistic inclination like hers. In the late 1950s, she learned that something was going on in New York: "I remember when I read that in *Time* magazine about Jack Kerouac, otherwise I'd've never known. I said 'Wow!' and split."[90] At the same time, many "weekend beatniks"[91] flocked to Greenwich Village and revelled in its climate of transgression.

A year after Kerouac's landmark publication, however, Ginsberg was living in the Lower East Side with his lover Peter Orlovsky. Both were fed up by the reporters who kept asking him about "Beatnikism,"[92] but in that rundown district they immediately discovered rampant amphetamine abuse. "Since 1958 it's been a plague around my house," Ginsberg recalled a few years later. "People that I liked or who were good artists, have gotten all screwed up on it, and come around burning down the door, stealing."[93] For many of those artists, speed was highly appealing because it could help introverted people become more at ease in certain social settings. On 31 December 1960, poet Diane Wakoski attended a party at Jones's new East Side apartment – he and his family had grudgingly relocated there after Jones was fired from his job following a trip to Cuba.[94] But Wakoski got so bored that she ended up in another poet gathering and gladly accepted a Dexedrine pill di Prima gave her, which made her "talk a mile a minute."[95]

But back in the Village, marijuana was fast becoming the choice drug for the Bohemians, such as Ellen Sander, who was delighted that it was so available in spite of its illegality. "Grass was a hushed scene then, but it was definitely around. You got high within hours of hitting the street."[96] According to di Prima, pot started to become more potent and commonplace around 1956. In fact, it was so powerful that a couple of years later she had her first visionary experience with it, during which she was temporarily transported to India. Around the same time, her gay friend living on Prince Street befriended a Black woman from uptown. Both worked as clerks on Wall Street and occasionally partied together in her basement apartment. There, guests could sit down on couches and smoke while watching TV. The black and white television set had the sound turned off while the host played some jazz, the guests could occasionally apply colour filters to the set, "and folks would talk a bit and sometimes dig how the TV was in synch with the music, or how it wasn't."[97]

Soon the coverage of the Beat subculture attracted impressionable teenagers like Ed Rosenfeld. Aged fourteen, Rosenfeld loved to take his drum to Greenwich Village and play all night. Eventually, he had his first experience with pot, but he did not find it particularly interesting. One day, however, the assistant headmaster of his school summoned him into his office because he strongly suspected that he was hanging out with the Village crowd: "and I said: 'Yes' and he accused me of hanging out with beatniks and I said: 'Yes.' And he accused me of smoking marijuana and I said: 'I tried it once, but I don't smoke marijuana.'" But the assistant would have none of it: "'You can't fool me; you're just like a marijuana smoker; I can tell a marijuana smoker!' And I left that meeting thinking: 'Well maybe I ought to give it another try!' [laughs]."[98]

Creative writer George Andrews (a friend of Ginsberg, Burroughs, and Corso) was one of the New Yorkers who had regularly smoked grass and resented the stigma attached to it. Thirty-five-year-old Andrews had been smoking it for more than three years and tried to discuss the matter with his father. Although he had read at length about drugs, his father sent him to a psychiatrist, who tried to talk him out of it with horror stories and the legal penalties he faced. The psychiatrist then asked him to stop smoking it for a week, but the next morning he had a joint before his appointment. The psychiatrist immediately told him that he looked in great shape since he had quit. For Andrews, this was further proof that the medical establishment was not qualified to judge his habits.[99]

By the end of the decade, grass had become the preferred psycho-active substance for the artistic and Bohemian crowds. A study on the Beat scenes suggested that pot smokers disproportionately outnumbered heroin users, particularly among the young.[100] Pot use soon moved out of Greenwich Village and reached "the worlds of advertising, radio-TV, college students." Some Village dealers were reported as selling weed in "fancy uptown East-Side bars" and in the suburbs, where the profit margins were substantially greater. Such was the importance of the increase in marijuana use that many school officials gave up on the policing.[101]

Crucially, the effects of marijuana were sufficiently close to peyote, which was now making inroads into urban Bohemia. Those who were interested in the cactus could easily procure it on the Lower East Side. One of the city's main dispensers at the time was Eric Loeb, who ran a store on East 9th Street that openly sold peyote, as well as mescaline and ibogaine, four days a week.[102] You could also buy peyote in pharmacies, and in some downtown Manhattan coffeehouses one could simply order coffee or peyote at the counter.

In June 1960, the Food and Drug Administration (FDA) raided a coffee shop operating at 306 East Sixth Street and seized approximately 310 pounds of peyote and 145 capsules of a cactus preparation. Although selling peyote did not run afoul of the New York State laws, the police invoked a city health ordinance regarding poisonous foods to discontinue the sales.[103] The capsules were manufactured in a basement by soaking the peyote in water, removing the liquid and injecting the resulting substance into capsules with a grease gun.[104] Turning the raw materials into caps was astute marketing because the cactus is extremely bitter and is known to induce nausea and vomiting. The drugs were mostly sold to Bohemians and college students for fifty to seventy cents a capsule, and the owner of the café claimed that users reported long and colourful experiences. For some of his clients, peyote became a lucrative business, and they advertised the capsules in the classified columns of some college newspapers.[105]

Folk musician Peter Stampfel, who had first heard about the cactus in "Howl," remembers acquiring some peyote in 1959 and offers a glimpse into the visionary experience: "The closed-eye hallucinations were the most beautiful shit I'd ever seen in my life. I was very fixated on the combination of blue and green, and had a long period of blue and green interactions which were of an awesome, devastating, constantly changing beauty. At a point it changed to purple and orange in a combination that I'd never really considered. It made all the great art I'd seen in my life seem second rate."[106]

Ed Rosenfeld had also heard about the cactus, and around 1959 he ordered a box of 200 buttons from Lawsons Cactus Gardens in San Antonio, Texas. "It was simple. It was like ordering seeds for planting flowers." He kept his stash in his bedroom closet in his mother's apartment, but she eventually threw it away, not knowing what it was. But in the meantime, he had managed to have about twenty experiences, using five buttons at a time, and he also shared some with his friends.[107]

That same year, di Prima also sampled peyote. One spring evening, Randy French, a gay mural painter and her next-door neighbour, invited her to try the cactus. She joined the other guests at French's, who were all sitting on the rug in his largest room, and began cutting and chewing a button – to her surprise, she actually liked the bitter taste. Nothing happened, so she bid everyone goodnight and went back to her place. Soon, she felt sick and threw up, and then she noticed that the floor of her apartment looked a bit odd: "when I looked at the usually horizontal plane under my feet it took some ultra-mathematical curve into another dimension and went straight *up* in a way that seemed to indicate that walking anywhere might be a dubious enterprise." Then she noticed a horse's skull on one of the chairs, laughing. Subsequently, she lay back on her bed and saw the universe unfold before her eyes. This was followed by a vision of the American western desert, "a vast expanse of crumbly, tawny sand, punctuated here and there by huge and human-sized cacti of various kinds."[108]

The ability of peyote to induce profound experiences took an intriguing turn when some users reported encounters with Buddhist iconography under the influence, most likely resulting from the popularization of Buddhism. The convergence of Eastern thought with drug use became far more visible in the 1960s when psychedelic drug users looked for frameworks to channel the spiritual awakening provoked by the psychedelic experience,[109] but even at the turn of the Sixties there were early signs. For instance, a man interested in Eastern spirituality and drugs acquired a peyote capsule in a coffee shop in 1958 and claimed to have "benefited from the insights and deeper understanding" of the experience, and he went on to acquire some more peyote through a friend in Texas.[110] Filmmaker Harold Naiderman also took the cactus once and reported an intimate encounter with the Buddha: "The very first image was of a stone Buddha picking me up, later after several other images passed before me I came back to the stone Buddha. He picked me up further and kissed me on the brow. I was relaxed and smiling. Towards the early part of the experience I sat up and saw myself as a stone Buddha. My last image of the experience was of seeing the great Buddha in Japan which has a white streak down it."[111]

Soon, the growing underground of psychedelic drug users discovered they could avoid eating the cactus by taking peyote's main alkaloid. Mescaline had remained a relatively unknown substance outside scientific circles, but it was quite easy to acquire. Delta Chemical Works and Bios Laboratories were located in the city and shipped mescaline through domestic and international mail order, and both firms often looked the other way when a lay person placed an order.[112] Long Island prison psychologist Art Kleps, for instance, easily obtained half a gram of mescaline from Delta in 1960.[113] Bios, meanwhile, did little to mention the dangers and contraindications on the labels of the chemicals sold.[114]

Annette Hollander was a medical student at Columbia when she tried mescaline in the early 1960s. Although she admitted that the conditions under which she took the drug were terrible, she nonetheless claimed to have acquired a new aesthetic sensibility: "Afterwards, I began seeing all kinds of relationships between the drug experience and everyday life experiences: from sunlight on the water to children's toys to a paper I hope to write someday on the visions of the romantic poets."[115] Audrey Beck, who had a keen interest in psychedelics, experienced it in Greenwich Village and found the experience highly rewarding but did not further investigate it because she was appalled that it was being used recreationally.[116]

Journalist David Solomon, who was then the editor of *Esquire*, was a huge fan of Huxley and his depiction of the mescaline experience. Solomon loved to hang out in Greenwich Village, and he was fascinated by drugs, jazz, and Black culture. His first psychedelic experience was with 400 milligrams of mescaline, during which he became intimately connected with reality and the material world.[117] By 1960, he had left *Esquire* and had become editor of *Metronome*, a magazine dedicated to jazz music. Solomon was acquainted with both Dizzy Gillespie and William Burroughs and used the latter's prose to condemn heroin use in the jazz scene.[118]

The better-informed psychedelic enthusiasts also heard about "morning glory" seeds (*ololiuqui*) that contain an LSA alkaloid with a chemical structure close to LSD, but their preparation was even more fastidious than that for peyote and their bitter taste and nauseous side-effects were not to everyone's liking. In May 1963, numismatist Robert Bashlow, who later co-published an anti-war book in 1967,[119] tried the ground herbs and initially noticed "the most wonderful sensations of color," but the pleasurable experience then made way for one of self-contempt. This was something he often went through with other drugs like cannabis or peyote but that he tried to counter by taking tranquilizers in advance. Under the influence of the seeds, however, he felt far more insane and tortured and ended up in Mount Sinai Hospital where he received tranquilizers.[120] Bashlow later ran into trouble with both the City Health Department and the FDA for having purchased ten pounds of seeds, which were being closely monitored following reports of recreational use.[121] Later that year, the New York City Board of Health asked suppliers to report the name and address of anyone trying to purchase an ounce or more.[122]

A year later, a reporter took some seeds in a New York apartment because he had previously sampled peyote and undergone a pleasant experience and he wished to further probe the depths of his psyche. It seemed, though, that the drug was becoming more and more popular because many of the stores he visited were out of stock. His trip had many ups and downs, but following a lengthy moment of introspection, he claimed to have found complete peace with himself and ultimately hailed it as his "first truly 'religious' experience." Weeks later, he felt more open and caring toward other people.[123]

While some New Yorkers were experimenting with morning glory and peyote, other drug users stumbled upon ibogaine, known to trigger intense visions that lasted much longer than peyote (close to thirty-six hours). The likeliest source of supply was the pharmaceutical company S.B. Penick, which was located in the city.[124] In 1962, nineteen-year-old

Howard Lotsof discovered the West African shrub thanks to a Staten Island chemist who had been involved in the early LSD scene of the late Fifties. Initially, Lotsof balked at the prospect of such a long trip, so he gave the sample to a friend, who enthusiastically reported back after taking it: "It's not a drug, it's a food. We have to tell Congress!" Months later, Lotsof secured more supplies and took ibogaine in his home in Greenwich Village. The result was a life-changing and colourful trip:

> The first thing I saw was a pulsating yellow screwdriver, which disappeared abruptly. And the next thing I knew I was walking up a ladder leading to a 10-foot diving board over a pool. As I was walking up the diving board, my bathing suit disappeared and I was naked. As I dived into the pool, my mother appeared beneath me with her legs open, and I was diving into her vagina. As I got closer, she changed into my sister, who changed into an infant. Then I went into the water, and that was it. The vision turned into a new one.

But the aftermath of the experience was even more significant. Back then, Lotsof had been a regular heroin and cocaine user, and three days later he realized that he no longer had a craving for narcotics: "I viewed heroin as a drug that emulated death; I wanted life. I looked down the street, at the trees, the sky, my house and realized that for the first time in my life, I didn't feel afraid."[125] Over the course of the next months, Lotsof gave ibogaine to nineteen other people, six of whom were using heroin, cocaine, and amphetamines simultaneously. But two of them went to look for the drug the next day because they actually enjoyed being addicts: "They have nothing else in their life … They like the excitement of being chased by the police. They like the excitement of going into little dark corners and buying heroin and getting home. It gives their life structure and form."[126] Additionally, Lotsof found that drug dealers had vested interests in keeping users addicted to opiates.[127]

The growing community of plant-users may well have discovered these new drugs in a relatively unknown but influential book by Robert de Ropp, *Drugs and the Mind*, which was first published in 1957. Both Solomon and Bashlow had greatly enjoyed this informative tome,[128] and for Rosenfeld and his friends it became their go-to text: "I remember the de Ropp book in particular being one that my friends and I talked about and referenced and read, because that seemed to be the only basis for authentic information." Later on, Rosenfeld also read Huxley's essays and fiction and then his letters, which were equally influential.[129]

At the turn of the 1950s, New York's psychoactive marketplace had significantly evolved from that of the previous century when New Yorkers were introduced to the opiates and cocaine. With the arrival of cannabis and speed, the meaning ascribed to the drug experience began to move away from the language of addiction, and the cultural avant-garde's productive use of these drugs suggested that they could lead to new insights and stimulate creativity. When vision-inducing plants like peyote and ibogaine became available, however, some New Yorkers believed that they had found an exciting new category of drugs. These would come to be known as psychedelics after English psychiatrist Humphry Osmond coined the word in 1957.

Yet this transition would not have occurred without New York's unique brand of Bohemianism that was bent on experimentation and the subversion of cultural norms. This was manifest in the Villagers' appreciation of bebop, which seemed to embody their quest for obliterating common frames of reference, as well as of Buddhism, which promised a more intimate form of spirituality than mainstream Christianity. New York's unique publishing industry and its influential newspapers and magazines played an equally important part by offering exciting accounts of psychoactive experiences.

The local media also helped New Yorkers discover Mexican mushrooms containing the psilocybin alkaloid. As the Fifties became the Sixties, psilocybin piqued the interest of a brilliant Harvard professor who believed that he had stumbled upon a drug that would change humanity forever. With Ginsberg's help, he began offering the psilocybin experience to anybody interested. A psychedelic movement was about to sweep New York's upper class and cultural vanguard.

2

Leary before LSD
Psilocybin, High Society, and the Birth of a Psychedelic Movement

In 1957, J.P. Morgan banker Gordon Wasson and his mycologist wife Valentina introduced New Yorkers to psilocybin by reporting on the use of hallucinogenic mushrooms among the Mazatec Indians of Mexico. Gordon's account was published in *Life*, and six days later Valentina published her own version in *This Week*, a magazine boasting a much greater circulation and that was part of the Sunday editions of major papers all over the country. Valentina passed away in 1958, but Gordon continued to study his cherished fungi, and a year later he organized an exhibit on mushrooms in New York's American Museum of Natural History.[1]

Thanks to Gordon's article, Ed Rosenfeld and his friends discovered that there were more drugs with similar effects to peyote,[2] while another New Yorker became interested in psychedelics as part of a broader quest for mystical enlightenment.[3] One woman responded to the *Life* piece by mentioning that she had been taking peyote for three years as a direct result of reading Huxley's "Doors of Perception."[4] In Greenwich Village, Beat writer Bonnie Frazer claimed that the news of Mazatec mushroom rituals had sparked an actual exodus: "one-half of the people I know who have gone to Mexico have made the thirty-hour trip into the mountains to get to Huautla [de Jiménez]."[5]

It took three years for the news of these thrilling ethnobotanical discoveries to reach Timothy Leary, the rising star of Harvard's Center for Personality Research who was destined for an accomplished career in clinical psychology.[6] At that time, though, Leary would never have even dreamed of dabbling with mind-altering mushrooms. Back then, his choice drug was liquor, and even throughout his psychedelic years, the High Priest of LSD never put down the bottle. "Timothy was really and always has been an alcoholic," laments Gerd Stern. "He allowed the drug world to become an additional layer on this alcoholism; he never gave up the alcohol, by the way. Alcohol and drugs are not the greatest mix in the world; they're destructive physiologically."[7]

Another unfortunate aspect of Leary's personality was his appetite for womanizing. In 1955, he had an affair with his project manager Mary della-Cioppa. But rather than file for divorce, his then-wife Marianne committed suicide in October, leaving him with their children Jack and Susan. Leary turned to della-Cioppa for stability and married her, but they soon separated after a few unpleasant months together.[8] Combined with his alcoholism, Marianne's suicide may go a long way in explaining Leary's flaws and his reckless behaviour.

Nevertheless, Leary's first contact with psilocybe mushrooms had dramatic consequences. On a personal level, it was a life-changing experience that toppled his world views and caused him to give synthetic psilocybin to influential people. Initially, he turned to urban Bohemia and the Beats, who seemed like ideal candidates for such a thrilling ride into inner space, but news of a Harvard professor handing out magic pills quickly reached the local upper class. As someone who loved being the centre of attention, it made him the go-to person for anyone interested in the experience.[9]

On a scientific level, the mushrooms seemed to confirm some of his intuitions as a maverick psychologist. In particular, he had come to believe that psychology's emphasis on returning patients to normalcy betrayed a white middle-class bias and that behaviour should be studied in everyday situations rather than in cold, clinical settings. More broadly, Leary was deeply dissatisfied with his discipline, to the extent that he had personally concluded that it did not work. As his research team kept track of changes in patient behaviour, "No matter what types of psychotherapy were being used, a third of patients would get better, a third would stay the same, and a third would get worse."[10] At long last, here was a drug that promised to transform individuals and eradicate mental illness.

In the larger history of New York psychedelia, Leary's psilocybin movement is an important episode that helped the transition from psychoactive plants like peyote to synthetic drugs like LSD. It also allowed a number of New Yorkers to get an early taste of the psychedelic experience and to form discreet congregations of intrepid explorers.

The Bohemian Connection

After securing employment at Harvard in 1959, Leary and his family found a house in Newton, a few miles away from the university. There he met a younger and charismatic assistant professor named Richard Alpert who seemed just as ambitious as he was. They got on well, and during the summer of 1960 they vacationed in Cuernavaca, Mexico, where they rented a spacious villa. It so happened that psilocybe mushrooms grew on the volcanic peaks north of the house, and one of their visitors, who had experienced them, suggested that Leary try them.

After some pondering, Leary's curiosity got the better of him.[11] As he recalled a year later, "Anthropologist friend arrived one weekend with a bag of mushrooms. Magic mushrooms. I have never heard of them, but being a good host joined the crowd who ate them. Wow! Learned more in six hours than in past sixteen years. Visual transformations. Gone the perceptual machinery which clutters up our view of reality. Intuitive transformations. Gone the mental machinery which slices the world into abstractions and concepts. Emotional transformation. Gone the emotional machinery that causes us to load life with our own role-ambitions and petty desires."[12]

Back in his office, Leary began to experiment with psilocybin and examine its effects on the human mind. He soon found the support of Aldous Huxley, then a guest lecturer at MIT. They took psilocybin in the fall of 1960, and as they were coming down they discussed how to start a global psychedelic movement. Huxley, who was diagnosed with throat cancer that same year, knew he had to pass on the torch to someone who shared his vision of a world free of suffering. However, the British philosopher cautioned Leary against an all-out revolution and advised him to carefully select his targets: "Work privately. Initiate artists, writers, poets, jazz musicians, elegant courtesans, painters, rich bohemians. And they'll initiate the intelligent rich."[13] For that, however, he would need the help of a street-wise Bohemian with such connections.

In November 1960, Leary received an enthusiastic letter from Allen Ginsberg, who had heard about his work at Harvard thanks to a New York psychiatrist. Ginsberg, by then, had experimented with nitrous oxide, ether, mescaline, peyote, and Ditran,[14] and he had just returned from the Amazon, where he had sampled the vision-inducing brew ayahuasca.[15]

Eventually, Ginsberg, his partner Peter Orlovsky, and his brother Lafcadio wound up at Leary's on 26 November[16] and had a memorable psilocybin trip during which the bearded poet reasoned that the drug should be at the heart of a peace and love movement. As Leary recalled, "It seemed to us that wars, class conflicts, racial tensions, economic exploitation, religious strife, ignorance, and prejudice were all caused by narrow social conditioning," which could be solved through widespread drug-induced deconditioning. Over the next few years, this is what they set out to achieve. But for all the talk of Ginsberg's "American egalitarian open-to-the-public approach," Leary did retain Huxley's advice to "train influential Americans in consciousness-expansion."[17] Thanks to Ginsberg's address book, they turned to New York City, which was brimming with such candidates.

Over the next two years, then, Leary carried on with his academic duties at Harvard and commuted to the city on most weekends to run psilocybin sessions. Through Ginsberg, he had no trouble connecting with Beats, jazz musicians, and the cultural avant-garde, who were naturally inclined to try his drug. But thanks to Huxley's writings and the seminal reporting from the Luce empire and other local news outlets, a much wider pool of wealthy New Yorkers were just as keen to experiment with the latest psychoactive sensation.

New York also had the geographical advantage of being close to New Jersey, where a Sandoz plant was making psilocybin and marketing the drug as Indocybin. It supplied it to researchers all over the country, and Leary knew that Sandoz had invested a lot of money and was eager for results because he had personally contacted Gordon Wasson. The amateur mycologist was on Sandoz's board of directors, and the company had also been one of J.P. Morgan's clients.[18]

Leary's New York campaign began in December 1960, and the first person he initiated was Neal Cassady, who had experimented with a great deal of psychoactive substances but not synthetic psilocybin. When Leary visited him in Newton, though, Cassady was appalled that the drug was being investigated in such a rigid academic setting and suggested that "hundreds of hip human beings hanging around New York City" would be most delighted to help him with his research. Leary accepted his invitation to run the session in his apartment, in a real-world situation.

In Manhattan, Leary found Cassady along with two women named Salinas and Patty-Belle. Back then, he knew very little about the local Beat scene, and the sociological differences were rather striking. "I'm particularly interested in how psilocybin measures relative to other drugs you've taken," Leary explained to Salinas. "Psychopharmacologists haven't yet been able to collect this kind of comparative phenomenological data." To which Salinas answered: "You mean, man, you want us to get high on your drug and then compare it with other stuff we've done?" After distributing the pills and factoring body weight, the four of them ingested the psilocybin, and Leary got the comparative description he wanted from Cassady: "This combines the good sides of every other drug with none of the bad ... More mellow and cozy than heroin, but you don't nod out. I feel more alive and wired and energetic than with speed, but not jangly. It's got the blast of cocaine, but it lasted ten times longer."

It is possible that this meeting caused Leary to realize that these substances had the potential to be used as adjuncts for spirituality. In this instance, he "was fascinated to witness the calm devotion, the almost religious commitment of the beatniks to the moment of in-gestion," and he was greatly intrigued when Cassady "folded his body into an oriental meditation posture and seemed to be concentrating on his breathing."[19] Of course, Cassady was already familiar with other psychedelics, which led him to appreciate similar substances that might expand his consciousness, but his religious approach to the drug likely came from the Beats' interest in Eastern spirituality.

Eastern religions seemed better equipped for psychedelia, but Leary and Ginsberg were about to discover that orthodox Christianity was far more ambivalent toward notions of drug-induced revelations. Next up on their agendas was Jack Kerouac, a Roman Catholic who had become infatuated by his literary success and had lapsed into alcoholism. Although Leary has recently been credited for "the invention and popularization of the concept of set and setting,"[20] a striking aspect of his time in New York City is that he was oblivious to the notion that environmental and psychological circumstances were an essential part of the experience. As a result, the limits of his naturalistic approach to the study of the effects of psilocybin on human behaviour were brutally exposed by the drunken Kerouac, and the inhospitable setting of Ginsberg and Orlovsky's "terminally dingy" Lower East Side apartment did not help either. For both Leary and Ginsberg, it turned into a harrowing trip, even though they did learn from it in the aftermath.[21]

Before taking the drug, a drunken Kerouac openly derided Leary's fascination for psilocybin: "So what are you up to, Doctor Leary, running around with this communist fagot Ginsberg and your bag of pills? Can your drugs absolve the mortal and venial sins which our beloved savior, Jesus Christ, the only son of God, [who] came down and sacrificed his life upon the cross to wash away?" They were about to find out.

They swallowed the psilocybin, but that did not stop Kerouac from overindulging in red wine and embarking on never-ending streams of consciousness. It was almost as if the powerful drug was having no effect on him. Leary, who by then had taken psilocybin with more than 100 people, had never seen such resistance from a subject, and it greatly affected his own trip. "He was imposing his saloon style on [the experience], and for me it was simply too much." This plunged Leary into his first negative experience, which was filled with religious thoughts. While he had also been raised as a Catholic, it was probably "Kerouac's French-Catholic gloom" that influenced him the most: "No kidding around, the world was a dismal dreary place ... It *was* folly trying to change human nature. Who was I to eliminate suffering when now, from my own soul, oozed a pus of despair. Yes, the Catholic nuns were right. This world was a vale of suffering. My life was a fraud."[22]

Ginsberg himself wasn't having the easiest of trips, but being more familiar with Kerouac's extravaganza, he coped with his endless monologues much better than Leary. The poet had taken fourteen pills, enough to undergo a powerful and intense experience. Soon, he felt nauseous and ended up vomiting, but he found the reassuring comfort of their part-time flatmate, Jeanine: "[I] went to her couch and lay down with her, my head on her breast, soft safe and sighed my fears away in her arms." As he remained there, he closed his eyes and experienced intense visions ranging from a "huge coiled organic cosmos" to Herbert Huncke "in hotel room recovering from junk sickness," followed by "Fiendish Angels with fangs of Judgment rushing thru the void over Atlantic Blakean Spaces to make meets with each other to take Conference over the future of Life."

As the distraught Leary retreated into the dark bedroom to find a semblance of peace, Kerouac rapped on. But although Ginsberg was having an intense ride, he eventually found comic relief in his ramblings. Kerouac "developed a very funny comedy of his own which was completely non-conspiratorial compared to mine." In particular, he somehow found great philosophical meaning in one of Kerouac's statements: "I think I'll take a shit out of the window." This, according to Ginsberg, Kerouac somehow achieved without ever moving from his chair. "See? Nobody complained."[23]

Eventually, Ginsberg found Leary on the bed, curled up in a foetal ball. He was prone to painful childhood memories and haunting visions of his late wife. Ginsberg's soothing presence lifted his spirits, and soon he was able to join the rest of the party. Back in Kerouac's presence, he drank wine and smoked cigarettes with him and eventually asked for his philosophical opinion of psilocybin. But once more, the writer was uninterested, and he bitterly concluded that "Walking on water wasn't made in a day."[24] Subsequently, Kerouac tried psilocybin again, but it simply wasn't for him. In spite of his distaste, he did send Leary a report three days later in which he conceded that the experience could be read along Buddhist lines: "It was definite Satori. Full of psychic clairvoyance (but you must remember this is not half as good as the peaceful ecstasy of simple Samadhi trance as I described that in Dharma Bums [a novel by Kerouac])."[25]

After the session, they took the subway uptown to meet with the Pulitzer Prize–winning poet Robert Lowell, an old-line Boston Brahmin from a well-to-do family who lived in a spacious apartment overlooking the Hudson River. Ginsberg, however, knew that Lowell was not the ideal candidate for the experience. His poetry betrayed a gloomy and troubled mind, and the psilocybin might be too much for him to handle (so Leary gave him a weakened dose – circa six pills). But the session went smoothly, and Lowell saw the experience as a valid way of revising the original illumination of Christianity: "Now I know what Blake and St. John of the Cross were talking about ... This experience is what I was seeking when I became a Catholic."[26] Ginsberg concluded that even a disturbed mind like Lowell's could undergo the experience in a supportive setting, but, perhaps more to the point, it contrasted greatly with Kerouac's own Catholic take on psychedelic spirituality.

Leary, Ginsberg, and Orlovsky then turned to the highly influential Barney Rosset. Through Grove Press and the *Evergreen Review*, Rosset was fast becoming the leading publisher of avant-garde and controversial material, such as the works of Jean Genet, Samuel Becket, and Henry Miller. Naturally, he was quick to fully appreciate the novelty of Beat poetry. As "Howl" was on trial for obscenity following its publication by City Lights Books, even an edited version of the poem was enough for Rosset to heap superlative praise: "This is the most radical thing I've read in America since I've come [to New York]."[27] For Ginsberg, Rosset would be a fantastic addition to their fledging movement: "If we can turn him on, we can illuminate New York and London."[28]

As the two Beats and the professor arrived at Rosset's townhouse, they realized that they had only enough psilocybin for two people and decided that Ginsberg would accompany the publisher. However, Leary had just received some mescaline from a New York company, and he and Orlvosky took it with Rosset's then-girlfriend, a twenty-year old woman named Zelda. But when Ginsberg came back to see how the mescaline was treating them, he anxiously reported that Rosset was struggling. In fact, Rosset had a history of mental illness, which had likely led him into "the gloomy thoughts department," worrying about politics, religion, his family and career.[29] At one point, he became obsessed by a painting hanging in the room that had been done by his first wife, Joan Mitchell. "Convinced it was actually coming off the wall, Rosset went over to the painting to push everything back in the frame where it belonged."

Years later, he did not remember Leary and his one and only trip fondly but credited Ginsberg for his presence: "Tim was not concerned at all that I was having a bad trip. But Allen was. He was absolutely there helping me."[30] It is unlikely that the experience had any long-lasting impact on Rosset's mental health and that it influenced his decision to republish de Ropp's *Drugs and the Mind* in 1961, along with a seminal collection on psychedelic art later in the 1960s.[31] What is more likely is that Rosset had the flair to realize that drugs were not only moving away from censorship and stigmatization following Huxley's publications but that their growing popularity meant that they could be added to Grove's catalogue of avant-garde books.

As for Zelda, Leary believed that she had found positive meaning in the experience because she was much younger. According to him, she subsequently moved away from Rosset, settling first in Ginsberg's apartment and then moving in with Leary and becoming his lover.[32] Leary was fond of bragging about all the young women he slept with, but in this particular instance, he conveniently forgot to mention a gruesome episode that reveals how careless he could be with these drugs.

The day after the drug session at Rosset's, the publisher went to work, but when he got back home, he found Zelda lying unconscious in a pool of her own blood after slashing her wrists. Rosset took her to hospital where she received treatment, and he blamed the strong mescaline dose she had received. It turned out that "she was a very upset person to begin with. A person on the verge of being psychotic anyway ... I thought that was extremely irresponsible of Leary." Weeks later, Ginsberg had a long conversation with Rosset and admitted that turning them on had been a mistake. But to add insult to injury, Rosset subsequently received a mimeographed questionnaire in the mail designed to assess the quality of the experience. Among the items were questions pertaining to sexuality: "Did it increase your sex orgasms by ten percent? Twenty percent? Thirty percent? Fifty percent?" Rosset was furious. Worse still, he had never received the pre-session questionnaire designed to screen candidates for prior histories of mental illness that Leary's institution mandated.[33]

After initiating Kerouac, Lowell, and Rosset, Leary and Ginsberg realized that they had not witnessed any radical personality change and wondered whether higher doses might have yielded more favourable results. As they continued to reflect upon these drug sessions, they replenished their psilocybin stash and set their sights on New York's jazz scene, where they would easily find more candidates. This time around, however, they went their separate ways.[34] By then, the poet was a respected figure in the city's cultural vanguard, and as a Beat he had long been drawn to Black culture and jazz. Moreover, both Ginsberg and Black jazzmen had a great deal of experience with psychoactive drugs, and in this respect he had little trouble bringing psilocybin to their attention.

It was fitting, then, that the first contact between Ginsberg and Dizzy Gillespie's legendary band occurred in Greenwich Village's Five Spot, which was then the indisputable meeting ground for Bohemians and jazz people. There he gave pills to pianist Thelonious Monk and paid him a visit a few days later to see if he had enjoyed them. The smile on Monk's face told its own story – he even asked Ginsberg if he had anything stronger. He then gave psilocybin to Gillespie, who was just as appreciative.[35] In April, Ginsberg took off for India,[36] leaving Leary alone to carry on their mission in New York.

As an Irish-American unfamiliar with the local avant-garde, Leary's connection with the New York jazz world was somewhat different. Although he would end up meeting some of New York's seminal Black musicians like Charles Mingus, his entry was made possible by a handful of wealthy white New Yorkers. At the same time, his Harvard credentials offered him a privileged access to psilocybin and allowed him to become the centre of attention among an informal but highly enthusiastic group of experimenters. These well-to-do socialites soon found themselves organizing group sessions in their respective homes, half a century after Mabel Dodge Luhan's peyote salon.

Turning on High Society

Sometime in 1961,[37] Salinas introduced Leary to Flora Lu Ferguson, the wife of Canadian trumpet player Maynard Ferguson, whom Ginsberg had just turned on.[38] After an underwhelming session at Harvard, Leary met with Flora at Charlie Parker's Birdland, where Maynard was playing with his band that night. Accompanying her was a young Moroccan model named Malaca. She had been married to a member of the royal family of Iran and was most interested in Leary's research.

After the gig, the four of them took a limousine back to the Ferguson's Tudor house in Riverdale. As they pulled up the gravel driveway, Leary noticed two Jaguars parked in front. Inside, he was just as stunned by the mixture of conspicuous wealth and hedonism. The massive living room had one wall "lined with electronic sound equipment and yards of record albums." Flora gave him a guided tour of the house and showed him his bedroom, which was full of furs, silk, velvet, and mirrors. In the master bedroom, he noticed some Tantric yantras, indicating that the Fergusons had an interest in Hinduism.

They all swallowed the psilocybin, and the Fergusons began teaching Leary eroticism. Soon after, he and Malaca connected. This was his first sexual experience under the influence, and a few days later he felt an urge to converse with Huxley about the matter. But the Briton immediately warned him "not to let the sexual cat out of the bag." Puritan Americans would have enough trouble accepting these new drugs and – for now – Leary put the association aside.[39]

Subsequently, the Fergusons introduced Leary to another well-off New Yorker: Uris real estate agent Bernard Friedman. Friedman first heard about Leary and psilocybin over some drinks with Maynard at the Birdland, and news of this mysterious drug easily piqued his curiosity. He and his wife Abby had been smoking pot for years – they were close friends of writer George Andrews, who had bestowed on them a bag of grass as a wedding present back in 1948.[40] Friedman certainly liked to drink, but he had reached a point where he wanted to go "beyond Scotch and Martinis."[41] More important, he was thinking about quitting his job to fully concentrate on creative writing, his main hobby. Psilocybin seemed to offer a deeply introspective experience that might help him reach a decision.[42]

In April 1961, Bernard and his friend George Rapée, a world-champion bridge player, attended a party at the Fergusons. There, Friedman was introduced to Leary, who gave him a handful of pills. As the psilocybin took hold and sent chills down his body, he became resentful of some of the guests and the way they spoke. In particular, there was a young aspiring top-model who could not stop rambling. "I was bugged by the overstylized jazz jargon," Friedman recalled, "particularly Melinda's. She seemed to be working at it harder than she had to. And that short-cut laugh. Like hah dig hah baby hah man hah." But eventually he found her way of speaking quite economical, and he came to realize that words could only have a very limited meaning under the influence.[43] In this particular instance, Friedman's insights were in tune with Huxley's writings in which he contended that the psychedelic experience takes the user to the confines of the human mind where words and abstractions become meaningless.

After his initiation, Friedman wrote to Leary to inform him that the psilocybin had helped him to become "freer, more relaxed" and that he would gladly repeat the experience. In return, Leary told him about his latest research project at Harvard: he was studying the effects of psilocybin on inmates in a Massachusetts prison, hoping that the psychedelic experience would be enough to reform them and have them released into the community.[44] Leary hinted that external funding for this study would be welcome, and, given his position at Uris, Friedman was happy to help, particularly if that meant more psilocybin coming his way.

Fortunately, Friedman was then working on lease agreements with a colleague who was the supervisor of the Uris Brothers Foundation, created by real estate tycoons Harold and Percy Uris. Better still: he was a Harvard graduate. So the news of Leary's exciting research at his alma mater thrilled him, and he pledged a $5,000 contribution.[45] The grant covered clerical expenses and the salaries of former inmates working in the community and was renewed in 1962.[46]

Over the next few months, Friedman enjoyed a privileged access to Leary's psilocybin and offered him colourful reports in return. In June, he organized a jazz garden party for about ninety people, but hosting made him nervous and caused him to overindulge in pot and scotch. But after taking some pills, he retreated into his inner space, away from the codes of social conduct. He reported no visions, insights, or physical reactions but "an extreme sense of detachment and distance." Subsequently, he realized the futility of entertaining so many people: "I stopped playing host, I stopped bothering to make introductions, I was alone, having a very good time, not needing anyone else, certainly not ninety anyone elses [sic]."[47] With the help of psilocybin, entertaining had literally become a form of entertainment.

Meanwhile, the local press was beginning to take notice of Leary's enterprise. In May 1961, David Solomon gave psilocybin to British journalist John Wilcock,[48] who along with Norman Mailer had been working at the *Village Voice* since 1955. The weekly paper was housed on Sheridan Square, just above the Stonewall Inn, which was a famous meeting place for gay people. The *Voice* epitomized Greenwich Village's spirit of avant-garde by pioneering "the kind of offbeat and subversive approaches that youthful journalists of the 1960s mimicked and amplified." Wilcock, though, quickly realized that his employers were looking for an innovative paper that would sell and not step over the boundaries of respectability.[49] Nevertheless, it attracted many talented writers who resented the narrowness of Cold War mentalities,[50] and throughout the Sixties it regularly featured articles on mind-altering drugs in New York.

Leary's Harvard credentials made Wilcock change his mind about psychoactive substances. "I'd resisted drugs for years," he remembered.

"Mailer had offered me marijuana, I'd turned it down. My friend who ran a jazz magazine said, 'Come and take these pills, it's an experimental thing!' I said, 'I'm not into pills.' He said, 'This guy's a professor at Harvard!'"[51] After giving in, he experienced a "pervasive feeling of goodwill" combined with "gusts of laughter" resulting from whatever topic they discussed. As they walked along 42nd Street, they saw a police officer approaching, but Solomon was quick to alleviate any fears of wrongdoing: "Dave took my arm to calm my paranoia and whispered in my ear. 'No law against laughing; no law against laughing.' It was an epiphany."[52]

Soon after, Wilcock tried LSD and mescaline, and the latter appeared in the pages of the *Voice* in July. Leary sent him some literature on psilocybin along with questionnaires, hoping the Briton might share his trip reports with him. In return, Wilcock sent him a draft of his column on mescaline,[53] which was published a couple of weeks later. In the article, he mentioned that he had greatly enjoyed the Huxley and de Ropp books, but he also issued a word of caution about mescaline, following the advice of a New York physician who had warned him that it should be taken under medical supervision only.[54] The following week, the *Voice* published an account of Wilcock's psilocybin experience, which openly endorsed Leary's research at Harvard and once again referenced the de Ropp book.[55]

As the summer of 1961 was coming to an end, the psilocybin scene was reaching other wealthy socialites in "a duplex maisonette on Seventy-first Street just East of Fifth Avenue." The hosts were a Ford Agency model by the name of China Girard and the influential theatre producer Van Wolf, best known for serving as promotion director for Mike Todd's 1956 *Around the World in 80 Days*. Both of them had met Leary thanks to the Fergusons, and they had privileged connections with just about every sphere of the metropolis. "Van seemed to know everyone," marvelled Friedman. "Models, jazz musicians, actors, pop artists, psychedelic artists, art dealers, drug dealers, café society, high society. A world of talent or money or both flower through the apartment in an almost continuous party of regular and transient guests who could be useful as theater-backers or Leary backers. Tim, a celebrity by now, added considerable luster to Van's gatherings." Wolf soon became one of Leary's supporters by organizing get-togethers at their place, hoping that other influential New Yorkers might sustain his psychedelic cause.[56]

Back then, Maynard was on tour, but that did not stop the Friedmans and Flora from experimenting with psilocybin on a regular basis, while Leary kept on studying the mysterious drug. There were times, however, when he wanted more than just raw data for his scientific research. Being introduced to New York's elite allowed him not only to extract favours and financial help but also to become the go-to man of this nascent psychedelic scene. The narcissistic Leary revelled in that role.

Early in September, the group was getting ready for another session. Flora served drinks, put on a Gil Evans record, and kept track of the time because Bernard was due to appear on Mike Wallace's pre-recorded "PM East" show to discuss housing.[57] She then asked Leary if he'd remembered to bring the pills along, to which he answered that he was going to Sandoz the next day to pick up a delivery. Flora probed further in a mournful voice, until he began shaking out his jacket pockets. "I love Tim," she whispered to the Friedmans, "but this is his least attractive game – making us beg. It's a power play." Eventually, the professor produced enough psilocybin for the four of them. Later in the evening, as Bernard's head was full of colourful geometric patterns dancing around, he noticed a Chinese-American woman in her thirties who told Leary that every psilocybin session should be recorded for scientific purposes. She was Gordon Wasson's secretary.[58]

The next day, Leary borrowed the Fergusons' white Jaguar to retrieve the psilocybin from New Jersey. He then picked up Friedman and drove to Wasson's uptown apartment that overlooked the East River. Wasson greeted them and introduced him to his secretary, Sylvia Pau, who took notes throughout the meeting. As they discussed the latest developments in psychedelic research and the conferences Leary had recently attended in Europe, Friedman got a little bored, and his eyes feasted on Wasson's living room: it was like being in a museum and a testimony of the considerable amount of knowledge Wasson had amassed over the years. "The shelves were full of books on mycology itself and botany in general, interspersed with such objects as ancient phallic Guatemalan 'mushroom stones,' fanciful toadstools, dainty porcelains, and small paintings and prints that had mushroom motifs. As far as I could see, the library was totally specialized."

Eventually, the discussion shifted to Leary's plans. He had hoped that this meeting would see the celebrated mycologist formally join forces with him, but Wasson remained "cold and distant" throughout and seemed thoroughly unimpressed. At this point, Leary had been giving psilocybin to hundreds of enthusiastic people like Friedman, but the 2,000 monthly doses he was getting from Sandoz were beginning to hinder his ability to satisfy everyone. He announced his intention to set up a research foundation that might manufacture psilocybin and that would have eminent people like Huxley and Wasson on the board of directors. The latter only answered with an embarrassing silence and soon indicated that the meeting was over.

Friedman seemed relieved to part company. It was obvious that Wasson was miles away from Leary's vision, and Bernard could "hardly believe he'[d] taken mushrooms" in the first place. The ever-optimistic Leary shrugged. "The behavior of a genius is unpredictable," he contended and reasoned that Wasson was probably still mourning Valentina.[59] But this was probably not the case. Back in May 1957, Huxley had visited Wasson, and although he had been just as impressed by his library, he had likewise described him as "odd," "solemn and humourless," and scornful of the other psychedelics.[60] In any event, Leary would have to work without his stellar endorsement.

The absence of this meeting from Leary's memoirs suggests that he did not digest this rebuttal well. In *Flashbacks*, he only mentions Wasson's visit at Harvard in spring 1961. The banker had allegedly come over to display his erudition, but he had no desire to collaborate with him. In this respect, Leary's hyperbolic comments probably say more about him than about Wasson: "They were *his* fucking mushrooms controlled from *his* Maker's Board Room. He seemed to view us as rivals. I made a mental note to phone Aldous about how to deal with the colonial competition."[61] Wasson, on the other hand, simply remembered how Leary – "an egoist of the first class" – had tried to persuade him to join the board of directors of his research centre in an ill-disguised attempt to add some celebrity gloss: "He would have made a great show of me, an exhibit; but I would only be the object of attention. I would not have anything to say."

Although these vitriolic statements uttered long after the Sixties by two men who occupy a central place in psychedelic lore may appear trivial, they are in keeping with two radically opposed understandings of the psilocybin experience. When Leary first tried the mushrooms in Mexico, he quickly made plans to turn on the whole world. By contrast,

Wasson liked to separate his occupation at J.P. Morgan from his research into mycology, even though some of his colleagues liked to probe him: "At lunch they would ask me. They would try to draw me out, inquiring about my experiences in Mexico. But I was talking about banking." The main reason for Wasson's resistance was that, unlike Leary, he "did not wish to get involved trying to educate people who were totally ignorant of the subject."[62]

Wasson was not the only celebrity to dismiss Leary's venture. That same month, the American Psychological Association (APA) held its annual meeting in New York and featured a symposium on consciousness-expanding drugs. Leary had convinced William Burroughs to take part, hoping to secure another major endorsement. By then, he was a major literary figure, thanks to the 1959 publication of his seminal *Naked Lunch*. Since Burroughs was one of the founders of the Beat movement and someone who had tried just about every mind-altering drug available, Leary was confident that he would enjoy the psilocybin. But when he finally connected with him in Tangier that summer, it turned out that Burroughs hated it.[63]

During the APA conference, "An overflow crowd spilled out in the hallway to hear Burroughs speak. Sprawled on the floor around the speaker's table, they strained to hear him as he read from his prepared manuscript in a low voice." To Leary's frustration, psilocybin was conspicuously missing from his presentation. Worse still, he subsequently published a letter denouncing Leary's research at Harvard in which he charged that Leary and his colleagues liked to "steal, bottle, and dole out addictive love in eye-droppers of increased awareness of unpleasant or dangerous symptoms." As Ginsberg later recalled, Burroughs believed that the whole peace and love movement was a joke and withdrew from Leary, even though the two would subsequently reconnect in the following decades and become close friends.[64]

Burroughs might have been another high-profile disappointment, but at least the conference drew some interested figures like psychologist Stanley Krippner (now a respected authority on the study of dreams), who had to sit on the windowsill because of the high attendance. He had first learned about psilocybin through Wasson's *Life* article, and he had immediately reasoned that this was "a marvellous psychological opportunity to learn more about consciousness and the human mind" and that he would be most interested in taking the mushrooms himself.[65]

Krippner had a friend who was taking his doctorate in Leary's department, and he soon travelled to Harvard to try the drug.[66] The conference was also attended by Virginia Glenn, who had long suffered from a debilitating form of diabetes, and it was only after listening to one of Alan Watts's taped lectures that she stopped contemplating suicide.[67] Like the Fergusons, Glenn enjoyed organizing get-togethers across the city where they could discuss altered states of consciousness and alternative spirituality. Through these parties and seminars, Krippner subsequently met influential scientists working on psychedelics.[68]

Meanwhile, the Friedmans received a package containing 100 Sandoz pills from Leary on 15 September. This time, however, Bernard decided that he would be travelling solo and reported a far more intense experience than the group sessions had offered hitherto. An hour after the ingestion came the visions: a mosaic of light, which soon shifted into a crab. Then the experience became both visual and physical. He turned into the crab and began exploring the inside of his own body. His organs soon assumed the quality of a landscape with hills and plains. He felt the sun crash into one of his eyes, and from the resulting gush of tears appeared a Viking ship and its crew. A little later, he was at the bottom of the ocean, surrounded by plants, fish, octopi, and crustaceans. Down there he felt at home and realized that the ocean was truth, far removed from the world of words. He came to the conclusion that death only concerned the end of one level of reality but that life was in fact eternal.[69]

Soon it became clear to Leary that the experienced Friedman could offer more than exquisite reports and that he was ready to initiate other adventurous New Yorkers. Probably because of the unmanageable number of volunteers, Leary started to give the drug away to those who wanted it badly enough, and some New Yorkers were fortunate to encounter psilocybin in the Village bars. Medical Doctor John Beresford, for one, was enthralled when a friend told him "about this 'mad Harvard professor' who had spread a handful of the psilocy-beans on the counter and said, 'Try these.'"[70]

One Bohemian who got hold of Leary's pills was LeRoi Jones, who by then was editing *The Floating Bear*, a mimeographed poetry newsletter, with Diane di Prima.[71] In Jones's autobiography, however, nothing suggests that Leary and his colleagues supervised his experience, and that might be why it was such a harrowing trip. "The shit made stuff seem like it was jumping around on my desk and in the house," he remembered. "Papers, pictures, furniture all would suddenly leap to another spot or jump up and down. After a while I began begging to come down (in my head)."[72] Unsurprisingly, Jones never tried psilocybin again.[73]

Friedman, however, recoiled at the prospect of giving the pills without proper supervision. After sending a trip report to Leary, the professor wrote back informing him that one Robert Rowe, a twenty-five-year-old stockbroker trainee with a background in physics, had heard about his research at the APA conference and very much wanted to try psilocybin.[74] "Would you be willing to meet this guy for a drink," Leary asked him, "size him up and then if you think he is swinger, make arrangements to give him mushrooms."[75] Friedman obliged but cautioned Leary that Rowe, who was undergoing psychotherapy, might not be a suitable candidate. While he was willing "to set aside one or two nights a month," he was not prepared to simply hand out the pills and let him experiment.[76]

Leary's next letter seemed to confirm Friedman's reservations about the future High Priest:

> We had a large meeting Sunday. Thirty people. Many gray beards and administrators present. A tricky dilemma. "They" offer help, respectability, support, medical school backing, etc. etc. if we narrow down and play the science game, that is, give up the social movement and play the academic game. This means, of course, no MRS [mushrooms] for you and Flo. My group here wants to go ahead on a broader basis – leave Harvard, change careers, etc. ...
>
> The issue in a few words: should we join the academic game or start a new game?
>
> ...
>
> P.S. So postpone the initiation sessions and enjoy your MRS.

Friedman greeted the news with a mixture of relief and annoyance: "I felt increasingly uncomfortable in the petty-powerful bureaucratic role of distributing mushrooms or, more often, *not* distributing them."[77]

After another psilocybin experience with Abby, Bernard enclosed what was to be his final official trip report in a letter to Leary. Though he told him he now wished to organize his mushroom material into a book or a long article, it is more than likely that he was also getting tired of him. Over the next months, the two of them continued to correspond, with Leary regularly inviting him and Abby to Newton. Bernard, however, was just too busy. He was writing his first novel while maintaining his duties at Uris, which was fast becoming one of the largest New York–based real estate corporations listed on the stock exchange. Fortunately, he was about to finally reach a decision about his career.

In spite of their deteriorating relationship, Leary continued to send the Friedmans more pills. By spring 1962, they had made new acquaintances who were invited to try the drug. Elizabeth was an Australian national whom Abby had met playing tennis and who represented her country at the United Nations. Along with her came her brother Arthur, who was an antique dealer, and the final participant was an old artist friend of the Friedmans, Jon. They all swallowed the pills and listened to a Modern Jazz Quartet record as they waited.

Things did not go to plan, however. Jon had not mentioned beforehand that he was seeing a psychiatrist, and soon he became prone to anxiety and paranoia. He insisted on calling his doctor, who in turn ordered them to the Bellevue Hospital emergency ward. Unsurprisingly, the medical professionals were unsure about the nature of his affliction. Eventually, Friedman suggested calling Leary for help, and he told them that he was collaborating with the professor for research purposes. Apologetically, the doctors woke him up in the middle of night. To their shock and to Friedman's, an irate Leary claimed that he was *not* part of his research team, and when pressed for a solution to Jon's torments, he simply told them that he was not a psychiatrist and hung up. Jon would have to spend the night under observation.[78]

The next day, Friedman was torn by guilt and chain-smoked through the morning while waiting for visiting hours. He called Leary for an explanation, but he angrily replied that it risked jeopardizing the whole program and that such a story would be ample ammunition for the conservative medical establishment.

In the afternoon, the anxious Friedman walked to Bellevue and found Jon in the visiting room. Jon looked splendid, much to his surprise. It was all the more puzzling, given that the poor fellow had been beaten up by two attendants under the influence. Friedman was thrilled and relieved. Though the circumstances were awkward, he felt the urge to tell him that this night had been beneficial for him: at long last, he was leaving Uris to become a full-time writer. He also advised Jon to try and not worry too much about his descent into to hell. "I'm sure this has been a nightmare," he conceded. "But I'm just as sure that, despite everything, you'll learn from the experience."

And days later, Jon was vacationing in Mexico, and in Fort Worth, Texas, he sent the Friedmans a telegram which read: "REGARD MUSHROOMS TOTALLY ACCEPTED STOP ONE OF MOST PROFOUND EXPERIENCES OF MY LIFE STOP LOVE JON." But in spite of the terrific news, Bernard still begrudged Leary: "I doubted his facile answers to my questions after returning from Bellevue and his loyalty to anyone but himself."[79] Friedman may have learnt a great deal from psilocybin, but if anything he was too charitable toward Leary, who could be very selective and very self-serving when it came to deciding what constituted legitimate research.

At the beginning of the 1960s, Timothy Leary started a veritable psilocybin movement that was inexorably moving away from Ivy League academia and into the realm of social movements. While civil rights activists were fighting critical battles in the South to end racial segregation, Leary believed he was going to bring about peace and love on a much greater scale – though exactly what would happen after everyone had turned on was always a topic for another day. His venture owed its support to favourable media coverage and to urban Bohemia's insatiable appetite for psychoactive experimentation.

In turn, psilocybin moved seamlessly into the jazz scene, which by then had lost some of its transgressive edge and was enjoyed by a wide pool of New Yorkers. Among them were wealthy socialites, who had found a pastime that was far more gratifying than cocktails, although the two were never mutually exclusive in that particular setting. From Leary's perspective, giving the drug to these influential New Yorkers made sense because they would then endorse his product and the revolutionary ideals he ascribed to the psychedelic experience. He believed it was only a matter of time before the cultural elite and the average drug user would converge to create a full-blown psychedelic movement. In the meantime, this was a unique opportunity to hang out with the local jet set.

The contrast between Leary, who went on to lose his position at Harvard, become the self-appointed High Priest of LSD, and be incarcerated in 1970, and the psychedelic adventures of the Friedmans is rather arresting. Bernard and Abby indeed tried acid in 1963, but the experience was somewhat underwhelming. As Bernard recalled, "although I enjoyed the high, I had already received the message I wanted from psychedelic drugs, mainly the resolution of my conflict between business and writing."[80] For Leary, it was the complete opposite, and his overindulgence in LSD seemed to magnify his personality flaws in a much stronger way. But it did not stop many of the New Yorkers who had been part of the first wave from maintaining close ties with him.

Just as psilocybin was becoming the latest sensation, the far more powerful LSD was also trickling out of the Sandoz plant in New Jersey and crossing the Hudson River into Greenwich Village. Within a few years, psilocybin had virtually disappeared from the psychoactive landscape, even though it had laid an important groundwork that allowed acid to freely permeate postwar New York.

3

Chemical Archetypes
From Experimental Science to Psychedelic Therapy

A puzzling aspect of Leary's time in New York is that little indicates that he ever attempted to connect with the metropolis' vibrant networks of science that had been studying the effects of mescaline and LSD for a decade. In particular, the idea that psychedelics could mimic psychosis in a temporary and controlled fashion ("psychotomimetic" drugs) found a favourable reception in the Department of Experimental Psychiatry of the New York State Psychiatric Institute at Columbia University.

The psychotomimetic hypothesis had some precedent in the scientific research into mescaline of the early twentieth century. In 1913, professor of experimental medicine Alwyn Knauer and neurologist and psychiatrist William Maloney presented their findings before the New York Neurological Society, and they claimed that the drug could induce a "transitory" psychosis to better understand the mechanisms of this disease. The visionary states they were plunged into made a strong impression on them, even though they referred to the experience as a form of delusion resulting from a poisoning.[1]

However, there were no references to these investigations when Max Rinkel, a Boston-based physician of German descent and a pioneer of LSD research, rekindled the psychotomimetic hypothesis after World War II.[2] During the 1950 annual meeting of the American Psychiatric

Association in Detroit, Rinkel's idea was shared by Paul Hoch, the leader of a team working on LSD and mescaline at Columbia and whose research, like Rinkel's, was bankrolled by the CIA.[3]

The psychotomimetic thesis was soon discarded by another psychedelic pioneer, Harold Abramson, who was also funded by US intelligence services. However, Abramson quickly realized that LSD could favour the recollection of material buried in the psyche. Gradually, psychoanalysts started giving the drug to their clients in an attempt to generate therapeutic breakthroughs, whereas classic analysis typically required rigorous commitment over the course of several years.[4] New York's long tradition of psychoanalysis certainly explains why psychedelic-assisted therapy became available locally, but more broadly postwar New York was struggling to effectively deal with mental illness,[5] which added incentive to look for ground-breaking treatments, particularly for schizophrenia.

Among those therapists was an extraordinarily brilliant psychologist by the name of Jean Houston, who immediately appraised the LSD experience through a Jungian framework and gave the drug to her subjects in order to release symbolic and mythic material. Even in her early twenties, she developed a remarkable expertise on the drug's therapeutic applications to a point where she soon became acquainted with Huxley and German-born Fritz Perls, a psychiatrist and psychoanalyst famous for developing Gestalt therapy with his then-wife Laura. Such was her faith in the transformative power of psychedelics that she co-founded an eclectic research centre to better understand them and guide New Yorkers through therapy.

New York's psychedelic psychiatry retained a strong experimental component, however. By the time LSD was making inroads into the analyst's office, a maverick psychiatrist began her own research into the psychedelic-assisted treatment of child autism in Queens. Lauretta Bender is best-known for her seminal Gestalt work, but her personal history of learning difficulties during childhood is probably what drove her to study these drugs in an attempt to help children cope with their disability. Moreover, Bender's story is significant because only a handful of researchers were exploring this possibility at the time[6] and, like Houston, she was a woman whose psychedelic legacy has been obscured by other male-dominated narratives.[7]

But the outstanding aspect of New York's medical history of LSD is its exceptional longevity. Beginning in 1950 with Hoch's research, psychedelic psychiatry managed to survive both the tighter regulations on clinical trials and the non-medical controversies of the Sixties. At the Spring Grove State Hospital in Maryland, "the longest, largest, most sophisticated, and most successful such program ever undertaken in the United States"[8] definitely led to seminal psychedelic research with far-reaching implications.[9] But over in New York, psychiatrist Charles Dahlberg began investigations of his own in 1959 and continued to use LSD in analysis while maintaining a steady flow of scientific publications on LSD and similar compounds into the late 1970s. In this way, the psychedelic history of New York City points to an important site of research that reveals that Spring Grove was not the only place that remained actively involved in the field after the Sixties.

New York's Early Psychedelic Research

LSD first arrived in the United States in 1949 at a time when it was easy for drug manufacturers like Sandoz to distribute their products to qualified scientists for premarket investigations. This meant that researchers could carry out studies on small groups of patients with little oversight and minimal funding and that they "could easily explore hunches, suggestions, and unconventional uses for drugs, and follow leads when they got unexpected results."[10] In New York, Hoch and his team became the first to study these drugs in a decidedly experimental setting.

Paul Hoch was born in 1902 in Budapest and migrated to the US in 1933 after completing his training at the University of Göttingen. By 1948, he was the head of the Department of Experimental Psychiatry,[11] and soon after his appointment, he and his colleagues James Cattel and Harry Pennes began their research into LSD and mescaline, which they obtained from Sandoz and Bios, respectively. Initially, they were interested in mapping the common responses to these drugs, and they were fascinated by the reactions of the "normal" patients whose reactions to both drugs included schizophrenic symptoms, which gave support to the psychotomimetic hypothesis of the time.

In those early days, Hoch and his colleagues did not see any therapeutic benefits in the drug experience. They barely paid attention to some of the patients' verbalization of mental content like traumatic memories, and it was hard for them to see any form of "condensed psychoanalysis" in the mescaline experience, as one scientist had already posited.[12] Yet some of their patients reported rich and colourful visions under the influence: one of them "saw dragons and tigers coming to eat him and reacted to these hallucinations with marked anxiety," and later on "He also expressed an ecstatic grandiose trend of having the feeling that he was God in heaven and then, however, had the feeling of suddenly being in hell."[13] Subsequently, these kinds of visions became quite commonplace and analyzed as part of a therapeutic process, but back then they were simply understood as the consequence of a drug increasing the schizophrenic mind's hallucinatory symptoms.

Eventually, Hoch's team experimented on patients suffering from depression, phobia, and anxiety. Under the influence, some patients released material pertaining to sexual issues and childhood memories, which often suggested that trauma was behind the symptoms. But in his final analysis, Cattel cautioned against a therapeutic line of analysis,[14] and this scepticism was most likely the consequence of the CIA's funding. Indeed, the main purpose of the research conducted at the Psychiatric Institute was to study new psychoactive compounds as part of a classified contract with the Army Chemical Corps in order to develop non-lethal chemical weapons and new means of interrogation.

With the blessing of the federal government, Hoch's team was free to test new mind-altering drugs with the knowledge that they could operate with hardly any red tape and certainly no ethical guidelines. In late 1952, professional tennis player Harold Blauer checked himself in to seek treatment for severe depression. On 8 January 1953, a few weeks before he was scheduled to be released following good progress, Cattel gave him several injections of MDA and DMA, two unknown mescaline derivatives, which had been directly supplied by the Corps. The fifth injection caused Blauer's heart to stop.

Rather than publicly acknowledge this tragic blunder, the doctors tampered with his medical records so that it transpired that Blauer had a pre-existing heart condition.[15] In a declassified statement made after Blauer's death, Cattel justified this carelessness with the problem of experimental science: "We didn't delineate all the possibilities of what might happen because then you contaminate your experiment." In fact, he openly admitted that he had no idea of the kind of drug he was giving to his test subject because of the covert nature of their testing: "We didn't know whether it was dog piss ... This was a secret. We weren't in on it."[16] It was only in 1987 that Blauer's real cause of death was acknowledged.[17]

For the time being, news of psychedelic-related deaths did not reach the New York press, which was only starting to monitor the nascent psychedelic science. However, a noteworthy aspect of these early accounts is that even the Hearst empire developed an interest in LSD research, and this was a far cry from the anti-drug campaigns of the 1920s. In 1954, the Sunday paper *American Weekly* (circulation: 9.1 million) told the story of a girl reliving childhood trauma thanks to the drug.[18]

In the meantime, psychedelic research broke new ground when Aldous Huxley and Humphry Osmond connected with Bill Wilson, a former Wall Street speculator best known for founding Alcoholics Anonymous. While this meeting did not lead to substantial breakthroughs in psychedelic science, it introduced the idea that this research should acknowledge the spiritual component of the drug experience, which Hoch and his colleagues had dismissed as a form of delusion.

Osmond had already pioneered the psychedelic-assisted treatment of alcoholism in Saskatchewan[19] when he met Wilson in the spring of 1955. Wilson was immediately taken by his idea of inducing a transcendental experience with mescaline on alcoholics because he placed great emphasis on encountering God for the recovery process.[20] Shortly after his first LSD experience in Los Angeles, Wilson started a salon in New York where he and others discussed the spiritual implications of the drug.[21] Both Wilson and Osmond then discovered New York's vibrant parapsychology circles, which played an intriguing part in the scientific investigations into psychedelics.

In the early years of the Parapsychology Foundation, Eileen Garrett's *Tomorrow* published articles on psychedelics,[22] and in 1958 she organized an international conference on the scientific implications of psychedelics on ESP.[23] Around that time, the foundation became involved in the funding of psychedelic research by giving Osmond and his team a small grant to investigate telepathy between twins,[24] and it also provided Leary and theologian Walter Clark with some funds to study the religious implications of the psilocybin experience,[25] an emerging line of inquiry in psychedelic science.

Harold Abramson, meanwhile, was using the CIA funds to move away from the experimental uses of LSD and mescaline. Born in 1899,

Abramson got his medical degree from Columbia and became a private practitioner in 1935. He quickly realized that he knew very little about his patients and how he might approach them as whole individuals. He then received training in psychiatry and psychotherapy, but he grew frustrated with the absence of pharmacology in those disciplines. Around 1950, he first heard about LSD and immediately saw an opportunity "to bring the laboratory and psychiatry together" in the first published papers.[26]

In contrast with Hoch's research, Abramson and his colleagues began examining the effects of LSD on animals in order to assess its pharmacology[27] before testing it on mentally stable adults.[28] Soon he began to understand the psychedelic experience as a form of ego-enhancement rather than a drug that could induce a temporary psychosis. This became manifest during a psychoanalytic interview with a woman who was struggling with fears of homosexuality.[29] Abramson undertook this investigation at a time when homosexuality was still believed to be a disease and at a time when McCarthyist politics were targeting gays and lesbians.[30] His work soon drew the attention of *Time*, which by then was closely following research into psychedelic compounds.[31]

Little suggests that Abramson treated his test subjects unethically or that he engaged in reckless experimentation like Hoch's team had. According to the published papers, his subjects were paid adult volunteers, including "graduate students, scientists, engineers, nurses, hairdressers, and housewives," and they had all been screened for prior histories of mental illness. Moreover, Abramson had quickly realized that the setting of the drug experience could shape its outcome substantially. As a result, he soon found himself running sessions in his Long Island home, away from the unannounced interruptions of colleagues.[32] By the end of the decade, Abramson had published dozens of scientific papers and administered LSD several hundred times. In contrast to Hoch's team, his patients found the LSD experience most rewarding. "It was very difficult for me to persuade people not to take it again," he concluded.[33]

It is most likely that New York's resolutely experimental and interdisciplinary research into psychedelics gave Lauretta Bender the freedom to launch her own investigations into the therapeutic possibilities of LSD. Born in 1897 in Butte, Montana, Bender experienced serious difficulties at school and had to repeat her first grade three times. Her teachers concluded that she was mentally deficient, but it turned out that she was acutely dyslexic.[34] This did not prevent her from receiving her MD at the University of Iowa in 1926 at a time when few women ever became physicians. Subsequently, she remained keenly interested in the study of reading and writing disorders, and arguably her greatest legacy is the Bender-Gestalt Test (also known as the Visual Motor Gestalt Test), a widely used tool she developed to diagnose learning difficulties among children.

In 1930, Bender started working at Bellevue Hospital, and a few years later she became the first director of the children's inpatient ward. She developed an interest in psychopharmacology and began using amphetamines to treat children suffering from hyperkinesia and other forms of mental illnesses. This approach departed from the main therapeutic understanding of Benzedrine of the time, which concentrated on the treatment of depression.[35]

In 1956, Bender was appointed director of research at the newly created children's unit at Creedmoor State Hospital in Queens.[36] She discovered LSD, and as someone subject to migraines she used the drug to treat her condition and "found it a very effective preventive."[37] By the spring of 1959, research into the effects of LSD on children with autism was already underway at Creedmoor thanks to one of Bender's colleagues, Eva Ebin, at a time when "there was no indication in the literature that the drug had been used with children elsewhere."[38]

Before Bender could initiate her own studies, however, she needed to convince Paul Hoch, who was now enjoying a much greater role in the entire field of psychiatry. By then, he had been appointed commissioner of mental hygiene of the State of New York, overseeing twenty-eight hospitals and approximately 100,000 patients.[39] Initially, Hoch balked at the idea of provoking a temporary psychotic episode among children,[40] and the most likely reason for his disapproval is that by the end of the 1950s he had come to the conclusion that LSD had no therapeutic benefits whatsoever. In 1959, Hoch chaired the first international conference on psychedelic-based therapy, which was sponsored by the CIA through the Josiah Macy Jr Foundation, and while many of the speakers pointed to their positive results with mescaline and LSD, Hoch stubbornly contended that these drugs were "essentially anxiety-producing drugs" and that they were "not especially useful" in therapy.[41]

By citing prior work, Bender managed to persuade Hoch that LSD would increase responsiveness to sensory stimulation along with skeletal and muscle activity by inhibiting serotonin. Her team started with low doses (twenty-five μgr) on mute children and children diagnosed with autism and schizophrenia between five and eleven years of age. They found that the majority of them were subsequently able to make contact with the medical staff and engage in motor play, which was accompanied by mood elevation. They gradually increased the dosage until they reached 150 µgr per day and noted "an improvement in their general well-being, general tone, habit patterning, eating patterns and sleeping patterns" within the autistic population, while some children improved their vocalization. The boys diagnosed with schizophrenia (without autism) "became more insightful, more objective, more realistic," even though they soon lapsed into depression because they realized that they were in a hospital cut away from their families. Bender and her colleagues came to similar "normalizing" results using psilocybin and the more obscure methysergide, better known as UML-491 and marketed by Sandoz as Sansert for the treatment of migraines.[42]

Following Hoch's promotion, Sydney Malitz became acting chief of psychiatric research at the Department of Experimental Psychiatry, and with his new team came a number of important changes. Gone was the CIA funding, and in its place Malitz secured a grant from the United States Public Health Service, which allowed him to initiate clinical investigations into psilocybin. Those trials bore little resemblance to the department's research of the beginning of the Fifties: here, students were paid to take the drug to ascertain its pharmacology. In one of their scientific articles, the researchers openly referred to the recent popularization of psilocybin and noted that "Only one of our subjects reported what might be described as a transcendental experience resembling the religious ecstasies observed by Wasson," but they were not surprised, given the clinical setting in which the sessions were conducted.[43] In another published paper, which hypothesized that popular literature on psychedelics had drawn some of their volunteers, Malitz's team offered clearer evidence of Huxley's growing influence through the report of a twenty-seven-year-old Asian-American student, who came out of the session with a great deal of prestige: "very few people have gone through this and I am in good company – people like Aldous Huxley."[44]

By the early 1960s then, New York was a site of broad research into the pharmacology of psychedelics, which was made up of several research groups with widely differing interests in these drugs. As the decade came to a close, there was enough knowledge to begin their integration into therapy.

Psychedelic Psychoanalysis

Even in the early days of experimental research into mescaline, another group was immediately interested in exploring these new substances along Freudian lines at NYU's Research Center for Mental Health, which was created to study the psychoanalytical theory of consciousness. In 1953, psychologist Robert Holt teamed up with George Klein, who until that point had been working with David Rappaport at the Menninger Foundation in Kansas, which Osmond subsequently introduced to LSD and mescaline.[45] Holt and Klein's investigations were highly meticulous, and by the time they had finished their investigations in the early seventies, they had been the recipients of three research grants from the National Institute for Mental Health.[46]

After receiving an initial batch of LSD, a couple of junior colleagues took some 100 μgr doses and found the effects quite interesting. Holt and Klein then invited every staff member at the Research Center to take part in the study and began gathering data during the academic year of 1958–59. Whereas most scientists turned to college students for subjects, they wanted to test the drug on mature adults, and Klein "hit upon a ready source of underemployed people: the theatrical union, Actors' Equity." The actors were screened for medical conditions and then went through a battery of personality tests during an entire day. On the day of the LSD experience, subjects were randomly given the drug or a placebo, and the thirty experimental subjects were each assigned a biographer, "being in principal charge of assembling, analyzing, and integrating the various available materials for personality assessment."[47] In one of their first publications, the researchers concluded that "The questionnaire was highly successful in differentiating placebo subjects from those receiving LSD-25, using either quantitative or qualitative measures."[48]

In contrast to this rigorously empirical research, the first mental health professional to undertake a large-scale administration of LSD outside the clinic was Jean Houston, who had a strong interest in altered states of consciousness that went right back to her childhood. She was born in Brooklyn in 1937, and her involvement in psychedelic research, which began while she was still in graduate school, might seem like a footnote in her otherwise outstanding career, during which she published more than fifteen books on psychology, religion, and human potential and during which she worked with anthropologist Margaret Mead and

Hillary Clinton.[49] Nevertheless, she was a major figure in the psychedelic science networks of postwar New York and one whose vision of the psychedelic experience was visibly shaped by psychoanalysis.

The most likely reason that Houston went on to offer such a liberal form of psychedelic-assisted therapy is that she discovered LSD in a Bleecker Street apartment. This occurred around 1959 thanks to Michael Corner, a neurophysiologist who was finishing his PhD and introduced her to psychiatrists who were conducting research into LSD. However, they were confronted by the puzzling recurrence of myths and symbols in their drug sessions for which their medical training had left them unprepared. Given that Houston was already an expert on these topics, they asked her to help them guide the subjects through the experience.[50] First, though, she had to try the drug.

After a life-changing LSD experience full of spiritual imagery, Houston decided to become a guide. As part of her preparations, she turned to the literature on altered states of consciousness, but she was particularly drawn to the symbolic meaning of Dante's *Divine Comedy*, which she understood as an embodiment of the psychedelic experience. Houston, then, saw her role as close to Virgil's by guiding subjects "to experience the interrelationship of this material within themselves."

Houston quickly realized that she could help patients release psycho-dynamic material by directing their attention to "seashells, stones, flowers, plants, and vegetables. I would open the door into the glorious cathedral within green pepper. Or I would surround my subjects with a cornucopia of fruits and vegetables and ask them to enter into a friendly relationship with them."[51] In this supportive environment, some gained insights on their past and their mental hang-ups several hours into the session, and others put forth new ideas and solved existing problems. "My subjects would often find themselves acting out myths and legends internally," Houston recalls, "and passing through initiations and ritual observances that appeared to be structured precisely in terms of their own most urgent needs."[52]

One of the reasons that she paid so much attention to context is that she had witnessed how LSD was being researched in the cold setting of the hospital. In one instance, a young medical student was told that he would experience anxiety and hallucinations just before an LSD session. "We were all sitting around in an antiseptic room," she remembers, "which is the worst possible kind of place, with everybody in white coats. The young man was very tense." As the drug took hold of him, the psychiatrist asked him specific questions pertaining to psychopharmacology, and later on he received an injection and an electroencephalograph, which made things even worse. By the end of the session, the psychiatrist had easily validated his hypothesis: "yes LSD is psychotomimetic."[53] Houston was mystified, but such an approach aptly reflected the clinical culture of the time, which was "increasingly focused on accumulating data, rather than honing technique and studying patient responses."[54]

Soon Houston's thoughtful LSD-based therapy drew the attention of interested celebrities like Fritz Perls. When she paid him a visit in his Central Park apartment, a distraught Perls confessed that he was suffering from mental illness and that he no longer felt qualified to treat his patients effectively. LSD was bound to help him. Houston listened to his afflictions carefully, but by the end of the interview she concluded that such a complex and struggling psyche was too much for a twenty-two-year-old to handle. It was only when the two of them reconnected at the Esalen Institute in California years later that Perls cheerfully told her that Leary had since offered him plenty of opportunities to sample the drug.[55]

In January 1963, Houston was graced by the visit of Aldous Huxley. By then, his psychedelic essays and his recently published final novel *Island* had become her scriptures, and it was with some trepidation that she opened the door to greet the dying psychedelic superstar. They sat down, and after reading aloud an excerpt from "Doors," they began discussing how flowers might offer a gateway into paradise under the influence of LSD, and for Houston it was striking that flowers and gardens had such an important place in so many of the world's myths. Huxley concurred and added that "Flowers can be the bridge between here and the beyond, for they exist in both realms."[56]

Another topic they broached was *Island*, which depicted an imaginary and Utopian society partly based on sacred mushroom rituals. However, Houston was deeply disappointed by the ending. Indeed, Huxley's fictitious society is ultimately crushed by an oil-hungry military regime, which brings an end to his enlightened society, and she had a hard time buying into this tragic conclusion. Huxley admitted that she was right and told her that a fire in his California home had destroyed all his manuscripts, including *Island*. The reason that he did not rewrite a longer story with a happier ending was down to his rapidly deteriorating health: "I haven't been feeling well recently, and I wanted to get the book out. I am afraid that I rewrote a shorter book in which the ideas were more important than the plot or literary development."[57]

Given the growing and broad interests in psychedelic drugs, Houston and Corner created the Agora Scientific Trust to better study the effects of psychedelics on mental health.[58] This interdisciplinary organization, located between Madison and Park avenues on 81st Street, was among the first centres in the country to focus exclusively on these drugs. Among the research advisers was *Playboy* executive Victor Lownes, and the trust could count on the financial support of Nassau millionaire Howard Teague, who bankrolled the organization by helping it acquire property and furniture. According to Stanley Krippner, Teague had a life-changing psychedelic experience and wanted to see psychedelics used legally.[59]

While few details about the internal functioning of the trust are known, Houston was in charge of a program designed to train guides. Here, psychiatrists and clinical psychologists had the opportunity to learn how to adapt their own techniques to include the management of a psychedelic experience. To achieve this, the trainees were given LSD or a similar drug, and this was usually enough to persuade them "that special methods were called for and would be well worth the learning." Moreover, Houston encouraged them to resist diving head-first into analysis and self-exploration. Instead, she instructed the trainees to fully appreciate the new sensory awareness triggered by the psychedelic, including the amazing experience of synaesthesia ("the hearing of color, the tasting of sound"). As well, Houston retained the use of objects, artworks, and fruit with the apprentices, who found symbolic meaning in them. For instance, "A sliced pomegranate became 'the seeds of anguish, the wounds of discontent,' which the subject then discussed in terms of a patient whose case he said was similar to his own."[60]

Another prominent guide and co-founder of Agora was John Beresford, yet another British immigrant who played a key role in the popularization of LSD and psychedelics. Beresford was fascinated by Huxley's explorations into inner space and first tried mescaline after ordering some from Hoffmann-La Roche.[61] Since he was still a professor at the New York Medical College, he acquired a large batch of acid from Sandoz, and he initially intended to study the effects of the drug on amoebas and conduct a series of experiments on bone marrow. But after a life-changing experience with the drug, he resigned from his professorship. He then joined Houston and Corner to take part in this exciting adventure and gave his LSD to the trust.

Roger Wescott, a Princeton graduate with backgrounds in linguistics and anthropology, was among those who took LSD under Beresford's supervision.[62] Although Wescott was enthusiastic, he "mistrusted the rigidity both of his personality and of his clinical technique." Early in 1963, he negotiated to schedule the session in the comfort of his own home in which Beresford gave the drug to Wescott and his fiancée. They both enjoyed the experience, but they felt that it would have been a different story had they not been together and inside the trust. More to the point, Wescott thought that they "could have had a much richer and freer experience with a more congenial administrant."[63] Sigrid Radulovic, on the other hand, had a life-changing experience with him in May of that year, which saw her shed her status of "a very successful, ambitious, competitive, antidrug, martini-swigging New York book editor" and become "a peaceful, barefoot, pot-smoking hippie single mom living in the Virgin Islands, working for the Black Liberation movement there."[64]

In March 1963, Beresford ran another group session in the apartment of the chairman of a Columbia department. A neurophysiologist had a "profound and wonderful" experience, which led "to a desire to study cultures of brain cells through the microscope," but another participant "got hung up at a nine month old infantile Freudian level, forgot his decorum and toilet training," and began fondling his penis, which caused a great deal of embarrassment for Beresford and the host. For the British physician, this infantile reaction was due to the complexities of life, which had become too overwhelming and had forced the subject to lock them away into his subconscious drawer.[65]

While LSD was the select substance to treat patients at the trust, psychologists could sometimes offer peyote to their participants. In one instance, three subjects, including a businessman in his late twenties, took it in an apartment, and after a while the businessman expressed the wish to explore New York under the influence: "The city, which had seemed from the window cold, grimy and slightly sinister, now was transformed into the wonderland I had envisioned when hearing fables as a child." Here too, peyote summoned arresting visions that echoed the non-medical uses that were already underway in Greenwich Village. As the evening went on, the guide indeed turned into "a kind of benign Buddha, making his own inner judgments of the people present."[66]

While Houston and Beresford were exploring psychedelics in such an eclectic fashion, Charles Dahlberg was likewise investigating the psychoanalytic potential of LSD by offering a similarly liberal approach to patient management. Dahlberg was an experienced analyst by the time he began working with LSD at the William Alanson White Institute in 1959. In fact, he candidly admitted that he had never done any research in the past, which probably explains why his work was so geared toward practical treatment.[67]

Like Houston, Dahlberg believed that LSD helped subjects to access potentially traumatic events and offered a form of "sensory deprivation" that allowed patients to focus on their inner realities, cut off from the outside. His technique involved the administration of doses that were under 100 μgrs on outpatients diagnosed with neurosis, and this was quite a bold move because many of his peers like Hoch were strictly opposed to releasing patients into the community after taking LSD.[68] To minimize potential dangers, however, Dahlberg had follow-ups on a regular basis, and he worked with a trained person who accompanied the patients to their homes at the end of the session and stayed with them until the effects had worn off.

A noteworthy aspect of Dahlberg's psychotherapeutic model is that he paid little attention to the setting in which the session was conducted because it ran the risk of distracting the patients: "Other workers [like Houston] have used props, music and blindfolds to encourage fantasy. I have not done so because, while it is true that fantasy and acting-out can be stimulated in this way, verbal communication, which is at the heart of the analytic process, is diminished by such means."[69] This approach departed from other North American research teams that made sure the location of the experience had several interactive features that might help the patients reach new insights.[70]

Outside the White Institute, most New York therapists were aware of the importance of a supportive environment. For instance, radical leftist Carl Marzani once took the drug under the supervision of a private practitioner. The room was darkened so that he could better focus on his inner self, and the doctor played some soothing guitar music on a stereo to help him loosen his thoughts. Marzani perceived the music as having a "Faustian" quality, to which the psychiatrist replied that the music depended on his interpretation: "the music is only a peg, as you are aware. These feelings are your feelings."[71] By probing further, Marzani managed to associate Faust with ambition and knowledge.

However, Marzani's psychedelic therapy was not confined to the physician's office. Sometimes, the doctor and the patient would take a walk outside in order to appreciate how different the world looked after taking LSD. And after roaming through his mind for about four hours, Marzani and his therapist went to Central Park, and there he noticed the differences: "The world is sharper, brighter than usual; trees, houses, faces, colors, textures, everything has a freshness, a sharpness, a clarity that is delightful." The doctor also showed him how the drug could increase the power of observation: "He plucks a leaf and holds it against the light: the minute tracery of the veins and structure has a distinctness I never would have noticed. The bark of a small sycamore is velvety in touch, the dappled browns and grays shading into a sensuous tapestry."[72] A few days after his LSD session, his perception of life seemed to have changed: "For the first time in months I pleasured in the life and activity of the river, in grass and trees, in breeze and flowing water."[73]

Later on, the psychiatrist suggested that as a political activist and an intellectual, he was trying too hard to change society and how people think. He reasoned that Marzani was suffering from restlessness because he was trying to achieve too much, without accepting failure or limited achievements. He managed to solve this after a third LSD session and found his self-confidence restored: "fame and glory ... are all very well, but even better is a simple meal shared in peace with an old friend." After his third and final LSD session with the psychiatrist, Marzani felt "friendship and affection" toward him, and the MD expressed something similar.[74]

Singer Ronnie Gilbert was suffering from acute depression, and in 1962 she found the help of psychiatrist James Watt, who offered a distinctly holistic LSD-based treatment that echoed some aspects of Marzani's own therapy. Under the influence, they visited art galleries, and Gilbert produced paintings that were "luminously nonobjective splashes of color and curiously pleasant." The aesthetic experience was likewise enhanced by walks in nearby Central Park, where she experienced "an atavistic sense of life around [her]." These experiences were supplemented with a spiritual component by going to churches. Her depression disappeared after six months.[75]

In late March 1963, a struggling Robert Cullen wrote to Leary to seek his help after reading a *Life* article about psychedelics. He had tried psychoanalysis in the past and had found the therapy helpful but insufficient. He still suffered from sexual disturbance and suicidal tendencies, which had been left unresolved.[76] But once again, James Watt came to the rescue by supervising Cullen's LSD experience in April, which had a tremendous effect on his mental health. "I will simply never be the same person I was, even after just one 'session,'" wrote Cullen. "The thought of suicide has become absurd to me. I will always think of you and Dr. Watt as two strangers I came to, who saved me from tragedy." While he wished to take the drug again, he was going "to delay a second LSD experience for some time in order to fully appreciate the remarkable effect it has had on [his] point of view." Cullen was so overwhelmed by his dramatic improvement that he immediately saw the drug as something more than just a medical technology: "I am convinced that the very future of the race may depend on what men like you and Dr. Watt are doing with LSD and similar 'drugs.'"[77]

Some liberal therapists were happy to encourage their clients' use of LSD outside their office, if they proceeded with caution. In 1961, millionaire Peggy Hitchcock had experimented with mescaline and was undergoing group therapy with Asya Kadis, best known for pioneering the application of psychoanalysis in groups. Hitchcock had just finished a long-term relationship with Allan Eager, a jazz musician addicted to heroin, and she realized that she needed to understand why she would want to get involved with an addict. As Hitchcock became increasingly taken to psychedelics, Kadis did not attempt to discourage her use and was instead very supportive of her "explorations of consciousness."[78]

Other doctors condoned even more uncanny forms of drug experimentation. A few years later, a journalist told the story of a mother who had taken acid before giving birth to her child in her own home and under the supervision of her physician. There were no issues with the delivery, and the mother stated that the drug had eased the pain. Yet she made it clear that the primary motivation had been "for the very intense, very personal, experience it promised" and later confessed that it had been the most meaningful event of her entire life.[79]

Some New Yorkers simply found therapeutic renewal after experimenting with psychedelics in non-medical settings. For example, a peyote user claimed to have improved his health as a result of his experimentation: after eating the cactus, he virtually stopped drinking alcohol.[80] Writer and visual artist Eve Babitz, on the other hand, was suffering from hypochondria: whenever she heard about a new disease, she would discover the symptoms in herself. The idea of going to the doctor's terrified her, even though physicians invariably found nothing wrong with her. But this disappeared altogether after some chemical explorations. "After my first session with LSD I was never afraid of doctors again," she claimed. "I wasn't even afraid of dying ... I am much freer now, with all those fears gone. It is such a relief. I feel like I can really live now, enjoy things, get involved in my work."[81]

As these multiple settings suggest, psychedelic science and LSD-based therapy seemed destined for a bright future in New York City. But in 1962, the federal government introduced a new piece of legislation that had a significant impact on study designs for everyone working in the field. Researchers now needed FDA approval to be legally permitted to investigate the effects of LSD on human subjects.

Regulating Acid

As research was blossoming in New York and in other parts of the United States, the country was rocked by a drug scandal that had nothing to do with LSD: thalidomide. This sedative, which was first marketed in West Germany in 1957, was used for investigational purposes, and for a time thousands of pregnant American women received it as an experimental treatment to alleviate morning sickness. "When the dramatic birth defects thalidomide caused were discovered in 1962, the danger of leaving the conduct of premarket drug research largely up to the discretion of researchers and pharmaceutical companies became starkly apparent." A bill was introduced to modify the federal Food, Drug, and Cosmetic Act of 1938, which resulted in the Kefauver-Harris Amendments of 1962.

As a result, double-blind placebo-controlled clinical trials became the norm, and given that the validity of psychedelic-assisted therapy was ultimately gauged through the psychological assessment of its subjects rather than through hard, biological data, this treatment model was fundamentally at odds with the new legislation.[82] In this way, the Drug

Amendments left no room for investigations with loose or non-existent study designs and prevented mental health professionals from freely administering obscure substances to unsuspecting patients or from offering Jungian psychotherapy in someone's apartment.

With the new legislation, research teams needed to submit their data to the FDA to show that a drug could be used on humans safely and with positive results, as well as the details of their study designs (qualifications, experience, facilities, etc.). Beresford, who had so easily obtained New Jersey acid a few years earlier, saw the writing on the wall. He had since connected with Leary, and in an April 1963 letter he expressed his skepticism as to whether any research into LSD could be undertaken without the Swiss firm's approval in the near future.[83]

Beresford's fears were confirmed a few months later. As the only legitimate supplier of LSD, Sandoz chose to sponsor research that was funded by the NIMH, state agencies, the Veterans Administration, and, a little later, the National Science Foundation. Hence, many privately funded research groups and private practitioners were unable to carry on their work with the drug. Even a well-respected scientist like Abramson could no longer have access to LSD.[84]

In the following years, non-medical drug use increased steadily. The federal government introduced the Drug Abuse Control Amendment in July 1965, which also translated into increased book-keeping and registration for the legitimate channels of LSD distribution. The FDA simultaneously created the Bureau of Drug Abuse Control (BDAC), which had staff and offices nationwide. However, the bureau had more pressing matters than hallucinogens: at the time, one congressman estimated that nine billion barbiturate and amphetamine tablets were reaching the illegal drug markets each year. The amendments, then, did not specifically prioritize psychedelic drugs, but they did offer provisions to add other substances deemed dangerous. It was only on 15 July 1966 that the FDA turned LSD into a controlled substance.[85]

In the spring of that year, Sandoz announced its withdrawal from clinical investigations into LSD and psilocybin, citing the black market and reckless proselytizers. As a result, research groups across the country were required to return their materials. Psychiatrist Paul Lowinger, who was running clinical trials in Detroit, openly denounced the firm's termination of valuable research into mental illness in a letter published in *Science*.[86] A reply soon came from the Sandoz Foundation in New York in which an executive pointed out that they had been generously supplying legitimate research for nearly twenty years free of charge and helping scientists with an up-to-date bibliography. While the Swiss firm contended that "the problems of preserving its reputation, policing of supplies, servicing law enforcement agencies, and keeping track of legitimate projects became too heavy a burden to carry," this did not mean the outright end of research into LSD. Rather, the supplies and responsibility were transferred to the NIMH, which continued to authorize a handful of government-funded studies.[87]

Jean Houston had already moved on by then. In 1965, she married sexologist Robert Masters, who had also worked at Agora, and during their honeymoon they wrote their classic *Varieties of Psychedelic Experiences*, which was given the front page of the *New York Times Review of Books*.[88] However, this landmark publication was their last involvement in the field. That same year, they started the Foundation for Mind Research to study non-drug-induced altered states of consciousness,[89] and as Houston wrote around that time, it was extremely difficult to obtain a licence to carry out research into LSD, which was no longer produced in the US and illegal to import. But by her estimates, there were still approximately twenty-two grams of Sandoz LSD in the country,[90] which were distributed among the last thirteen groups of researchers working with federal or state grants.[91] By 1966, however, there were in fact a total of seventy sanctioned research groups in the country, though that figure eventually dropped to nine.[92]

Charles Dahlberg, for one, was allowed to continue his work, and he responded to the heated exchange in *Science* with an optimistic letter. As Masters and Houston were finishing their book manuscript, Dahlberg's team received a substantial grant from the NIMH ($166,251; $1,447,750 in 2021) "to assess, through a longitudinal, double-blind investigation using psycholinguistic, psychometric, and clinical indices, the effect of LSD-25 upon ongoing psychotherapeutic interaction" at the White Institute's Psycholinguistic Laboratory of the Research Department.[93] The process of negotiating the grant had been surprisingly straightforward. "To my delight," Dahlberg wrote, "when [colleague] Joe Jaffe and I went to the NIMH to talk about the project, I discovered that they were almost as happy at our meeting as I was ... Our association with

NIMH has been instructive, helpful, encouraging, and remunerative."[94] Dahlberg agreed that adverse media coverage had impacted psychedelic research significantly, but at the end of the day he was just happy to continue his exciting research.[95]

Dahlberg's subsequent research at the White Institute continued to explore the therapeutic applications of the drug using the same psychoanalytical framework, and in spite of the tighter regulations on psychedelic science, patients could still go home with an attendant immediately after the session.[96] However, they were now required to fill in an FDA consent form as well as several questionnaires for rigorous screening of prior conditions, but most of them saw this as a reassuring proof of the scientists' seriousness against a backdrop of widely advertised non-medical LSD use.[97]

Against the tide, then, the White Institute carried on its research into medically sanctioned LSD, and the scientists working at the Research Center for Mental Health likewise continued to publish scientific papers into the early 1970s. A probable reason that they were largely unaffected by the change in legislation is that they had long been interested in carrying out studies using a highly empirical methodology that sat better with the new regulations than Masters and Houston's own eclectic model.

By the mid-Sixties, they were attempting to map the common subjective responses to LSD through a questionnaire that was created specifically for this purpose,[98] and they continued to use a placebo group of test subjects for their studies.[99] In all the papers that they published in the late Sixties, nothing indicates that the researchers were paying attention to the controversies and the gradual curtailing of psychedelic science, and it was only in a 1972 book summarizing their contribution to the field that they lamented the "confused public and governmental response" to LSD that distracted from its usefulness as an investigative tool to study human behaviour.[100]

Most researchers in New York were not as lucky. After 1966, they could only publish prior findings and scientific papers offering reviews of the state of the field, while lamenting the controversies and Sandoz's decision. Among those was Sydney Malitz, who had grown tired of those debates: "Few subjects, save religion and politics, have evoked such heated discussion as the use of LSD-25 and mescaline in psychiatric treatment."[101] Another team led by Herman Denber, who had been investigating the clinical potential of mescaline at the Manhattan State Hospital,[102] could not pursue its clinical work either, and their final contribution to the field was a 1969 paper criticizing "Efforts to limit laboratory and carefully controlled clinical studies" with psychedelics.[103] In the latter part of the Sixties, Abramson published a review article on the clinical applications of LSD on children in 1967,[104] but he had become quite vocal in his criticism of the dire state of the field, both in a subsequent publication[105] and a popular magazine.[106]

Amid the controversies, Masters had to briefly come out of his retirement from psychedelic research to chime in. In their 1968 collection on psychedelic art, he and his wife openly stressed that further research was warranted because these substances had "value in psychotherapy, but also for research in many areas outside medicine and therapy – for example, philosophy, psychology, anthropology, religion, scientific problem-solving, and the arts."[107]

But in private, Masters was furious at the public outcries surrounding LSD, and as the director of research of his new institution, he told his colleagues that he was no longer prepared to let politicians and the media orchestrate a smear campaign without fighting back: "I, for one, am fed up with all this bullshit. Now I am going to tell some unpopular truths about psychedelics."[108] This meant publicly discussing the effects of LSD on sex in *Playboy*,[109] with material that had been omitted from *Varieties* for fear of bringing controversy to psychedelic research. But given that it had come to a near standstill, that no longer mattered to him.

Lauretta Bender and her team could have turned to the NIMH for supplies, but by then there were rumours linking LSD with irreversible chromosome damage. Three years later, her last known involvement with psychedelic science was to publish a paper that did not corroborate those reports after she had closely examined their eighty-nine child subjects.[110] For Krippner, Bender purposefully withdrew from LSD in order to protect herself and preserve her reputation as a medical doctor, even though she was very enthusiastic about psychedelics.[111] Nonetheless, she managed to have her New York State licence to administer psychedelics renewed on 1 July 1971,[112] although what she did with that licence is not known.

That same year saw the passing of the Controlled Substance Act, which epitomized the Nixon administration's war on drugs, and under this new piece of legislation, LSD became a Schedule I drug, considered to have a high potential of abuse and no value for medical applications. Two years later, one of the NIMH's prominent scientists and a veteran of psychedelic research concluded that psychedelic therapy was "no better than other therapies," and in 1974, the institute officially put an end to the funding of LSD research in the United States.[113] By the end of the decade, investigations had come to a close, and the thousands of academic papers that had been published over the course of almost three decades were a powerful reminder of the enthusiasm the drug had generated in the postwar years.

Throughout the Seventies, Dahlberg and his collaborators published their findings on the effects of LSD on speech – a largely unexplored area in psychedelic science – in rigorously empirical study designs. In two investigations co-sponsored by the New York State Department of Mental Hygiene, they found that LSD slowed down patients' monologues,[114] and soon afterwards they examined the effects of the drug on verbal interaction during psychotherapy.[115] Sometime in 1978, Dahlberg transferred from the White Institute to the Department of Communication Sciences at the New York State Psychiatric Institute to continue his work. His final string of publications revealed that LSD increased the use of novel figurative language[116] and that patients made more personal statements and were less inclined to use explanation[117] during psychoanalysis.

Given those somewhat moderate contributions, it is unsurprising that Dahlberg's legacy has been overshadowed by undoubtedly more significant psychedelic research on alcoholism and end-of-life anxiety. Dahlberg's involvement in the field, which ran over the course of two decades and which took him from psychoanalysis to psycholinguistics, nevertheless reveals both the longevity of psychedelic research in New York and the influence of the city's robust psychoanalytical tradition.

The story of psychedelic science in New York City offers an almost microcosmic synthesis of that history on a national level. The early focus on the ability of LSD and mescaline to induce a temporary psychosis quickly shifted to a more therapeutic understanding of these drugs. By the early Sixties, LSD-based psychoanalysis was widely available both in the offices of private practitioners and within the walls of the White Institute and of the Agora Scientific Trust, one of the first, if short-lived, psychedelic research centres of the country and perhaps the entire world.

New York's psychedelic scientists also made more modest contributions by studying the effects of LSD on child autism and by pioneering research on LSD in the realm of psycholinguistics and parapsychology. And as in other parts of the country, New York's psychedelic research has a darker history with the tragic involvement of the CIA, even if this covert funding for Cold Warfare undoubtedly benefitted a well-regarded doctor like Abramson. These diverse medical settings enabled hundreds if not thousands of New Yorkers to undergo the psychedelic experience, and it is unlikely that these early experimenters refrained from sharing their chemical explorations with their relatives and friends.

By the mid-1960s, this new therapeutic culture seemed to be gaining a foothold in postwar New York, regardless of the legislation and regardless of the regulatory concerns about safety and efficacy. For instance, one doctor, who had tried the drug in a non-medical setting with a very positive outcome, claimed that he knew "a lot of therapists and three or four doctors who are using it,"[118] and Dahlberg confirmed that some therapists were indeed using LSD illegally "as last-ditch attempts to do something with resistant patients."[119] Psychedelic research in New York, then, partly explains the non-medical acid wave that swept the city in the 1960s.

It should not come as a surprise that New York's lively scientific networks hardly paid any attention to psilocybin and its belated arrival into the postwar pharmacopeia. The early focus on both mescaline and LSD meant that there was little incentive to start examining a new psychoactive drug following its 1958 synthesis. In this way, this near-absence of studies on indocybin (CAP) in the city makes Leary's own undertakings all the more unique because they allowed a synthetic drug to make an almost direct transition from the laboratory to the streets.

4

New York on Acid

At the beginning of the 1960s, New York boasted a growing psychoactive marketplace and important scientific research into the therapeutic effects of mescaline and LSD. While working-class neighbourhoods continued to harbour heroin and amphetamine consumption, New Yorkers ranging from real estate agents and psychoanalysts to Bohemian poets and journalists had discovered the mysterious category of psychedelics that promised highly rewarding mind-altering experiences.

But while many favourably experimented with peyote and psilocybin, it is easy to see why LSD quickly became the choice drug of that category. Acid was a potent mind-altering substance that could offer life-changing experiences, but it also had highly appealing characteristics. It had no physical side effects, and a minute dose was enough to produce a colourful psychedelic experience that could last nearly twelve hours. More importantly, the drug had no legal status, and it had to wait for the second part of the decade for non-medical use to be effectively prohibited. When LSD entered the drug scene, it was just another substance among the battery of drugs available to Americans in the golden era of psychopharmacology.[1]

Once more, the local media played a significant part in the popularization of LSD. In 1956, Aldous Huxley spent an entire day giving radio and TV talks that the New York Academy of Science had scheduled for him.[2] In 1963, two members of the Anglican Orthodox Church learned about Leary's research during Richard Alpert's presentation at David Susskind's "Open End Television Show."[3] A year later, Alpert gave another talk on a WMCA radio show hosted by the famous Barry Gray, and for a thirty-two-year-old biophysicist, this was "a most engrossing discussion" on LSD, which spurred his desire to try the drug.[4]

The Luce empire continued to offer favourable reporting. Luce and his wife Clare had enjoyed their multiple experiences with the drug, and their candid enthusiasm reached both the pages of his magazines and his staff. At a 1964 annual ball, a *Time* and *Life* executive was shocked when Luce openly endorsed LSD in one of his speeches.[5] The media mogul, who exerted a strong influence on his magazines right until his death in 1967, reportedly gave copies of a book on psychedelics to the managing directors. Even when LSD became more controversial in the second part of the decade, *Time* and *Life* offered balanced coverage by cautioning its readers against indiscriminate LSD use, while simultaneously extolling its medical benefits. Some of his employees soon developed a keen interest in psychedelics.[6]

In this favourable context, LSD use steadily increased throughout the decade. After championing psilocybin for more than a year, even Leary had to admit that acid was the real deal. But this time around, his influence on the dissemination of LSD in the metropolis was more limited, and by the time he had discovered the drug in 1961, it was already part of New York's growing psychoactive bazaar. Unsurprisingly, LSD first arrived in Greenwich Village, but very soon it started to appear outside the capital of urban Bohemia, which was undergoing important changes at the turn of the 1950s. Slowly, psychedelia moved across Lower Manhattan and started to settle on the Lower East Side, where it enjoyed a tense relationship with the local working class.

The Early Days of LSD

Before creating the Agora Scientific Trust, John Beresford met a growing circle of psychedelic drug users, including Eric Loeb, who was still running his store,[7] and Michael Hollingshead, who has gone down as a legend in psychedelic lore for being the man who introduced Leary to LSD.[8] While the Harvard academic was getting psilocybin through Sandoz, another acquaintance of Beresford, Chuck Bick, was conducting a similar operation with LSD by distributing it to "bankers, lawyers, doctors, teaching staff from New York and Columbia Universities, writers, musicians, painters, playboys, clergymen, prostitutes" in Manhattan. The whole process of obtaining the drug was just as easy. He simply phoned the company and told them that his assistant would be picking up another vial of ten milligrams.[9] Ed Rosenfeld was one of those who tried the drug in its early days, and he remembered that "There was a little coterie of people who were interested in exotic drugs" in Greenwich Village.[10]

The young Jeff Perkins was also introduced to acid at the turn of the decade. In 1960, he moved to New York from Massachusetts to attend art school where he befriended a student from Detroit named Tony Watkins, who was half-Asian and half-Black. They both liked to hang out in a little bar next to Washington Square Park. One night, they were drinking beer and listening to the juke box when they were approached by a Black man who seemed to be under the influence of something quite powerful. "Do you want to get high?" he asked them. Perkins was game, but the man wanted to be sure, "and then he said 'do you want to get *really* high? Do you want to get *very* high?' And I said 'well, yes. I do.' And so he gave us both a sugar cube ... And this was LSD." A little later, Perkins and Watkins went outside and walked around Washington Square Park, which was covered in snow: "And I remember we were falling in the snow. It wasn't really a very strong LSD experience, but it was high. You got very beautifully high."

Perkins was keen to try LSD because he had been smoking marijuana on a regular basis. "And pot was kind of similar – but LSD had this ultra-perception associated within the physical experience."[11] Likewise, a twenty-year-old singer and actress became interested in LSD after sampling cannabis in the Village.[12] For Rosenfeld, who had experimented with peyote, LSD was a lot easier to manage. "Cleaning the peyote buttons, cutting off the buttons, taking the strings out, chopping them off, getting them down – LSD was much simpler."[13]

Like Perkins and Rosenfeld, clergyman Michael Itkin had experimented with psychoactive plants before discovering LSD but over a much longer period of time. Beginning in the mid-1950s, he tried just about every known psychedelic as well as the less commonplace Hawaiian Baby Woodrose (*Argyreia nervosa*) and buffoteine.[14] Moreover, Itkin had been through extensive Jungian psychotherapy, which he believed prepared him "in some way, for the experience [he] underwent with L.S.D." This happened in the fall of 1962 in the context of an uncontrolled experiment with the drug. For a religiously inclined person like him, the experience was "most revealing about [his] innermost life, etc., as well as having brought to a full realization the truth of the Christian faith."[15]

That a devout Christian had found great meaning in acid might come as a surprise, but a brief look at his life and times suggests that his interest in psychedelics was likely the result of his liberal world views. Itkin was licensed to the ministry in 1955, but he was considered a radical in religious circles. Long before Unitarian minister James Stoll's watershed "coming-out tour" that began in September 1969,[16] this independent Catholic openly admitted his homosexuality and championed the integration of gays and lesbians in church, while actively campaigning for social justice in the following decades.[17]

Moreover, Itkin's experimentations occurred at a time when New York was undergoing deep spiritual transformations. In the summer of 1957, Evangelical preacher Billy Graham announced that he was setting out to turn New York into a holy place, and his revivalist crusade drew impressive crowds all over the city. As well, Graham acknowledged New York's religious pluralism and condemned the strands of anti-Catholicism and anti-Semitism that had long plagued Protestant Evangelicalism.[18] Hence, psychedelic spirituality matured in a generally favourable climate of tolerance toward unorthodox beliefs (such as spiritualism). Religion in New York did not completely reject doctrine, but it "became a religion of meanings and significances, superseding religions of doctrines and decrees."[19] In doing so, it left the door open for psychedelic drug users to interpret their experiences along those lines.

A few months after trying LSD, Itkin contacted Leary, who was actively looking for clergymen to participate in his research.[20] In the meantime, however, the Harvard professor had met Hollingshead. The Briton had suffered a profound existential crisis following his first LSD experience in his Village apartment and sought Leary's counselling. Eventually, Hollingshead managed to convince Leary to try LSD, and somehow his first acid trip was even more profound than his initial psilocybin trip. As a result, he carried on his psychedelic mission in the city while moving closer and closer to early academic retirement.

Around that time, the psychedelic movement received a major boost from the local upper class in the person of Peggy Hitchcock.

As a millionaire and heiress to the Mellon family who saw herself as a "trust fund baby," she led a carefree life away from professional duties, and she became fascinated by Leary and LSD. Throughout the centuries, the New York wealthy typically formed close-knit communities, and as the local middle class grew in numbers and threatened to climb the socio-economic ladder, the upper class remained aggressively focused on the "relentless pursuit of privilege." But affluent New Yorkers were nonetheless more inclined to meet new people and explore new ideas than people in any other American or European city,[21] and this might explain why Hitchcock chose to become involved with Leary.

In any event, she discovered LSD at a time when she longed for a more exciting life, in spite of her stupendous resources. "I found myself very bored with my 'nice' upper class milieu," Hitchcock admits. "My friends at the time were mostly artists and musicians, with whom I felt much more at home." She discovered Huxley's literature, which made a strong impression on her, and soon afterwards she took mescaline in the apartment of a painter during the summer of 1961.

Hitchcock was a friend of the well-connected Van Wolf, and when he told her that he had met two Harvard academics working on psilocybin, she believed it might improve her mental health. She met Leary, and in the winter she finally took the drug in Richard Alpert's office and subsequently attended several other psilocybin parties at the Fergusons. In 1962, she finally tried LSD at their place,[22] and in the following years she became Leary's part-time lover and a major financial backer of his psychedelic movement.[23]

Over the next few months, more New Yorkers sent Leary expressions of interest and support. A PhD who had taken peyote with some friends in 1955 was thrilled to hear about his research and asked him how he might become involved with his group.[24] Another experimenter was just as delighted and claimed that Leary's scientific commitment to prisoner rehabilitation and the creation of enlightened psychoactive communities was "almost too good to be true." But the supporter also warned that controversy would never be far away, despite the stellar endorsements of Huxley and Allan Watts.[25] It is unlikely that this warning sank into Leary, who by then knew that his future was outside academia.

However, there was still time to initiate Alan Harrington, a novelist known for his black humour and social criticism and a veteran of the Village scene. In April 1963, Harrington underwent the LSD experience accompanied by Ralph Metzner, a young graduate student and one of Leary's close collaborators. As the drug took hold of him, the writer alternately sobbed and laughed. He came to realize the absurdity of the world surrounding him and found the whole universe so bizarre that "It was almost humourless."[26] But in the aftermath of his trip, Harrington believed that the ego-shattering acid experience had possibly saved his marriage. He and his wife were no longer getting along, and under the influence he realized that he deeply loved her.[27] Another remarkable aspect of his experience was his spiritual awakening. Harrington was self-described as an atheist, but in this instance he returned to his ordinary consciousness with a strong metaphysical connection.[28]

For others, however, the acid experience had the opposite effect. Linda Sontag, a seventeen-year-old college student, resented religious dogma under the influence. One day, she ingested a strong dose and wandered around Greenwich Village. Eventually, she sat in the back of a church and watched the Christian faithful light candles and kneel before statues. To her, the rituals were outdated and devoid of authenticity: "I felt the emotionless expressions of devotion as they repeated words of prayer, the meanings of which they no longer remember ... I thought, how sad, they can't or won't see that the power they sing to, pray to, kneel before is asleep within them – every one of them."[29]

For Jeff Perkins, the LSD experience likewise allowed him to bypass orthodox religion: "These words – spiritual, religious, Divine – they all have these associations of imagery that I know very well. The Virgin Mary and St-Thomas, and Jesus Christ and God ... They are iconic images. None of these things ... apply to that experience at all." Instead, he was left with an extraordinary feeling that was hard to describe: "If anything, I mean, the feeling was that I was God. Or I was Divine."[30]

After 1963, Leary and Alpert's appearances in New York became much rarer. Halfway through the spring semester at Harvard, Leary abruptly took off for California and asked a secretary to hand out reading lists to his students. It was only when he appeared in the West Coast media that his employers learned he was no longer fulfilling his teaching obligations. In May, he was fired for abandoning his job and so was Alpert for giving LSD to an undergraduate student.

While this scandal was not enough to make the news across the entire country, it was nonetheless picked up by the *New York Times*,[31] and it signalled that psychedelics were inexorably moving out of the scientific realm and spilling into the metropolis. For local artist Martin Carey, however, learning about their dismissal was cause for celebration. "The '50s were such a dull, sleepy time, and school was dull and boring and inoffensive. The people who had trouble in school were usually more intelligent, so they got bored." So seeing the two professors being dismissed "was like a light shining into all that boredom."[32]

Fortunately, Leary could count on the stupendous resources of the Hitchcocks. That same year, Peggy's twin brothers Tommy and Billy bought a 2,500-acre estate in Millbrook, New York. Leary had given LSD to both of them, and they graciously invited him and his followers – including the Fergusons – to move in to carry on their experiments.[33] For a couple of years, New Yorkers saw little of Leary, but he nonetheless remained an influential presence in the city, thanks to a widely read psychedelic guidebook.

In 1964, Leary, Metzner, and Alpert published *The Psychedelic Experience*,[34] which was based on the *Tibetan Book of the Dead*. Though in retrospect he found the book a little naive, Ed Rosenfeld initially believed the adaptation was very good because it had successfully used an Eastern spiritual framework to channel the insights of the psychedelic experience.[35] David Mancuso, who went on to become a legendary disc jockey in the 1970s, tried Sandoz acid that same year, and consulting their guidebook significantly shaped his interests in psychedelics. "The book blew me away," he remembered. "It became my bible and I started getting involved with [Leary]." By 1965, he was regularly organizing limited group sessions with LSD in his loft using the book.[36] A year later, a bisexual user, who saw psychedelics as spiritual enhancers, wrote to Leary to let him know that he greatly admired his guidebook.[37]

In other parts of the city, some spiritually inclined LSD users carefully structured their drug sessions with religious texts and Leary's guidebook, while paying critical attention to the setting. In a Brooklyn apartment, for instance, a room was decorated and arranged in a way that recalled Jean Houston's therapeutic protocol. It featured candles, burning incense, and objects such as a fragment of driftwood, an oval stone, some coral, and a ball of glass that could break the light into several patterns. These objects had been purposefully left on the table "to be touched, scrutinized, mused over."

The five people – a thirty-seven-year-old photographer and host (Ben), a thirty-four-year-old engineer, a twenty-three-year-old secretary, a twenty-four-year-old student at an acting school (Michael), and a twenty-year-old (Kathryn) who worked for a suburban newspaper – sat quietly on a canvas mattress and meditated, hoping to undergo a positive spiritual experience. The host had taken acid three times in the past, but he refrained on this occasion in order to control the session and act as a guide.

The host produced the *Book of Tao* and read excerpts to give the LSD experience a mystical dimension: "Tao is a vast immeasurable void … Looked for, it cannot be seen; it is invisible. Listened for, it cannot be heard; it is inaudible. Reached for, it cannot be touched; it is intangible … it is the greatest mystery." Later, two participants went to sleep, but Michael became restless and panicky, so Ben told him to rest his head against his leg to establish a physical contact and tried to reassure him by reading excerpts from *The Psychedelic Experience*.[38]

As these spiritual understandings suggest, some New Yorkers were liberally borrowing from several religious traditions, and at the heart of their rituals were the acid-induced altered states of consciousness. Notwithstanding Graham's revivalist crusade, this was also in keeping with the broader spiritual awakening in the US and in most parts of the Western world.[39] Americans became less interested in rigidly following scriptures and instead longed to attain the Divine through brands of religion that were more personal and experiential.[40] Though this awakening was the result of several factors, psychedelics certainly played a modest part in it.[41] In a supportive environment, taking psychedelics could trigger a blissful feeling of unity that was in turn interpreted as a very personal experience with the Divine. God could now be reached from within and without the help of religious institutions.

East of the Village

Leary's movement certainly allowed a broad range of New Yorkers to become interested in the spiritual import of the psychedelic experience, but while he and his crew were experimenting, acid and psychedelics started to appear all over the city, away from Greenwich Village.

By the early 1960s, the Beat culture had become a nationwide phenomenon, and the Village was struggling to accommodate the newcomers in search of authentic lifestyles. The pressure on local real estate was such that for the most diehard aspiring Villager, the only hope of finding a place was to comb through the *Village Voice*'s classified ads first thing in the morning and rush to a pay phone to make enquiries. But even then, it was usually too late, as NYU student Lynn Gingrass quickly discovered. So he and a friend conjured up a mean trick to beat competitors whereby one of them stood in line by the *Voice*'s offices on Sheridan Square waiting for the paper while the other disconnected the microphone of every pay phone in the area. The other house-hunters furiously vented their frustration on the idle phones, and "They just stared in disbelief when somebody actually got a phone that worked – I'd surreptitiously slipped the thing back on. And then sort of at my leisure I called three or four places and was obviously the first person to go to each one of them, and I found this incredible place."[42]

The rents were going up because of the Village's popularity, but the newcomers were also starting to bother the locals, and the tensions soon crystalized in Washington Square Park. At the turn of the Fifties, di Prima loved to hang out there, particularly in the summer, when the park seemed like an endless party scene. "You could hear the drumming blocks from Washington Square, and when you stepped into the crowd around the fountain, you saw the young men barefoot and naked to the waist, and the young women, their skirts held high, stomping and dancing together in the heavy night." Back then there were no curfews in effect, so once all the folksingers and gays had left the area (usually around 2:00 am), people like di Prima simply crashed on the steps of the fountain.[43]

In April 1961, however, the parks commissioner banned the performance of folk music, a genre that embodied the Village's cultural transformations in the Sixties.[44] The ban was soon lifted thanks to local protests spearheaded by the owner of the Village Vanguard,[45] but there were more battles ahead. A few years later, the commissioner proposed revamping the park following years of debating and planning. The plan was allegedly designed to "discourage beatniks and other 'undesirable elements' from congregating there," partly because of complaints logged by local property-owners.[46] Additionally, the park had become an important place to acquire drugs, which remained a distinct feature throughout the decade and the Seventies.[47] Over on the Village's streets, the Department of Licenses started to enforce stricter regulations, which led to the temporary closing of three off-Broadway theatres and the suspension of readings at Le Metro, a popular place for Beat poetry. In turn, some of the most prominent Bohemians like Ginsberg and di Prima organized to defend their right to read poetry.[48]

Gradually, urban Bohemia began moving across Manhattan to the northern part of the Lower East Side. Just as the white middle class was leaving the city for the suburbs, working-class minorities from the South and from Puerto Rico settled in the area, looking for economic opportunities. But instead of finding prosperity, the city's ongoing deindustrialization left them in a state of poverty. During that period, these newcomers remained largely unrepresented in local politics, and by the mid-Sixties Blacks were five times more likely to suffer from police brutality than whites. All this occurred in a larger context of a manufacturing sector on the decline, which in turn was illustrated by the high unemployment figures for Black and Hispanic New Yorkers.[49]

Di Prima and Ginsberg had been early pioneers in that respect, but in the early Sixties most Greenwich Villagers would never have entertained the thought of living there. Suzan Rotolo, who was then dating Bob Dylan, considered the area off-limits. "Broadway was considered no-man's-land, dividing Greenwich Village from the Lower East Side."[50] In 1963, radical activist Osha Neuman nonetheless moved to the area from the suburbs to start a painting career. It is easy to see why Rotolo had reservations about the grimy neighbourhood.

> People here could not afford the manicured distances favored by the middle class. They brushed up against each other, breathed in each other's faces, and woke each other up at night playing the radio too loud or fighting with the window open. The streets were all stains and clutter. They smelled of piss, mildew, roach powder, and rotting garbage. Refuse and filth blanketed the empty lots. Weeds sprouted between middens of mattress springs, rusting car parts, old clothes and beer cans ... The floors in the railroad apartments groaned beneath layers of cheap linoleum. The ceilings were heavy with peeling paint. Roaches overran kitchens. You could hear the rats scurrying at night in the walls.[51]

In spite of the atmosphere of decay, the neighbourhood was attractive because it was cheap and it seemed like "the symbolic antithesis of postwar suburban society." Soon it was no longer seen "as the old neighbourhood of ethnic diversity but as the site of cultural protest and alternative lifestyles."[52] The East Village was born out of these transformations.

Initially, new psychedelic enclaves sprouted just west of the area. By 1963, di Prima and her family were living in an apartment on Cooper Square – another unofficial border separating both Villages, according to LeRoi Jones[53] – and on New Year's Eve she received a call from a friend offering sugar cubes saturated with LSD. Someone then just dropped off the four cubes wrapped in aluminum foil with instructions to fast beforehand. For di Prima, this was another wonderful experience: her apartment glittered with light and energy, and she experienced the Eastern philosophies she had been reading about for years.[54]

A few blocks south, Ed Rosenfeld moved into a ground-level loft at 21 Bleecker Street sometime around 1962 or 1963, and he put together the sole edition of the *Ecstasy Review*, which featured essays, stories, and poems about psychedelics. He also started writing literature for his syncretic Natural Church, a religious institution he set up to provide a legal framework to use psychedelics as sacraments. While New York State is known for its long history of religious communes and alternative spirituality,[55] Rosenfeld's spiritual endeavour reveals that New York has likewise harboured similar eclectic religious movements.

By the end of the year, Rosenfeld had officially incorporated the church and was running it at 52 Bond Street. He charged $100 for a session for which participants were required to attend a pre-session meeting before coming back for the actual drug experience.[56] To structure the drug sessions, Rosenfeld borrowed freely from Eastern literature. "I used to guide people using the I-Ching," he recalled, "and we guided people on trips and there were three of four of us who were associated with the church ... the reason I used the I-Ching is because it seemed to me to be the fusion of Daoism and Confucianism – Daoism being extremely spiritual in its insights and Confucianism having to do with how people organize themselves." Rosenfeld had reasoned that incorporating as a church that turned psychedelics into sacraments might protect their use of psychoactive drugs.

His Natural Church did not last long, however. In 1965, he was raided by the police, who confiscated all the materials. He left soon after, but outside his church, the neighbourhood was brimming with drugs, Bohemians, and artists. On Bleecker Street lived dancer and choreographer Daniel Nagrin in another loft, and on Bond Street lived Herbert Huncke, who was still hustling and shooting up, and jazz musician Charles Mingus, who by then was a keen acid user. Smack dealer Stanley Gould, an early admirer of Charlie Parker and occasional junk connection for Burroughs, found a loft on 2nd Avenue below 8th Street.[57] As Rosenfeld reminisced, "Many people of that type were experimenting with pot and other stronger psychedelics" in that area.[58]

At the heart of the East Village, however, some of New York's psychedelic Bohemians were greeted with open hostility. Jeff Perkins was in a Broadway loft for Thanksgiving when he took LSD. A young Black girl became attracted to him, and she proposed that he accompany her to a party in the Village. "And I remember going in. They were all black kids. And I was the only white guy there. And I was high. And sensitive. Though I'm not uncomfortable with blacks. I've lived with black people. Most of my friends in high school were black kids." But gradually, the situation made him feel uncomfortable. And indeed, the girl soon asked him to leave the party because her friends didn't like the presence of a white guy with them.[59]

But as more and more New Yorkers like Perkins made incursions into the area, it became increasingly obvious that psychedelia's future was there, and this sense of transition was strengthened by the inception of a psychedelic news platform in the summer of 1965: the *East Village Other*. The EVO was at the forefront of a growing wave of "underground" newspapers that appeared all over the country and in several parts of the world during the 1960s. These papers "appealed to self-styled cultural outlaws: freelance intellectuals, dissenters, artists, and folk and jazz musicians, who clustered in taverns and espresso houses in low-rent neighborhoods."[60]

Among the paper's founders were Walter Bowart, an artist who had been doing illustrations for the Committee to Legalize Marijuana earlier that year, poet Allen Katzman, who had been running readings in East Side coffee houses since 1961,[61] and Harvard drop-out and part-time publisher Dan Rattiner, who joined them to put together the second issue.

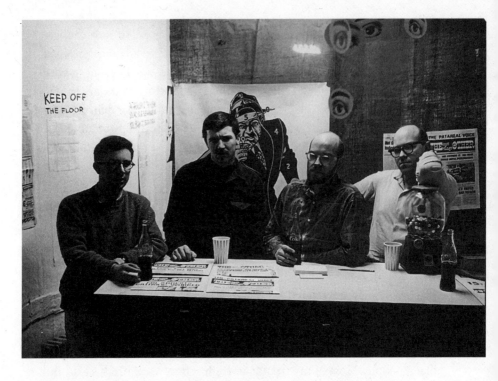

Figure 4.1 From left: Dan Rattiner, Walter Bowart, and brothers Allen and Don Katzman, 14 January 1966

When Rattiner first visited Bowart, he was living in a loft of a tenement located on Avenue B and 2nd Street, and the rundown area "had been [recently] renamed The East Village by some enterprising artists." Bowart, Katzman, and Rattiner pooled their resources, and months later the paper had its own offices on Avenue A and between 9th and 10th Streets, in front of the dilapidated Tompkins Square Park.

Rattiner typified the geographical shift that was underway in New York's Bohemian culture: "I was the 'straight man,' as people said. I came, every morning, on the cross-town Eighth Street bus from the cool, beat world of Greenwich Village on the West Side to the mean, filthy streets of the wild-eyed East Village. I got off at St. Marks Place and Avenue A. And I walked up a block and a half."[62] John Wilcock was another who joined the fledging venture after spending the previous ten years writing for the *Village Voice*. At the EVO, he wrote columns for a few months before leaving for Japan, where he joined a Tokyo underground newspaper.[63]

Along with the potent scent of marijuana, a feeling of pioneering filled the paper's offices. In the very first issue, the *EVO* bombastically announced that it had a duty to cater "'to the new citizenry of the East Village.'"[64] This did not really happen in the second part of the decade, but the *East Village Other*'s statement nonetheless cemented the sense of imminent change in the area, while simultaneously signalling that psychedelia was to play a critical role in the transformations.

Following the lead of the *EVO*, several shops soon opened in the area and began selling LSD users a whole battery of paraphernalia like posters, records, books, pipes, and colourful pieces of clothing. These places, which were known as "head shops," became important locations for acid heads because they helped them enhance their trips with various psychedelic items and provided them with space to meet like-minded people. As well, they allowed some New Yorkers to earn a living through a kind of business operating on the fringes of legality. By selling objects that were explicitly connected to the drug world, head shop owners and employees proved that psychedelia had employment opportunities outside the laboratory.

In 1966, Jeff Glick opened the Head Shop on 9th Street with merely $300 worth of merchandise bought on consignment. By the following year, it was selling "psychedelic art posters, bright-colored paperweights and diffraction jewelries – silvery disks that radiate colors of the spectrum and which can be worn as cuff links, earrings or pasted on the forehead like a third eye."[65] The store quickly expanded into two branches and planned to open a "psychedelic department store." One of the owners boasted that the necessary funds to open that store had been easily raised and that he had to turn down potential investors. His customers (between 200 and 500 daily) were mostly young and middle-class, and some of them turned up in a chauffeured Cadillac.[66]

Several other stores followed suit. The Electric Lotus sold the usual artefacts, along with sitar records, Hindu water pipes, and "DayGlo" posters, while the Underground Uplift Unlimited on St Mark's Place offered buttons with psychedelic messages.[67] These head shops embodied the eclectic nature of psychedelia by selling products that allowed some New Yorkers to explore new commercial avenues but that also helped "people to alter their minds – and even their societies – through meaningful drug use."[68] For Stanley Krippner, these places provided an important platform that allowed psychedelic art and culture to find their way into many East Village apartments.[69]

In 1967, the rising hip quarter had its own psychedelic nightclub, the Electric Circus. The venue featured "lights, slide projections, mime, rock, strobe effects, dancing area, and band projection," which were carefully combined in a way that no single elements took precedence over another. The visuals were masterminded by light-show artist Tony Martin, and they combined a series of abstract kinetic images with "floating" images that were accompanied by the pulsating strobe lights.[70] Krippner also attended the venue and was taken by the installations and the atmosphere. As he recalls, "Many people were tripping when they came into the Electric Circus and danced."[71]

By then, some astute observers had noticed that psychedelia had developed its own language and began to parody it. In 1967, Ken Shapiro and Lane Sarasohn launched Channel One at 62 East 4th Street. There, patrons sat down in a theatre equipped with three television sets. As Shapiro explained, "We concentrate on humor, psychedelic satire. The heads are a gorgeous subculture, with their own language, their own jokes – and since so little of it can be broadcast over regular media, drugs and sex and such, it gives us a whole world of totally new material to work with. We like to think we're providing heads with their own CBS."[72]

How to Turn On

As Shapiro's venture indicates, LSD use had given birth to a distinct psychedelic subculture[73] with its own codes of conduct. In New York's dense and competitive urban setting, several acid users positioned themselves as expert drug users, while looking down on those with little or no experience.

The story of Bob Friede, who used his parents' house in Manhattan for drug parties in the early months of 1964, is a fitting illustration of the internal dynamics and competition of this subculture. Parties involved around thirty to fifty people and had several rooms dedicated to drug use. A one party-goer remembered, "People were smoking pot in one room, using mescaline in another. Just the atmosphere of that place was a kind of high." But in spite of his hospitality, Friede was derided by most of his guests for being unhip. "I know lots of kids with lots of bread [money]," one party-goer claimed, "and most of them are more or less accepted. Friede never was. He wanted so desperately to be hip, and he didn't know how." Another offered a clearer explanation as to why he was mocked. "Friede wouldn't go out and 'cop' the stuff himself … He always had someone go out for him. He wouldn't go through the street scene. He thought he was superior. How could we accept him? He never paid his dues."[74]

Psychedelic subcultural capital[75] was critical for anyone to be recognized as genuine, and ingesting a great deal of LSD was another way of positioning oneself within the psychedelic hierarchy. But some dubious psychedelic experts seemed too far-out to be taken seriously. During a 1967 gathering in Central Park, one acid user claimed to have taken a 1,500-microgram dose of LSD (about ten to fifteen times the standard dose), but the reporter was unimpressed and contended that this was the "first acid head you ever saw who had an ego, to speak of."[76] Indeed, most acid users tended to be leery of those who bragged too much about their drug use.[77]

Likewise, acid could sometimes be taken under peer pressure if a person wanted to avoid being branded a coward, and some of the younger users would "dare" their friends to take it because of the risk and deviance associated with it. On one occasion, an eighteen-year-old took the drug on a dare because his friends told him that he "wouldn't be able to take it," but because the young man was allegedly unstable, the experience was a negative one. Competition and prestige were important among this group of students: they bragged that they could have LSD delivered to their school and that they knew fifteen to twenty fellow students who had taken the drug – including a "well-known politician's son."[78]

With the increase of acid consumption came ethical guidelines designed to serve and protect users, and in this respect drug dealers were expected to sell quality staples only. "You have known [the dealer] for a few years," claimed one user, "or maybe as little as six months but you know that he'd never give you a bad count or sell you acid or mescaline which he had not tested first. He may have even tripped you out for [the] first acid trip (the type of cat who used to make sure that everyone who got his acid could handle it … well the first time round)."[79] One dealer followed this rule and refused to sell his materials indiscriminately: "I would never sell it to anybody I thought was at all psychotic … If I have any doubts whether they can handle it, I tell them I'm out of acid."[80]

One of the reasons that drove acid heads to think carefully about the ethics of acid use was that there existed significant risks associated with the drug that required guidelines to maximize the LSD experience and minimize risks of adverse reactions. *Village Voice* rock critic Richard Goldstein liked to have an experienced and drug-free individual on hand to guide the session and avoid any mishaps – "a 'guide,' a kind of designated driver who could talk me down from a panic attack or give me Valium if all else failed."[81]

Most users agreed that it was important to carefully plan sessions by paying attention to spatial environments and by being in the right frame of mind. For instance, a chemical engineer and his wife took LSD on a regular basis and sent their children away, re-arranged the furniture in their home, and sometimes visited museums and galleries under the influence.[82] According to a woman who was writing a cookbook on mushrooms featuring a chapter on psilocybe fungi, a prepared body and a prepared mind were crucial for the outcome of the trip. Indeed, she once took a small dose of mushrooms, and she thoroughly enjoyed the experience because she had fasted beforehand and "was feeling great to begin with."[83]

For others, difficult trips might occur when they were unprepared, like a twenty-two-year-old from Greenwich Village who needed psychiatric treatment after taking LSD: "I ran from the room sobbing, it was pure panic. I ran, or I think I ran, for miles before I regained some control. Then I walked for hours praying I wouldn't die."[84] A twenty-three-year-old Welfare Department social worker also reported sensing a split in his identity during his LSD experience: "My sexual identity became female and I knew what it was like to be a woman." The sensation frightened him, so he took some thorazine to counter the effects.[85]

Managing these difficult moments often depended on one's age and past experience with these drugs. Older users, rather than teenagers whose egos and personalities were still being built, often found themselves better equipped to deal with the powerful attacks on the psyche. Hence, the more experienced users could sometimes help their younger peers with these disquieting moments. Teenager Amelie Edwards once had a tough trip and felt the need to withdraw from people, but a woman in her early twenties calmed her down and helped her to manage that difficult moment.[86] Jean Houston had also realized that teenagers experimenting with these drugs were more likely to develop adverse reactions and that taking LSD after the age of twenty-five was critical to maximize its benefits.[87]

Some young New Yorkers were attracted to the drug simply because they had heard about it and reasoned that they should try it. One seventeen-year-old from Forest Hills was drawn to it because he wanted to experience ecstatic visions: "I'd heard so much about it, that you could see all the wonders of the world right in your own mind, and I figured I had to try it." Another important incentive was the states of self-introspection LSD could cause. A nineteen-year-old student from the City College of New York who was undergoing therapy dropped acid because he "wanted to find some meaning to life – find the direction in which [he] was going."[88] And a young commune dweller reported a similar experience with the drug: "I think that acid is very good for finding out a few things about yourself and the feelings around you. I would say that some people don't need it but that everyone should try it once, because there might be something hidden within themselves that they could find out."[89]

However, teenagers were far from the only New Yorkers who were interested in LSD, and the drug drew a wide pool of experimenters. They could include CEOs, lawyers, bankers, engineers, market researchers, teachers, TV executives, actors, clerical workers, social workers, construction workers, and gas station mechanics. A twenty-seven-year-old stockbroker, who had taken the drug once, was surprised to learn that many of his fraternity brothers (all with high-profile jobs) were users. For a twenty-three-year-old Welfare Department social worker, LSD use was a form of risk-taking and as a hobby no different from mountain-climbing or sky-diving.[90] And for liberally minded parents, acid could be a family affair. Indeed, activist Peter Stafford once attended a lecture during which participants discussed the appropriate age for a child to take the drug, and some of them were open enough to admit that they had already given the drug to their children.[91]

In the aftermath of their trips, several experimenters found that their lives had changed as a result. For instance, one user reflected on his drug use that had begun in 1963 and revealed that he was more inclined to sexual experimentations than before and that he had become interested in men.[92] For others, LSD seemed to offer them new insights and capabilities to a point where some claimed to have improved their grades in school thanks to psychedelic drug use.[93] Paula Sherwood was another whose life was changed and who found a new career as a direct consequence of her experimentation. She had dropped out of a teachers' college in Ohio in 1961, and she then took on several jobs in advertising and publishing. After trying LSD, she realized that she was better suited to teaching small children, so she went back to college to complete her degree.[94]

Regardless of the varying motivations for psychedelic experimentation of these New Yorkers, all depended on the city's distribution networks. But presenting a clear geography of LSD dealing is not an easy task. While the distribution of physically addictive drugs like heroin is typically linked to space,[95] these new drugs were harder to track down, as one narcotics agent admitted. "With heroin or the pills you can find them on corners, or at least in certain areas. They stay together near the supply, which is usually in Harlem or in Brooklyn or maybe in the Village." Whereas the use of heroin was correlated to geography and poverty, the use of LSD was, if anything, correlated to class, a much more difficult parameter to take into account in order to locate suppliers. However, because LSD hits were dosed in micrograms, transporting and storing them was much easier.[96]

In fact, the sources of supply were manifold in this well-connected city. Many students brought acid back from their holidays in Europe – one firm in Italy could still legally manufacture the drug in 1963. This momentary influx of LSD caused the prices to drop to fifty cents a dose in some parts of the city, but as the academic year resumed, the prices went up again. Europe aside, Canada and Mexico had a steady flow of the drug available. Domestically, major LSD factories were rumoured to have been set up in New Jersey, Boston, Iowa, and Kansas, while the San Francisco Bay area likewise became a psychedelic hub. Finally, some of the city's acid was reportedly manufactured within the five boroughs in small makeshift laboratories or in larger facilities.[97]

According to a local journalist, the prices tended to fluctuate depending on the level of publicity the drug received. Before the crackdown on non-medical distribution, he could purchase an acid hit for as little as $2. But government attempts to regulate the drug increased media exposure, and this created a profit incentive that caused the street prices to jump to $5 and $15 in some instances.[98] A *New York Post* journalist likewise gathered substantial information on the world of illicit drug distribution in 1966. Most dealers were college drop-outs between twenty and twenty-five years of age who operated in their apartments and usually sold a single dose for $3 or $4 (one could also buy vials or bottles for larger quantities). Typically, a dose would be a mixture of powdered LSD and distilled water fixed on a tab or a sugar cube, and it would contain around 100 or 200 micrograms of LSD.

LSD and psychedelics differ from addictive drugs in that they allow less room for substantial profit margins, and dealers typically sold acid to friends or to make a little money on the side. For instance, one writer made ends meet by dealing,[99] and another smuggled $20,000 worth of the drug into the US from England, intending to use part of the money for his living expenses and his college tuition.[100]

But some dealers sensed that they could still make good money and became "pushers," who encouraged people to buy their materials in a more aggressive way than the average dealers. Pushers, who could be found in Washington Square Park, Tompkins Square Park, and Morningside, rarely used the drug and often dealt other substances; so LSD was treated like any other staple. For example, two pushers from Harlem often went to the East Village with diluted acid, and one young man purchased $250 worth of LSD in powder form, but it turned out to be baking soda.[101]

Gradually, a divide began to grow between the psychedelic and heroin subcultures. In November 1965, one reporter noted that acid was the drug of choice among the Greenwich Village teenagers he interviewed. If LSD was unavailable, they might take amphetamines or drink alcoholic beverages, but they stayed clear from junk.[102] Another user admitted that the tendency was to avoid these kinds of addictive drugs.[103] As Ellen Sander concurs, smack users could not be trusted. "Some of them were musicians, mostly jazz leftovers, and they were terrifying. They seemed amiable enough, but if you turned your back on one of them he'd steal you blind."[104]

This growing split also became apparent in the New York jazz scene where successful musicians appeared to be moving away from heroin after discovering LSD. After Leary introduced Charles Mingus to the drug, he became moderately involved in his acid movement, and as he recalled in 1963, "When we started out we used to do heroin on the lower east side, and we used to say 'Oh man, how hip we are.'" In the early 1960s, however, they became enthusiastic LSD users: "me, Monk and Miles buy our acid by the jar." This turn to acid also corresponded with a period of economic prosperity that most likely explains this transition: "Now we're making over a $100,000 a year, each. Miles lives in a renovated Russian Orthodox Church."[105]

In the first part of the Sixties, LSD joined New York's lively psychoactive marketplace and immediately stood out from the other mind-altering drugs available in the city. Leary's psychedelic movement certainly played a part in this popularization, but far more New Yorkers developed their own ways of using the drug and their own understanding of the psychedelic experience. Soon there were elaborate psychedelic scenes in Lower Manhattan, which had a strong spiritual undercurrent that borrowed freely from various traditions. Initially, LSD appeared in Greenwich Village, and gradually psychedelics moved eastward and to other parts of the city.

In the second part of the decade, psychedelia featured a far more revolutionary edge that culminated in the creation of a psychedelic counterculture that used the insights of the LSD experience to openly criticize postwar America and its culture of conformity and consumerism. In the process, it boosted the transition to the East Village and turned the neighbourhood into the city's psychedelic hotspot, as the *East Village Other* offered a clear voice to this radical fringe that believed LSD had the power to completely revamp postwar society and bring about peace, love, and understanding to one and all.

5

Building Utopia
Nina Graboi, the East Village, and the Psychedelic Counterculture

By the mid-Sixties, Timothy Leary had left academia to fully dedicate his life to psychedelia and to promote LSD as a magic bullet that would end human suffering. At first glance, this radical outlook may seem like the product of non-linear thinking coming from a flawed individual. But in fact, this line of reasoning became far more prevalent in the second part of the decade, which saw many acid heads question the social norms of postwar America and form a utopian psychedelic counterculture.[1]

It would be tempting to connect the rise of radical psychedelia with the seminal progressive movements of the time, but LSD and politics enjoyed a deeply uneasy relationship.[2] On the one hand, acid allowed some users to meditate on the injustices of the world, like the two men discussing the horrors of the Vietnam War as they were coming down from an acid trip in 1965.[3] For many New Left activists, on the other hand, drug use discouraged protest and was equated with selfish hedonism when the US government was dropping bombs in Southeast Asia.[4] In 1967, socialist David McReynolds was outraged when Richard Alpert proposed boycotting the 15 April Spring Mobilization Against the War in Vietnam because "some people are going to burn their draft cards there and it will be bad public relations for the psychedelic community to be involved in that kind of thing." This led McReynolds to publish an open letter condemning Alpert's cowardice that prioritized drugs over real-world issues.[5]

Given this mutual ambivalence, it is ultimately hard to assess how much of the broader climate of protest spilled into New York's psychedelic counterculture. What is perhaps much clearer is that the unique pharmacology of LSD played a crucial part in its inception. Indeed, the acid experience could challenge the users' relation with reality at such a basic ontological level that it seemed to thrust them into "instant childhood." This reconnection with the early stages of infancy devoid of any cultural programing was a fundamental aspect of the psychedelic experience Huxley had pointed out a decade before when he had realized "what Adam had seen on the morning of his creation – the miracle, moment by moment, of naked existence."[6]

Following such a comprehensive disconnection from mundane reality and the material world, "the palm of one's hand, the leaf in the tree, the fabric of one's jacket acquired as much significance as one's parking space, the Dow Jones index, one's spouse."[7] As a result, many deconditioned acid heads had trouble connecting with postwar society. A sixteen-year-old LSD user illustrated this in an explicit fashion: "When I'm high I see people's games, the smiles that don't mean anything, the useless conventions. I realize I'm not the only boy who feels unsure, who wants to cry. And now I'm happier because I know I don't have to hide anything."[8]

A more fitting illustration of the transformative properties of LSD and like drugs is the story of Nina Graboi, a middle-class woman who was deeply unsatisfied by her life in the sleepy Long Island suburbs and by the gender stereotypes she was reluctantly enforcing upon herself. Like many American women whose positive psychedelic accounts have often been obscured by the stories of their male counterparts,[9] her experiences allowed her to see through the cracks of conformity and to dramatically change her way of life. Her time in New York, then, goes against the idea that the counterculture of the 1960s was strictly a man's world and that it was devoid of any form of feminist sensibility.[10]

Graboi's personal odyssey is also significant because her involvement in New York was part of the psychedelic counterculture's quest to nurture space in order to engage with the outside world. To achieve this, she became the director of a religious organization Leary had created in an attempt to connect psychedelics and spirituality. However, the Center for the League for Spiritual Discovery quickly became a flagship for radical psychedelia while occasionally bridging the divide separating young drug users from their concerned parents. Other acid heads helped the local counterculture by organizing exhibitions and setting up crash pads to assist the young flocking away from the suburbs. In the process, the East Village became the new capital of psychedelia, epitomized by the growing role of the *East Village Other*.

The story of New York's psychedelic counterculture, then, reveals that idealistic drug users did far more than just criticize the society they lived in and retreat into their inner space. Rather than simply withdrawing from postwar America, they set out to create institutions and opportunities through "active social engagement and community-oriented hard work."[11] This occurred at a time when radical undertakings were spilling into outdoor spaces in several US cities (particularly in San Francisco), whereas the Beats' prior involvement had remained largely literary and poetic – indoor-oriented activities indeed.[12]

From the Third Reich to Greenwich Village

Nina Graboi was born in Vienna at the end of World War I and brought up in the thriving Jewish community of Leopoldstadt. After narrowly escaping the Nazis, she and her husband Michel reached New York City in the summer of 1941. As they searched for business opportunities, Michel discovered that he could apply waterproof coating on toddlers' articles of clothing and stuffed toys so that they could be easily cleaned with a sponge. The Fifth Avenue stores liked their samples enough to place several orders, and before they knew it, they were renting a downtown loft and employing some sixty sewing machine operators.

Soon after, the Grabois had their first child, Daniel, in 1944, who was followed by Nicole fifteen months later. Eventually, they had enough money to buy a corner lot on Long Island and to commission two architects to draw plans for a fourteen-room house. With such a stunning change of fortunes, Nina had to pinch herself.

But something was amiss. Graboi became both a model housewife bent on conspicuous consumerism and an admired socialite known for her lavish parties. Boredom and emptiness slowly settled in, and the widespread sexism of the time[13] became painfully apparent during these social events. Over the next few years, she took on theatre production, but she became disillusioned by the fakery of the glamorous theatre world. At the same time, she began to reflect on her marriage and realized that Michel was not really the man she hoped he was. Suicidal thoughts started to creep into her head.

In the mid-1950s, she began a quest to find something better than the suburban way of life. One day, she picked up a magazine in the dentist's waiting room and read about a housewife who had been hypnotized and turned into an eighteenth-century Irish woman. The idea that a person could have her consciousness so dramatically transformed was a fascinating perspective. Excited by the implications, she became a member of the American Society for Psychical Research housed on Fifth Avenue. For the next year, she voraciously read books dealing with ESP and parapsychology.

A little later, a major breakthrough came when she got her hands on a Hindu philosophy book. "It was like a blow to my solar plexus;" she recalled, "it jarred me awake … The teachings were logical, unsentimental, yet filled with the spirit of non-harmfulness, compassion, understanding, love."[14] By the late Fifties, she was meditating on a regular basis and attending classes of Hindu philosophy and comparative religion at the New School for Social Research.

In the early 1960s, she read about some fascinating psilocybin research in the pages of *Time*. That year, Walter Pahnke, a graduate student of Leary's, gave the drug to ten divinity students in a Boston chapel in a double-blind controlled setting, with nine of them subsequently reporting mystical or religious experiences.[15] Could psychedelics be the key to attaining the exceptional states of consciousness she had been reading about? As she considered the proposition, she read Huxley and Watts, who "spoke eloquently of the dimensions the psychedelics open up."[16]

Graboi edged closer to psychedelia in the spring of 1965 when she attended a seminar on Tibetan Buddhism in Pennsylvania and connected with Virginia Glenn, who soon invited her to the weekly get-togethers. There, Graboi met Watts, Stanley Krippner (who was then collaborating with Glenn in a study on dreams), Masters and Houston, as well as George Peters, who was running a volunteer-based "LSD Rescue Service" to assist distraught acid users in the Chicago area.[17] Listening to all these highly articulate experts, Graboi concluded that psychedelics might be able to bridge science and religion.

But before taking the leap, she had to deal with her broken marriage. Having lived through the 1950s, which placed such a great deal of faith in monogamy and the nuclear family,[18] her fears were understandable. What she could not have known at the time, though, was that American marriage was in a state of transition and that divorce rates were sharply increasing: by 1964, an estimated 36 per cent of contracted marriages ended in divorce (compared to roughly 5 per cent just after the Civil War). The breakdown of the type of marriage that was prevalent in the 1950s can be explained by the erosion of a gender-based division of labour, and another likely explanation aptly illustrates her quest for greater meaning: "In the United States these changes occurred in a culture that has long trumpeted the virtues of individual choice and, more recently, personal freedom and self-actualization."[19] Her next move could not have been closer to the mark.

Graboi's interest in parapsychology and altered states of consciousness drew her to Abraham Maslow's humanistic brand of psychology, which came to be known as the "third force." As an alternative to psychoanalysis and behavioural psychology, it was more concerned with helping people become better individuals – precisely through self-actualization – than with looking endlessly for mental hang-ups. Maslow rose to prominence thanks his 1962 best-seller *Toward a Psychology of Being* and eventually became president of the APA as well as the head of the Brandeis University Department of Psychology.[20]

Graboi was already corresponding with Maslow when a friend of hers suggested that she open a lecture bureau to both further her interest and address her vocational concerns. At the time, Michel and Nina were renting a studio apartment a few blocks away from Washington Square Park in a desperate attempt to rekindle their lost passion. But instead, the studio became the site for The Third Force Lecture Bureau, and soon it was a hub for forward-thinking people interested in humanistic psychology, parapsychology, altered states of consciousness, and the connection between psychedelics and human evolution.[21]

One morning, Glenn called her at the bureau. Timothy Leary was giving a talk at the Hotel Albert in Greenwich Village, and would she like to come along? Graboi had a largely unfavourable opinion of Leary, but during the conference she was impressed by his coolness and focus in spite of all the agitation coming from the young crowd. In her eyes, he turned into a person "who crackled with energy and good spirits."[22]

112 | PSYCHEDELIC NEW YORK

After being introduced to him, she also met his public relations man, Larry Bogart, an early critic of nuclear power and subsequent founder of the Anti-Pollution League. Bogart offered her office space at 866 United Nations Plaza for her bureau, which soon received enthusiastic letters of support from Maslow and Huxley's widow Laura.

Little did Graboi know that she was about to see a lot more of Leary. In December 1965, he and his family were arrested at the Texas border after agents had found them in possession of cannabis. But rather than plead guilty, Leary used the upcoming trial to show that the marijuana laws were unconstitutional and that as a practising Hindu he could invoke the First Amendment to justify his habit.[23] Back in New York, Billy Hitchcock used his connections to help him with his legal defence. After he was found guilty on two counts and sentenced to a total of thirty years in prison in March 1966, a local Timothy Leary Defense Fund (TLDF) was set up to raise monies for the appeal.[24]

Leary was now back in New York on a regular basis, but his presence was a far cry from the fervour he had displayed in the early part of the decade. Whenever he stopped at the bureau for coffee, he always seemed preoccupied by his legal matters. By then, the two had grown fond of each other, even though Graboi always had mixed feelings about his mission. While she came to believe in the transformative power of the psychedelic experience, she did not think that LSD should be distributed indiscriminately but given to a select few only.[25]

Soon her connection with the acid guru became a problem. Her husband Michel strongly disapproved of it, as did several people who were part of Glenn's informal group. After publicly announcing that Leary, Alpert, and Metzner had joined the bureau, she received several letters of complaint, including one from Maslow himself.[26] This disavowal should not have come as a surprise given how ambivalent he was toward the counterculture of the Sixties in spite of his popularity within radical circles. It is ironic, for instance, that Abbie Hoffman had thoroughly enjoyed Maslow's teachings at Brandeis in the previous decade but that Maslow subsequently dismissed the radical leftist as a clown.[27]

Nevertheless, Graboi was inexorably moving away from her life in Long Island. In the Manhattan offices of the TLDF, she saw young acid heads happily volunteer for administrative tasks like writing letters and making phone calls. In Greenwich Village, she spent even more time with them and learned about their countercultural inclinations. "Now I went to Washington Square Park to sit with them around the fountain or on the grass," she recalled. "I listened to their music and to their talk and discovered that they came much closer to my own way of thinking than my circle of suburban friends."[28]

At last, Graboi was ready for her first real glimpse into the world of mind-altering drugs. Through Glenn, she learned about an LSD conference that was scheduled in June at Berkeley. By then, she had befriended Watts, and he invited them to stay on his houseboat in Sausalito. One evening, they visited some of his friends, who were passing joints around. While most smokers saw pot as a mild psychedelic, Graboi had an unusually powerful experience that was surprisingly close to the effects of LSD: "I was spinning backwards through evolution, my awareness of myself as a woman with a name, a past, a family, an address, gone. I was ape, lion, tiger, horse, dog, rabbit, fish, insect, and then a primitive organism that scrabbled out of the mud onto dry land."[29]

Graboi returned to the East Coast a changed woman. If anything, marijuana had been a door-opener that made her hungry for more. On 27 July, two weeks after her return from California, Metzner invited her to smoke diethyltryptamine (DET), a short-acting psychedelic. Metzner was only a block and a half away from her apartment on 12th Street, and he lived with his then-girlfriend Gray Henry, whom he had met at Van Wolf's salon.[30] Henry had attended Jean Houston's course on "The Varieties of Psychedelic Experience" at the New School and had taken LSD under Houston and Masters's supervision.[31]

Metzner and Gray greeted her in a high-ceiling room where they had been burning incense, while "candles threw mysterious shadows on the wall" and they played a Judy Collins record. Metzner prepared the dose by filling a glass pipe with dried parsley to conceal the awful taste of the white powder. Graboi picked up the pipe, inhaled deeply, and fell back.

The DET thrust her into another dimension full of otherworldly encounters like Pan, the Greek god of the wild, who danced around her while iridescent gems cascaded from his hair and his mouth. Later on, she had a vision of her duplicate self, struggling with buried trauma, which she found hilarious. At this point, she realized that she could conjure up just about anyone and deal with them in a very casual way. Next up was Michel, whom she thought she hated, but in this instance he materialized as a mere toddler who buried his head in her lap, clinging on to her skirt. She summoned him to go, and finally he disappeared. The final test was the ultimate evil, Adolf Hitler: "Instead of brimstone he smells of glue and I see that he is a puppet. Glue oozes from his joints." The visions were interspersed with "sparkling towers, mosaic-laden mosques, gothic spires. A row of dancing girls. No, dancing atoms. No, energy. Wavelets of energy, dancing to an inaudible rhythm."[32]

After this overwhelming experience, Graboi finally tried LSD at Millbrook, which completed her transformation. Initially, though, she marvelled at the new reality that lay bare before her eyes and reflected on the life she had left behind: "Returning from Millbrook after that weekend was like stepping into a familiar scene with new eyes. What I had once taken for reality now looked like flim-flam. The hypocrisies and delusions in which I, like most people, had spent my life stood naked before me."[33] Now it was much clearer to her why Leary thought LSD was a godsend. As she was still digesting the acid experience, a friend from her previous life invited her and Michel to a party. She accepted hesitantly, but as she prepared to go out, she realized how absurd socializing had become: "As I apply make-up I think of the lovely faces of the Millbrook women, so innocent of make-up except when they paint them for the fun of it."[34]

In fact, this was the last party of the kind she ever attended. Following her experimentation with these drugs, she was now ready to fully embrace the local psychedelic counterculture where she could both integrate those life-changing experiences and mingle with like-minded individuals who would understand her. And little did she know that Leary was about to entrust her with the leadership of his new religious organization.

The League for Spiritual Discovery

With an appeal pending at the US Supreme Court, Leary devised a risky legal strategy based on the contested spiritual import of the psychedelic experience. He formalized the connection by incorporating the League for Spiritual Discovery as a religion, and in doing so, he followed the path of Ed Rosenfeld's Natural Church that had made a similar case two years earlier with just as little success.[35] The outstanding difference between the two organizations, though, was Leary's mastery of media attention, which immediately gave it the publicity it needed to thrive.

On 19 September 1966, Leary announced the inception of the league during a press conference at the New York Advertising Club on Park Avenue. He appeared before the journalists wearing a button that read "Legalize Spiritual Discovery," and he told them that the church would make a case for inward-directed psychedelic spirituality.[36] According to him, the league had 411 members and a fifteen-member board of guides, who all lived at Millbrook and had quit their jobs to dedicate themselves to the new religion.[37]

By the time the High Priest had made his announcement, LSD and Leary were already notorious. Where Rosenfeld's sect had drawn only a handful of clients, Millbrook was overwhelmed by letters and phone calls from New Yorkers eager to join.[38] One of them was Janah Loprest, who was thrilled by the idea of finding God within rather than in scriptures and sermons. But in spite of her interest, she made it clear that she did not wish to join the league to sample LSD but rather "to experience into depth divine love."[39] Another was Joel Levine, a Hunter College student who was just as impressed by the league and who believed that it would bring some kind of balance to the Western world.[40]

Although the experimental commune continued to be an important focal point until its termination in the final part of the Sixties, it was actually in Greenwich Village that the league set up shop and soon became a shining light for New York's counterculture and a local incarnation of "the spirit of Millbrook."[41] To achieve this, however, Leary needed a highly capable director who would know how to connect with both radical psychedelia and the outside world while operating on a shoe-string budget.

One day, Leary and his latest girlfriend Rosemary Woodruff came down from Millbrook to attend a party at Billy Hitchcock's Manhattan penthouse. They were staying at Graboi's, and as they got prepared, he told her he wished to open a New York Center for the League for Spiritual Discovery. With his trademark smile, he proposed that she become the director. By then, Leary had seen her conversing with many young drug users, and it was obvious that they trusted her. "You often talk about how important it is to prepare them for the trip," he told her. "Well, here's your chance."[42]

Graboi was both astounded and honoured. On the one hand, she believed that non-medical LSD use was only going to increase and that more and more wide-eyed kids were going to be found wandering around the city streets aimlessly. Her new role would allow her to make a difference. On the other hand, she realized that it would spell the end of the Third Force Lecture Bureau and that her association with Leary was bound to cause an uproar among her relatives and friends.

Although her husband had refused to entertain the idea of divorce, he was now forced to take a radical stand that played into her hands. "Choose between me and the Center," Michel threatened. On New Year's Eve, she packed her bags and partied with her Millbrook friends.[43] She relinquished her bank account and moved into the 12th Street apartment. Although she hated housecleaning and had lived the past fifteen years with a maid, formally moving in with a new frame of mind allowed her to view this routine under a different light, as if her home was inhabited by a holy presence: "Now cleaning it was no longer a chore," she marvelled. "It was a prayer and a dance."[44]

Graboi then began looking for the centre's home, and soon she found a rundown storefront at the corner of Perry Street and Hudson Avenue on the same block as the famous White Horse Tavern. It needed a lot of work, but it had potential and charm. At first, the landlord refused to commit after Graboi mentioned Leary's name, but she immediately made it clear that *she* would be in charge and that no drugs would be allowed on the premises. The league had its headquarters.

As the refurbishing went on with the help of volunteers, their presence in the neighbourhood soon drew animosity from the locals, but Graboi's calm and diplomacy was a match for any kind of outrage. One day, an angry salesman from a carpeting firm walked in and shouted at her for supposedly teaching kids how to fry their brains. She smiled back at him and simply pointed to the young men "cheerfully wielding screwdrivers, hammers and saws." Upon learning that the centre was not a place to use drugs, he asked her for her guidance. He had caught his son smoking pot, and he immediately saw Graboi as the ideal counsellor. Even better, he donated carpet square samples, which "became an important feature of the Center's decoration. We laid them out in geometric patterns, and the problem of the floor was solved."[45]

Another issue Graboi had to face early on was Leary and his cult of personality. By then, she knew very well that he loved being the centre of attention, but behind the wit, smiles, and charms, he had a temperament "that could cut like broken glass." This became acutely apparent when she learnt that he was seriously thinking about relieving her of her duties at the centre in spite of her dedication. Apparently, he wanted her to actively supervise the renovations, whereas she saw herself as "the calm center of the Center" that could do much to connect the counterculture with the outside world in a productive and meaningful way. Moreover, he had angrily suggested that she donate her belongings to decorate the centre, just as he had told Woodruff to give away her record player after working through a whole bottle of champagne.[46]

In a strong letter, she told him that she could see very clearly through his megalomania. "People close to you inevitably find themselves involved in a power struggle," wrote Graboi. "You manipulate them, build them up, then tear them down." Moving forward, she stressed that their relationship should be based on mutual respect and that he would be well advised to reflect on his eccentric lifestyle before judging hers. "If you decide," she went on, "that I am of value to you, remember this: my way of life is <u>mine</u>, and that includes my beautiful apartment, my 27 years with Michel ... – just as your champagne drinking, your fancy restaurants and hired cars are yours." And ending on a note of sarcasm, she made it very clear that she was not prepared to surrender the little material comfort she had in her home in the name of dubious anti-materialism: "I will maintain this luxurious style of life on the $75.00 a week I draw from the Center, and will not tolerate any attempt on your part to make me feel guilty about it."[47]

Without much surprise, this episode is not mentioned in Leary's memoirs, nor is his entire collaboration with Graboi for that matter. What it does reveal to an extent, though, is that her psychedelic experimentation had been so liberating that even the power-tripping Leary was unable to subject her to his will. After this unfortunate argument, the two of them continued to be friends and carried on their effort to make the centre a stronghold for New York's counterculture.

Later that month, the centre was finally inaugurated through a series of lectures. For the opening, Leary, Alpert, Metzner, Ginsberg, Orlovsky, Burroughs, and Gergory Corso all gave talks. Among the attendees was Don McNeill, a *Village Voice* journalist who tragically drowned a year later under the influence of LSD. His colleague Richard Goldstein remembers that McNeill was a homeless journalist who had invaluable insider knowledge of the local counterculture. "He was covering people who lived in crash pads. And he had a bed on the top floor of our office that he slept in at the time, when he was on the streets ... And it was from him that I learned a lot about the counterculture in New York."[48]

At the centre, McNeill was struck by a poster-sized portrait of the High Priest on one of the windows[49] that clearly indicated that he was the leader of this new unorthodox religion. Another reporter subsequently noticed the presence of Eastern elements such as "the whining of the sitar, the ringing of the tabla, the smell of incense, the droning voices in another room." One meditator was sitting perfectly still with his legs tucked away, his eyes fixed on a Buddha statue. All six participants seemed to be "trying to lose their identities and achieve a sense of unity with their environment."[50]

Subsequently, the centre hosted weekly discussions on psychedelics, meditation, and Eastern spirituality by prominent figures of the psychedelic movement, and Graboi met a lot of kids who reported religious experiences resulting from acid use. For instance, one user had taken LSD during his freshman year and was determined to become a saint,[51] while another claimed to see light around individuals when using the drug. He also told Graboi he had undergone uncanny out-of-the-body experiences.[52]

Not every attendee looked East for spiritual frameworks, however. To assist Graboi, Leary sent over a young seeker from Millbrook, who was fascinated by Native American Indians. At the centre, he could spend hours perusing books on Indian art until Graboi directed him to the literature pointing to the similarities between Native American and Buddhist rituals.[53] Around that time, scholars of religion were wondering whether there might exist a universal core of the religious experience resulting from drug use, and some anthropologists investigating psychoactive plant-based rituals across the world were attempting to demonstrate the universality of the psychedelic experience.[54] Some of these academics were sympathetic to the counterculture, and it is possible that Graboi's liberal comparison was the consequence of the debates of the time.

The centre also became a meeting place for talking about topics like sexuality, which was going through important changes in the 1960s. Graboi spent a lot of time there discussing this and realized that "the boys loved [sex]. The girls pretended to, but under a thin veneer of hipness, most of them wanted one man, their man, instead of the one-night stands that were so common among them."[55] Certainly, many in the 1960s saw the "sexual revolution" as an excuse for promiscuous and violent sexual relations.[56] But Graboi nonetheless felt that LSD was instrumental in developing new patterns of sexuality.[57]

Goldstein likewise remembers how casual sex had become the norm within the counterculture. "You could see on Washington Square people fucking. It was going on all over the place. There was no consciousness of any diseases ... You went to a park and did it. You'd lie in the grass and do it." But there may have been a connection with the higher states of sensory awareness, as his vivid description of the sexual experience on LSD with another man illustrates: "Just the experience of touching for hours and this sort of aura. I also remembered discovering – a dry heat rose from the body, when you were aroused. Like a wood-burning stove. And it's the same quality of dry heat which I've always thought was the indicator that you were having a good experience ... Not sweat. Something more like steam, but not steam. More like the way heat radiates from a stove. A tile stove."[58]

Jeff Perkins also had a gay friend who understood the psychedelic experience in a similar fashion. But to him, a strong connection with the Divine occurred simultaneously. "And his saying was 'I feel like I'm fucking God.' And it had two meanings: physically fucking God and just fucking as a metaphor, an adjective ... So the feeling is extraordinary."[59]

On a day-to-day basis, the centre was mostly a hangout for young, carefree acid users. "They look at the books and brochures, sit on the floor reading, talking, playing the guitar. Most of them are young, under 25. Their clothes are in varying degrees of disrepair. You have to look funky – neatness is what separates the straights from the hip."[60] Soon Graboi grew tired of clearing up the litter after them and thought of putting up a sign, but she realized that she would have to be creative to maintain a modicum of order without undermining the radical edge of the centre. So one staff member drew a "psychedelic goddess" and wrote "DON'T BE A LITTERBUG" underneath the drawing to devise a rule that was in keeping with the transgressive atmosphere of the place.[61]

A greater challenge she faced was her appearance and age, which could be cause for suspicion. As a counsellor on altered states of consciousness, Graboi, who typically sat behind her desk by the entrance door, had to look trustworthy to those seeking information. One day, a young man in his late teens, who had been experimenting for the previous two years, approached her and asked for her opinion on LSD. "I'm on a trial," she immediately realized. "I'm middle-aged, wear lipstick and straight clothes."

Yet this deficiency in countercultural capital was compensated for by her experiences with psychedelics. "Acid?" she replied. "It can take you on a trip to heaven, or on a trip to hell. I've been to both. How about you?" He grinned and told her he'd been to both. The young man was favourably impressed: "I passed the test. He sits on the floor."[62] In fact, the young man could not have sat on a chair if he had wanted to because purchasing some 200 chairs for the audience would have been too costly for the league's finances. Fortunately, the audience did not mind, since it was made up of people "to whom chairs are as much a badge of the straight world as short hair."[63]

Occasionally, unsympathetic visitors showed up, like a middle-aged passerby wearing an overcoat and a tie. The kids were engaged in a calm discussion about spirituality, and the scene was so baffling that he forgot he had come there to complain in the first place. Regathering his composure, he pressed Graboi to admit that acid could be dangerous, which she had no trouble doing. He felt that his son had changed, and he believed that psychedelic drugs were the culprit. But she discussed these issues with him in a friendly way, and following this productive conversation he regularly dropped by to say hello. On another occasion, she even gave pamphlets about LSD to a policeman who was sweeping the centre for illegal drugs. Two weeks later, he came back for more. "Interesting stuff," he conceded. "You know, all we hear about LSD is the bad stuff. I'll show these to some of my colleagues."[64]

According to Krippner, who believed that Graboi and her volunteers were doing good work, the police were closely monitoring the group to entrap league followers, a tactic commonly used to arrest marijuana activists.[65] "They would send decoys in that pretended to be on the verge of taking LSD," he remembers, "but they didn't arrest anybody because nobody was ever saying 'yes this is where you can get LSD; yes you should take it.' ... They left it up to the people to make their own decisions. They were basically giving information and counselling."[66]

But even though Graboi had made it clear that no drugs were allowed on the premises, that did not stop people from showing up under the influence. Volunteers had to run the centre on a twenty-four-hour basis and set up an emergency line to assist those who might be undergoing a difficult acid trip. They would be taken to the meditation room to calm down, but the more severe cases ended up in a small room where Graboi or a volunteer would sit with them and talk them down. Soon it became an open secret that the centre was the go-to place when an acid trip went wrong.

Moreover, the league followers were encouraged to discriminate between the psychedelics that could offer meaningful spiritual experience and the other psychoactive substances that could lead to addiction: "We made a clear distinction between psychedelic substances and drugs like heroin, cocaine, amphetamines, alcohol, etc.," remembered Graboi, "and as a general rule, the regulars of the Center shunned these drugs."[67]

Eventually, Graboi met Murray Levy, who like her believed that the psychedelic counterculture needed a lot more visibility. To that effect, he proposed setting up a psychedelic storefront where they would present psychedelia to the outside world. Graboi found the idea eccentric but liked it.[68] She was wary of the counterculture's sometimes confrontational approach and felt that more people could be reached by making personal contact.

The psychedelic showcase, as it came be known, appeared on Madison Avenue and 92nd Street on 12 January 1967. A series of stands were connected with rainbow-hued fabrics and sold psychedelic artefacts like jewellery, paintings, books, and various pieces of craft. It was run on a volunteer basis, and according to the official brochure, it had attracted artists, writers, philosophers, and religious figures who were keen to present their work and share their views on psychedelics.[69] In the rear, Graboi set up a booth to represent the League for Spiritual Discovery and provide the attendees with information. The atmosphere was in keeping with the meditation room of the center: "We brought Timothy's carpet, the Buddha, cushions, Indian bedspreads ... candles, incense and music."[70] In this way, the league increased its visibility even further on the streets rather than remaining indoors.

The showcase drew curious folks who were invited to sit down with Graboi and her circle of youth to discuss LSD. At first, they were ill at ease, but they soon opened up a great deal: "the intelligent answers our kids gave as well as their sincere desire to build a bridge for those alienated, worried parents made a real exchange possible. It was rewarding to see faces loosen up as we discussed our differences without anger, without noise, without hostility."[71] Some of these outsiders came back to see them at the centre, and by the end of the showcase, Graboi had walked away with a couple of handsome donations.[72]

Levy and Graboi then went separate ways and enjoyed markedly different fortunes, but both continued to reach out to the outside. By then, the league was receiving requests to give presentations, and on one occasion Leary passed on an invitation to talk about the new psychedelic religion at the Riverside Church, close to Columbia. As Graboi walked into a small, sixty-seat-capacity room, the sight of the crowd made her nervous, but the feeling quickly disappeared. "Until a year ago I was a law-abiding citizen," she joked. "Then I smoked marijuana and became a criminal." After she had extolled the benefits of chemically induced ego loss to minimize the fear of death, some of the attendees were convinced enough to ask her where they could get their hands on LSD.[73]

Levy, meanwhile, attempted something far more ambitious by opening the New Consciousness gallery-store on Carmine Street. But in spite of his good intentions, he seriously underestimated the local atmosphere of the area. As he started moving in, there were already signs that a nearby Catholic church, mostly attended by Italian Americans, was openly hostile. The store was broken into several times, and once a neighbourhood gang attacked them in broad daylight. The hoodlums had acted on the orders of a local mob figure, who gave Levy seven days to clear off. The police were oblivious to his afflictions, and when he decided to temporarily close the storefront, thieves cleared it entirely.[74]

A few months later, however, the centre was also forced to close down because its finances were at a record low. That summer, Graboi went to Millbrook hoping that Leary might have a solution, only to find an empty mansion and a grim-looking High Priest. In July, forty people had been arrested on flimsy charges, and Leary had narrowly escaped using Billy Hitchcock's private plane. Upon returning to Millbrook, they had moved into the woods,[75] and even a trustworthy friend like her was not allowed on their campsite for fear of bringing more heat there. "Maybe it's time to phase out the Center," Leary suggested to Graboi, who was choking back her tears.[76]

Combined with Levy's hardships on Carmine Street, this was another sign that the future of radical psychedelia was not in Greenwich Village. 1967, then, was the year when the psychedelic counterculture completed its migration across Lower Manhattan.

The New Village

The East Village (or the Ninth Precinct) is delineated by the East River to the east, 14th Street to the north, Broadway to the west, and Houston Street to the south. Contrary to the capital of urban Bohemia, it was still a residential area that offered very little in the way of entertainment and shopping. As Don McNeill noted, "Until recently the roster included only a number of boutiques, several bookstores, a few restaurants, and a lone discothèque."[77]

One of the reasons that the Village life had not changed much over the decades was its relative geographical isolation resulting from Manhattan's vertical transportation grid. As a result, many Bohemians initially saw it as a distant place. When writer Michael Stephens moved there, his poet friend Andrei Codrescu remained in Greenwich Village, and they started a new correspondence. For Codrescu, it was as if they had "moved to different countries ... It seemed like they were different worlds."[78]

Young acid heads, on the other hand, were more interested in getting high than in comparing both Villages. With affordable rents and a sense of pioneering expressed in the first issue of the *East Village Other*, intrepid drug users started appearing locally, often with little or no means of supporting themselves. This was the case of nineteen-year-old Fred, an NYU dropout from Long Island whose parents had disowned him. With no more money to pay the rent, he was evicted from his place on Avenue B, and his furniture ended up on the streets – a convenient way for other Bohemians to furnish their own homes for free. Eventually, his three boxes of possessions could fit into a shopping bag. However, "He does have a place to sleep, food to eat and, somehow, drugs when he wants them."[79]

Others leading similar carefree lives found sanctuary in communes. Around that time, thousands – probably tens of thousands – of such places appeared all around the country, but this historic wave extended far beyond countercultural enclaves only and epitomized the climate of protest and spiritual rebirth of the Sixties.[80] In the Village, several communes appeared locally and became havens for both runaways and psychedelics.

Amelie Edwards was one of the teenagers who shunned her middle-class comfort of Westchester County. Edwards was fifteen when she first went to San Francisco on a family trip and had her first glimpse of urban Bohemia. When she got back to New York, she started going to Washington Square Park every Saturday, and there she befriended a girl from the Bronx who was about her age. Together, they discussed the possibility of moving away from their respective homes.

Following a misfortune near the park, she found it difficult to go back to her parents and moved into a commune on 6th Street. There she took a lot of acid, which was freely available to those on the premises. It helped her to create even more distance from her upbringing. "Well, when I started using drugs," she recalls, "I wanted to cut myself off completely from anything I had known in the past ... I remember I had a gold ring that my parents had given me with my initials on it. I gave that to someone, because it ... wasn't important to me. Gold rings just seemed like part of this capitalistic society that I didn't want to be a part of any more."[81]

Around that time, Mayor John Lindsay was trying to rejuvenate the entire city through ambitious cultural policies designed to help New Yorkers reclaim public space. A 1962 survey had indicated that New Yorkers were afraid to use their parks, and in 1966 the Lindsay administration set about to turn Central Park into a bastion of artistic happenings that emphasized play and spontaneity rather than gazing passively at works of art.[82] This attempted transformation of "fear city" into "fun city"[83] may have struck a chord among teenagers like Edwards, who liked to play games in the streets: "We used to walk around bare-foot. We ... used to go pan-handling. And we used to play with toy guns in the street. Water-pistol type guns."

Eventually, she met Michael, who became her boyfriend, and together they spent their free time drawing, making up stories, and attending poetry readings. They liked to hang out with David Johansen, who subsequently founded the proto-punk band New York Dolls and had an impressive collection of records they listened to on acid. Michael also dealt a little LSD, which he believed was the key to a better world. As a result of their psychedelic experimentation, they cast a resolutely critical gaze on the outside world, making "remarks to people about their 9 to 5 jobs and their business suits ... We would tell people 'Smile!' like 'How come you look so unhappy?' 'Why don't you smile?' that kind of thing."[84]

Peter Lefcourt of the *Village Voice* noticed a similar suspicion of New Yorkers lacking obvious countercultural capital. Once he took two young panhandlers for lunch in the Village after they had asked him for some change. In spite of his generosity, he still looked a bit dodgy because he had played Simon and Garfunkel on the jukebox rather than the Doors or Bob Dylan, who by then were the among the leading rock acts. To gain their trust, he first displayed his "roach clips" (a cannabis cigarette holder), but sensing this wasn't enough, he had to convince them that he was part of the scene: "I make up an elaborate story about my last acid trip and throw in a little bit of East Village gossip. In time they start warming up, and pretty soon they're rapping away like teletype machines [about their own drug use]."[85]

Lewis Yablonsky conducted ethnographic research among the local commune dwellers and likewise noticed the connection between psychedelics and the rejection of conformity. For instance, twenty-two-year-old Sonny believed that his experimentation with drugs had made him happier. Sonny came from a wealthy Roman Catholic family, but in spite of his material comfort, he had attempted suicide several times, mainly because his parents had picked his life for him. His first LSD experience was life-changing and allowed him to see past the flaws of the modern world.[86]

For these new Villagers intent on psychedelic experimentation, the closest source of supply would have been a local head shop that embodied both the eclectic nature and the idealism of the counterculture. The Psychedelicatessen had grown out of an art gallery run by Susun Weed, her husband, and his brother. Weed was a mathematics major who had left the University of California at Los Angeles and moved to the East Village in 1965 in pursuit of LSD. She first took the drug in late 1966, and that trip convinced her that she wanted to drop acid as often as possible. She did not want to buy it off the streets, so she hired a chemist to make pure LSD for her.

One night soon thereafter, Weed and her friends were looking for rolling papers, but none of the local head shops stayed open so late. So they decided to open a 24/7 head shop on Avenue A, one block from Tompkins Square Park, which was fast becoming the heart of East Village psychedelia.[87] The Psychedelicatessen sold psychedelic paraphernalia like pipes, incense, and posters, but it quickly became a marketplace and a commune for artists and craftspeople like candle makers, costume designers, jewellers, and others.

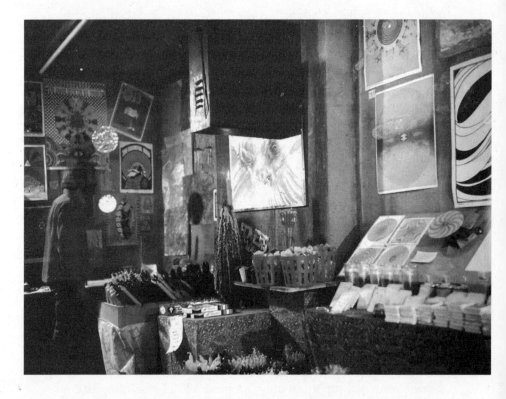

Figure 5.1 Inside the Psychedelicatessen circa 1967–68

Meanwhile, Weed and the members of the Psychedelicatessen commune were taking LSD every second or third day, thanks to their chemist named Peter (a member of the commune). Because sugar cubes, which were the usual vehicle for a dose of LSD, were cumbersome and easy to identify, Susun and Peter decided to put the doses on blotter paper. In fact, during a raid, the police saw nothing suspicious about fifty blank pieces of paper, though they actually contained tens of thousands of doses.

After setting up the lab, Weed also began a correspondence with Albert Hofmann himself. He helped them to change the solvents used as part of the manufacturing process, just as access to safe ones was becoming ever more difficult, and he sent them powdered LSD in the mail because, like her, he wanted people to take pure LSD only. At the Psychedelicatessen, LSD was given twenty-four hours a day or sold to offset the production costs of the lab. With a weekly ad in the *Village Voice*, the store thrived, supporting and connecting the growing number of acid heads enjoying the local psychedelic scenes.[88]

LSD might have been plentiful in the Village, but taking the drug in this rundown quarter was not to everyone's liking. In the fall of 1966, Trina Robbins had also come over to New York from Los Angeles, and a few months later she took some acid with her boyfriend and wandered around the Lower East Side. "As the acid took hold," she recalled, "everything started to look weird, and not in a good way. It was a case of 'people are strange when you're a stranger,' even though the song had not come out yet. Faces came out of the rain and they looked ugly." In a state of panic, they arrived in Tompkins Square Park, and Robbins immediately saw a beacon of hope: the offices of the *East Village Other*.

Inside, they collapsed onto an old sofa while Allen Katzman tried to help them mellow out. "And then something wonderful happened," she remembers. "As he calmed us down, Allen turned into a rabbi! It wasn't too hard for him, because he was already Jewish and bearded, but his beard grew and got darker and he became the kind of rabbi you see in Woody Allen movies, yarmulke and all. Then as Allen continued to talk, he would slowly morph back into Allen Katzman, and then after a short while, he'd become that rabbi again." After this memorable trip, Robbins drew "a kind of proto-comic" to say thanks and slipped it under the door of the offices. It was printed in the next issue, and so began her career as an illustrator.[89]

Beyond improvised psychedelic assistance, the EVO assumed an even greater leadership for the acid counterculture and attracted more and more journalists. However, the paper did not stay long by Tompkins Square Park: in the spring of 1966, Peter Leggieri joined the EVO, and a year later he negotiated a "barter" lease with the Village Theater at 105 2nd Avenue. This allowed the paper to move into a 5,000-square-foot area in exchange for advertising space and in turn to acquire the necessary equipment to make their publication even more psychedelic.

In November, Leggieri became publisher and editor-in-chief after Bowart, who was now involved in a serious relationship with Peggy Hitchcock, left the paper, while Katzman remained the paper's editor. Far from destabilizing it, this new partnership ushered in a new "golden era" that lasted almost two years, during which circulation almost doubled while bills and wages were paid on time. In January 1968, the Village

Theater filed for bankruptcy, but within a couple of months West Coast rock impresario Bill Graham had bought it back and turned it into the Fillmore East. The advertising-for-space agreement did not change, and the journalists got an even better deal: "free, live music, performed by the world's greatest rock bands in airshaft stereo."[90]

The *EVO*'s growing influence became subtly apparent during the 1967 Central Park Easter Be-in, which some enterprising New Yorkers organized following the success of the initial San Francisco happening. During the event, the most striking "drug" available was dried banana peels, thanks to a group of fifteen people moving around the park to promote this new "high."[91] A few weeks before the event, *Village Voice* journalist Marvin Garson had written about this new sensation after experimenting: "After a few hours of oven-drying, the scraped peels of two bananas yielded me enough residue for two Camel-sized cigarettes. It looked a little like pipe tobacco, and it smelled a lot like bananas. Frugally smoked, it was identical in its effects to about half a joint of second-rate pot, i.e., it got me just barely high enough to suspect I was high."[92] Over in the East Village, "dealers" of dried banana peels could be found on street corners, and a group of radical leftists even organized a "Banana Be-in" in a corner of Tompkins Square Park.[93]

Given that bananas were sold over the counter in most stores, Garson safely concluded that prohibition was unrealistic: "what legislator would dare affix his name to 'The Banana Control Act of 1968?'"[94] But banana abuse became widespread enough to appear in the pages of *Time* and *Newsweek* and to warrant an official FDA investigation. By the end of May, the agency concluded that the high was the result of a placebo effect rather than a hitherto unknown alkaloid. The whole fad, it turned out, was the consequence of a silly hoax.

The story of the rise and fall of banana-peel smoking illustrates how fast such rumours could circulate in the subterranean press through the coordinated efforts of New York's counterculture. While the hoax originated in California and spread through its local underground papers, the first reference that connected bananas and getting high appeared back in 1963 in the pages of poet Ed Sanders's *Fuck You* magazine, which he edited on the Lower East Side. The rumour received an important but totally coincidental boost from British pop icon Donovan, who released "Mellow Yellow" in November 1966 but who eventually confessed that the song referred to a yellow electric dildo.

In New York, the *East Village Other* had played a decisive role in the dissemination of the hoax. In their Tompkins Square offices, Bowart, Katzman, and Wilcock had created the Underground Press Syndicate (UPS) in June 1966, which pooled nationwide reports from the country's underground papers.[95] Six months later, twenty-five new papers had been founded across the United States, and they had all joined UPS. Partly through this unique channel, the hoax had easily moved around countercultural venues in cities like Dallas, Washington, Chicago, Austin, Detroit, and Los Angeles.[96]

Within the *EVO*'s offices, marijuana and LSD remained the drugs of choice, and they significantly influenced the paper's identity. Early in 1967, art editor Bill Beckman was drawing "Captain High," a psychedelic superhero whose mission it was to get high and stay high. Kim Deitch learned about Captain High and the *EVO* through a friend who thought that his work could be as good Beckman's. Eventually, he came up with a new character, "Sunshine Girl," who immediately found her place in the pages of the paper.

By way of financial compensation, however, Beckman could only offer Deitch a job as a pot dealer. "So I started doing *Sunshine Girl* and dealing dope," Deitch recalls. "I wasn't the greatest dealer in town, because I was dealing a lot to my friends, and of course your friends want bargains, but I was making a little money, and I certainly had all the dope I wanted to smoke for free."[97] This changed after Joel Fabrikant, a hard-nosed businessman and a Republican, became the publisher and got Deitch on the payroll in the spring of 1968.

Captain High was in fact one of the first cartoons of the era to have an explicit connection with psychedelics and the counterculture. Beckman went on to publish the early work of Gilbert Shelton and Robert Crumb, but Katzman turned down Art Spiegelman's first comic strips and "advised him to get some actual experience with drugs and sex first." In 1969, the *EVO* released the first issue of a monthly comic tabloid, *Gothic Blimp Works*. From the second issue onward, Deitch edited the paper, and soon everyone wanted to be part of it, including West Coast cartoonists. As a colleague recalled, "By July, he had amassed so much original art that he decided to stage a show in a storefront at 335 East Ninth Street. Joel Fabrikant got paid for some weird deal with a giant bag of … LSD that week, he recalled, so he was enjoying it on a daily basis and sharing it with his comic museum visitors."[98]

In fact, pot and acid were so commonplace that the staff was often high when the paper was put together. In 1970, they received the visit of Robert Hughes, an influential Australian art critic who had arrived at *Time*'s offices in 1969.[99] Hughes had the opportunity to witness the weekly paste-up nights at the EVO and saw the process as a rekindling of Dadaism. The laying out of the paper certainly had a chaotic element to it, but it was the product of psychoactive excess rather than a tribute to that artistic tradition. As one cartoonist recalled, "the joints and acid tabs were the payment for a good night's work. Someone routinely emerged from the editor's office around 8:30 p.m. with a shoebox full of the stuff, as well as with the night's layout assignments, which included at least three pages of 'intimate' classifieds. The layout crew would help themselves to grass (the acid was saved until after the session was over) and manuscripts, find their tables, select their decorative ruling tapes and transfer type sheets, and settle down to 'design' pages."[100]

Contrasting with the EVO, Greenwich Village's *Village Voice* was initially far more conservative with regard to drug use. In spite of its coverage of the topic, booze was the drug of choice on the premises, according to Goldstein. "When I came to the *Voice* in 66," he remembers, "it would have been more of a drinking scene. And anybody who was using marijuana wouldn't have done it in the office." The major difference between the *Voice* and the EVO was that the latter was explicit about its countercultural intentions and its sympathy toward LSD and psychedelics. "The *Voice* was a newspaper whose editors ran an enterprise and made it very clear they were interested in whatever was out there … So the temperament of the *Village Voice* initially was to sort of sit back at your desks smoking a pipe and just say 'OK, this is happening.'"[101]

Soon after the EVO had moved into its new offices, it was joined by the Group Image merely a block away. This eclectic group was made up of idealistic acid heads, and their loft was meant to be a crash pad, a hangout, an artistic hub, and an underground media outlet rolled into one.[102] There, Lynn and Freeman House were running the *Innerspace* psychedelic newsletter with the help of Martin Carey, who did the artwork.[103] *Innerspace* offered a platform for psychedelic enthusiasts to share their ideas, and although it was based in NYC, it appeared in other major American cities and featured contributions from psychedelic activists like Peter Stafford and Lisa Bieberman (who opened a Psychedelic

Information Center), as well as the better-known celebrities.[104] Although the outreach of the newsletter paled in comparison with the influence of the *East Village Other*, its mere existence, combined with the Group Image, strengthened the notion that psychedelia had effectively moved to the East Village.

New York City's psychedelic counterculture was the result of a number of individuals whose experiences with mind-altering drugs had obliterated their ontological certainties and left them asking important questions about the way they should lead their lives in the light of their revelations. For some of the young commune dwellers, it meant dropping out of the boring suburbs and embracing anti-materialistic hedonism. But for many psychedelic radicals, it was all about creating new spaces like the psychedelic showcase and influential institutions like the *East Village Other* in order to underscore the counterculture's power to actively engage the community.

Nina Graboi's account of her experimentation is a fitting testimony of this transformative power and of the way psychedelics enabled her to peer through the veil of postwar conformity. As a result, she became passionately involved in radical psychedelia, and her time in Greenwich Village was marked by an attempt to reach out to the outside world rather than remaining confined in a psychedelic bubble. Just about anyone collaborating with Timothy Leary in challenging undertakings struggled to adapt to his narcissistic personality, and Graboi was no exception, but her psychedelic experimentation was so empowering that it allowed her to effectively carry on her mission on Hudson Street regardless of his influence.

In the larger history of LSD and psychedelics, Graboi's legacy resides in the short-lived Center for the League for Spiritual Discovery, a hybrid religious institution that could offer a platform for the local counterculture just as much as it could reach out to the outside world. Perhaps more important, it offered an early form of harm reduction and counselling that most likely limited the incidence of adverse reactions to psychedelic experiences in downtown New York.

6

Kaleidoscope Eyes
Isaac Abrams, Psychedelic Art, and Multimedia Light Shows

While idealistic acid heads were using the insights of the psychedelic experience to fuel a revolutionary outlook on postwar America, others realized that LSD could open the door to otherworldly aesthetics. Among them was Isaac Abrams,[1] whose life story offers a unique window into New York's drug underworld. Abrams had never drawn anything before his first psychedelic experiences, and for him drugs were directly responsible for his launching a career that has spanned across two centuries. Moreover, he was probably the first person to come up with the concept of psychedelic art, and the inception of the new medium was formalized when he and his then-wife Rachel organized the first ever psychedelic art exhibition. Incidentally, the combined testimonies of Rachel and Isaac offer a rare glimpse into the shared psychedelic experiences of a married couple.

This connection between psychedelics and artistic innovations was just as manifest in multimedia light shows.[2] Though Thomas Wilfried had pioneered the medium in his "Lumia" compositions in the 1920s,[3] it was greatly enhanced in the 1960s, thanks to highly creative acid users. Multimedia artists devised complex installations usually based on light and sound to create a strong feeling of disorientation among the audience, and many described the process as an attempt to reproduce the psychedelic experience without any drugs. By the end of the decade, light shows had become so successful that they were moving out of psychedelia.

The development of this experiential psychedelic art occurred at a time when Mayor Lindsay's cultural politics were strengthening New York's position as a leading capital of the arts by encouraging its citizens to participate in local artistic endeavours. Some of the most fitting illustrations of his promotion of New York art occurred in 1966 as the Lincoln Center for the Performing Arts was nearing completion. Lindsay had appointed art historian Thomas Hoving to implement these new policies, and Hoving organized a series of happenings in Central Park that allowed New Yorkers to interact freely with several installations. Later that year, Allan Kaprow created the "Towers" happening, which allowed New Yorkers to climb around stacks of used tires covered in plastic sheets. Tellingly, he believed that spectators should be turned into participants and should actively engage in the artworks.[4] As an emerging genre originating from drug use, psychedelic art remained on the fringes, but the fluidity of the boundaries separating works of art from the viewers nevertheless became its central feature.

Another striking aspect of psychedelic art was that it was by and large apolitical, in contrast with other art forms like Black theatre, Beat poetry, abstract expressionism, and anarchist theatre that were part of New York's artistic vanguard.[5] While activists protested against the war in Vietnam and campaigned for civil rights, Gerd Stern and the other artists from his multimedia art collective USCO had realized the bankruptcy of politics through their LSD use.[6]

This, however, did not prevent light shows from briefly flirting with radical psychedelia when Leary and his crew created a series of plays with the help of multimedia artists Jackie Cassen and Rudi Stern. First and foremost, these shows helped to generate money to finance the League for Spiritual Discovery, and they were a success in that respect. But the plays were also meant to re-enact the lives of visionary figures like Jesus Christ, the Buddha, and George Gurdjieff under a distinctively psychedelic light.[7] By operating at the crossroads of drug activism, spirituality, the arts, and technological innovations, Leary's "Psychedelic Celebrations" were among New York psychedelia's most sophisticated cultural productions. A good measure of their historical significance is not just the favourable critical reception they received but also the attention they drew from the world of cinema.

By the end of the decade, multimedia art and total environments had evolved into a highly interactive nightclub called Cerebrum. As a place that sold no liquor and that concentrated on stimulating the patrons' five senses while emphasizing the importance of play and reconnection with lost childhood, Cerebrum was a place that does not elicit easy qualification but one that nevertheless reflected both Lindsay's ambitious art policies and psychedelia's culture of rejuvenation.

Becoming an Artist

Isaac Abrams was born in 1939 into a Jewish family of Romanian and Moldavian descent that had prospered thanks to a shoe polish business. It was another success story based on waterproof coating, this time around for the US soldiers fighting in Europe and the Pacific. When Isaac's father turned forty-seven, he sold the business and told his son not to worry about making loads of money like he had. With this piece of advice in mind, Isaac became a lot more open-minded and was always on the lookout for interesting things and people.[8]

In 1956, Abrams got a job in a music store. The owner was a white saxophone player who had created vinyl records featuring drums, bass, and piano only so that fledging sax players could practise. They got on well, and soon the two of them were going to the Birdland and other jazz venues to see the most prominent jazz musicians on a regular basis. Around that time, he told Abrams about mescaline, which Isaac found fascinating. A year later, Abrams went to college to study history and graduated in 1961.

One day, he stumbled upon a little art gallery where he saw some lovely collages made of wood and paper. Robert Rauschenberg was then the main artist associated with such mixed-media assemblages, which came to be known as his "Combines," the medium that bridged the abstract expressionism of the Fifties and the pop art of the Sixties[9] and used both paint and the material objects of everyday life. Rachel and Isaac bought one of the collages that had been made by Jerry Jofen, the grandson of the Great Rabbi of Warsaw and an artist who was interested in painting, film, performance, and mixed-media.

It turned out that Jofen had some Harvard psilocybin in his possession. When he brought the subject up, Isaac remembered his former boss's description of the mescaline experience, and he felt he was now ready to try psychedelics. So in February 1962, Jofen and the Abrams took the drug in their apartment on Atlantic Avenue near Brooklyn Heights. It was the first time they had taken a psychoactive drug of any description – they had yet to try marijuana.

As Isaac recalls, the whole apartment began morphing under the influence. It had a tin ceiling, "and all the tin squares in the ceiling started moving." They both thoroughly enjoyed the experience, and for Rachel it was "like the most amazing joy-ride." Eventually, Jofen took them to the Charles Theater in the East Village, which showed experimental film. The three of them sat down to watch some hand-painted films and films by Jack Smith, a seminal underground filmmaker known for his cheap, tacky, and occasionally controversial flicks.[10] These films made a huge impression on Isaac, but Rachel was too overwhelmed by the drug and struggled to concentrate on the cinema.

Soon after, the Abrams had their first experience with mescaline. On this occasion, Jofen and the Abrams went to the country, where Rachel's parents had a house. The mescaline helped them to experience nature on a different magnitude. "Walking barefoot and experiencing the whole sense of walking barefoot, in a way I'd never really felt before," remembers Isaac. "I could feel the energy of the earth and all the details of the earth." Rachel also experienced a deep connection with nature. "Like, just sinking into the earth," she recalls. "I felt that I was just part of the earth." Down the road lived a man who farmed snakes for venom. Rachel had always been afraid of snakes, but by then she had read Huxley's *Island*, and she remembered that the book advised you to visualize your enemies to make them friendly: "So I visualized snakes sitting in a rocking chair. Knitting! [laughs] with an apron on. And … my whole fear of snakes just disappeared."

Subsequently, Isaac got a job as a bookkeeper on 23rd Street, and he regularly hung out with Jofen, who had a loft on 20th Street. There he met other important characters of the jazz and heroin underground like Herbert Huncke, saxophone player Jackie McLean, and tuba player Ray Draper. Jofen, however, immediately cautioned him against speed and junk. Although Abrams tried both drugs, he quickly realized that psychedelics were far more interesting, and he drew the line between that category and "drugs."

Through Jofen, Abrams met several underground filmmakers and visual artists who were experimenting with mixed media. "And they shot movies at the huge paintings. Some of them introduced tar and broken glass, and big iconic figures painted … [Jofen] was well known for doing things like a performance piece, which consisted of him crawling across the stage for half an hour." In this troubling but undoubtedly creative setting, Abrams became involved in underground film and met Jack Smith and other artists.

Rachel and Isaac continued their psychedelic explorations with Stanley Krippner, who introduced them to the highly potent DMT. Isaac first smoked DMT with Krippner in Woodstock, New York, where they both experienced being carried away by a swooping owl. Rachel eventually tried it with her husband in someone's flat in the city, but she found it too scary. "There was an oriental carpet on the floor," she remembers. "Whatever happened, I felt like I was melting into that carpet and disappearing." The presence of other people made it even worse because she did not want "to be the weird one, the scared one." Isaac, on the other hand, had several meaningful DMT experiences full of uncanny encounters like "Meetings with beings or elfish – you might interpret them as elves or gnomes or something."

At the time, LSD was less commonplace, and in those days DMT was a staple among knowledgeable business people, according to Isaac. "Guys with wide-rim glasses were running around with DMT. It was one of the first things that was available in New York." It was dubbed the "businessman's high" because a trip lasts less than thirty minutes and could fit into a tight corporate schedule. Visual artists were soon drawn to the drug's ability to "punch holes in the senses."

The DMT was most likely coming out of a clandestine Brooklyn lab operated by Nick Sand. Sand was born in 1941 to Clarence Hiskey, who was caught spying for the Soviet Union while working on the Manhattan Project. Sand had his first mescaline experience in December 1962, which was followed by several peyote sessions.[11] Like other Greenwich Village Bohemians, he travelled to Mazatec country to meet curandera María Sabina, and in the summer of 1963 he set up a makeshift laboratory in his mother's attic. In the process, he became most likely the first chemist to cook DMT.[12] Soon the demand increased, and eventually he rented a two-storey commercial building where he continued to manufacture psychedelics on an even greater scale, using "Bell Perfume Labs" as a cover. By then, he had discovered that the free-base of DMT could be smoked, and this made DMT more appealing to those who flinched at the idea of injecting it.[13]

In 1963, Isaac met Howard Lotsof, who was experimenting with mescaline and ibogaine in his Brooklyn lab. On one occasion, they were at someone's place close to Tompkins Square Park and decided to take 500 mgr of ibogaine each. For a while, nothing seemed to happen until Abrams stood up: "And when I stood up, my body flew out of my body. Like one of those telescopes that opens up. There's 8 or 9 sections. Then my body that flew out of my body, flew off the body that flew out of my body. And again, and again, and again. And suddenly I was extraordinary tall."

Confused by the sensation, the two of them reasoned that they should go back to Lotsof's place, which was close by. This was easier said than done, however. The ibogaine was so powerful that they could no longer identify the colour of the traffic lights and spent ages waiting to cross until they finally followed the lead of a woman with a baby carriage who unwittingly guided them to safety. When they arrived at Lotsof's, Abrams sat on the bed and soon noticed that the venetian blinds started looking like a TV going out of phase. It was so overwhelming that he ended up collapsing on the bed:

> And when I did that it was like I tumbled down into this whirling, whirling kind of – almost like a whirlpool. And down and down and down. And I literally felt myself flowing down through this thing and I landed in this place and I realised I was inside my head. Inside my subconscious. And it was warm and it was wet. And it was sticky. And in there, there was all the people in my life. My father, a whole bunch of people came in this place. And there was all kinds of things happening. Conversations. And it went on and on like that.

After that, he was able to sit up and walk out of the room, which was full of a vibrant, electrical energy. This feeling lasted almost three days, during which Abrams had to go to work still under the influence. "At the time I was operating a book-keeping machine," he recalls, "but it was still a problem. I could do everything, but I was at the same time existing in this other place. People looked different ... And I was in a corner and I could see all these ley lines, geometry, all this kind of business."

Following such dramatic and visionary experiences, Abrams began to wonder whether these otherworldly voyages might be translated into meaningful artworks and whether there might be such a thing as psychedelic art. The answer came at the end of 1964 after Rachel and Isaac's first experience with New Jersey LSD. For both him and Rachel, it was another ground-breaking experience, and Rachel believes that the superior quality was responsible for the positive outcome. Isaac, meanwhile, concluded that there *was* such a thing as psychedelic art and began painting.

While he was developing his own vision of psychedelic art, other artists were likewise drawn to the vision-inducing experience. Arlene Sklar-Weinstein was one of many to be impressed by those vivid aesthetics, and when she took LSD under the guidance of a psychologist, it was enough for her to radically revisit her art. As she recalled, "work prior to LSD, developed over a twenty-year span, was competent but largely derivative since there was no clear center of emanation."[14] Dave Roman similarly experimented with the drug in the mid-1960s and realized that studying in an art school had been a waste of time because of the stifling directions imposed on the students. Ever since, he had been able to find spontaneous inspiration, and for the first time in his life he genuinely enjoyed the act of drawing.[15]

These psychedelic artists were developing their skills just as closely related genres were gaining traction in the New York City art world. For instance, Brooklyn chemistry professor Gerald Oster had a meaningful experience with acid and began to paint as a direct result. He first heard about psychedelic drugs through Huxley's writings, and as a leading authority on the scientific appraisal of moiré patterns he was particularly intrigued by those visionary states. In December 1964, he presented his findings in front of a crowd of artists and psychologists at a staff seminar of NYU's Research Center for Mental Health, and he noted that the illusions of the moiré patterns curiously resembled the LSD experience.[16]

In February 1965, Museum of Modern Art curator William Seitz organized the first exhibition of optical art. Like psychedelic art, the colourful and undulating "op art" was profoundly experiential, and the hypnotic patterns on display had an unsettling quality that likely prepared the artistic avant-garde for the more explicitly mind-altering genre of the next few years. Op art had been covered in a favourable *Time* article a few months before the exhibition (which considered that moirés qualified as op art),[17] and while it stopped short of calling it psychedelic,

Seitz was nevertheless the first to draw the connection, "commenting that these optical effects 'are increased … under the influence of the drugs like mescaline and LSD.'"[18]

Psychedelic Art Is Coming

In this favourable context, psychedelic art was reaching a boiling point. That year, the Abrams rented out space at the Coda galleries on East 10th Street and started renovations to turn it into an art gallery. They were going to organize the first ever psychedelic art exhibition, and they advertised the event on the *Village Voice* bulletin board. The ad, which remained there for two months, ambitiously announced that "Psychedelic Art Is Coming."

The Abrams made these plans just as the Millbrook crowd was becoming more and more interested in exploring the artistic import of the LSD experience. By then, Isaac was aware of Leary's controversial research and decided to pay him a visit upstate. When he arrived there, Leary was sitting in a tree, thirty feet above the ground. Isaac shrugged and climbed up to tell him about his art gallery and that he was looking for artists to be part of an art exhibition. The High Priest liked it. "I think you have a really good idea," he told Abrams. "We would like to help you. A lot of people up here are artists, like Allen Atwell and some other people, but Allen in particular."

Abrams had tremendous respect for Atwell, an art teacher at Cornell University who had studied Eastern spirituality, had lived in the Far East, and believed that the psychedelic experience had profoundly changed his work and made it "more apocalyptic."[19] As early as 1964, he had painted "monstrous forms – daemonic, fantastic beings, clusters of eviscerated organs, and other horrors" over the walls and the ceiling to turn his Upper East Side apartment into a "psychedelic temple."[20] Subsequently, Atwell painted the outside walls of the Millbrook mansion as well as Van Wolf's apartment so that it looked like the inside of a human body during a psychedelic trip.[21] Atwell's art, then, was an early indication that the highly experiential genre would not remain confined to canvas and paper.

The fifth of June 1965 was quite possibly the most important event in the entire history of New York psychedelia. First and foremost, the occasion was a massive get-together for acid heads rather than an exhibition

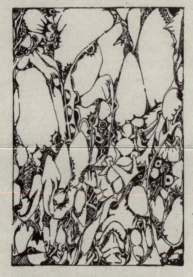

Figure 6.1 An invitation to the Abrams' psychedelic art exhibition

proudly announcing the birth of a new genre in a world capital of the arts. More than 2,000 reportedly attended, to a point where the police were forced to close off the streets at both ends to divert traffic. "Suddenly there were people doing face-paint, wearing top-hats, even some people with long hair appeared magically," recalls Isaac. That evening, and as the gallery remained open in the following months, many scrutinized the works of art under the influence.

The exhibition, which drew the attention of celebrities like Andy Warhol and Rauschenberg, also featured a panel discussion on the implications of the psychedelic experience. Most artists made it clear that LSD had the ability to open up the senses and new avenues of artistic awareness but that artistic work remained challenging.[22] For the psychedelic movement, on the other hand, it was another chance to extoll the benefits of the acid experience, and Rachel remembers that "the street was filled with people come to see the gurus." Among those who took part in the enterprise was Michael Hollingshead, who exhibited some of his paintings[23] and read his poetry, which Isaac found "epic and important and undecipherable." While he read on, two DEA agents turned up and showed them their credentials in order to get in without paying the fee they charged at the doors.

Leary was another to speak, and unbeknownst to him he met his future fourth wife, Rosemary Woodruff, on that occasion. At the time, he was still married to Nena von Schlebrugge, a Swedish top-model who frequently appeared in *Vogue, Mademoiselle,* and *Harper's Bazaar.* Much like Peggy Hitchcock, Woodruff was bored with the New York jet set, and she had found something far more exciting in LSD and Leary.[24] She had taken some acid earlier that day and arrived at the gallery in great spirits. As she listened to him talk about "audio-olfactory-visual alterations of consciousness," she felt an immediate connection. "He was didactic, oracular, self-aggrandizing, and very amusing. Afterward we walked to the corner for a drink."[25]

The exhibition, then, was a good measure of how quickly the non-medical use of LSD and psychedelics had created its own culture – it was almost irrelevant that the Abrams never sold any artworks throughout the entire six months of the exhibition. The psychedelic gallery paved the way for similar places in the second part of the decade, as Rachel recalls: "When we started the Coda gallery there was – I remember –

I think his name was Jeff [Glick], and he started the first head shop ... He wasn't far from the gallery."

The gallery soon attracted other figures of the artistic avant-garde like Ronnie Tavel and John Vaccaro, who were both known for their experimental theatre called the Playhouse of the Ridiculous. Both of them had drawn a great deal of inspiration from Jack Smith's flicks (Vaccaro had played in his controversial *Flaming Creatures*), and Tavel had occasionally acted in and directed some of Warhol's movies.[26] He was also acquainted with LSD, and during a conversation with Isaac, the latter told him that he was ridiculous. "I love that!" was Tavel's answer. Soon thereafter, he and Vaccaro founded the playhouse,[27] and Tavel's *Shower* was performed at the Abrams' gallery.[28]

Meanwhile, Isaac was enjoying a spectacular rise as a psychedelic artist. His first canvas, *Hello Dalí*, was a tribute to the Spanish painter. After finishing his painting, which is five feet wide and seven feet high, he put it in a van and took it to the St Regis Hotel, where Salvador Dalí was staying at the time. Upon seeing his work, Dalí immediately applauded. But by the time Abrams had gotten over this incredible endorsement, Dalí had gone back to Spain, and the aspiring painter realized he would have to continue to self-teach,[29] even though he briefly studied with the visionary artist Ernst Fuchs in Vienna and then underwent psychoanalysis to better integrate his experiences.[30]

Six months later, Isaac painted his landmark *All Things Are One Thing*, a highly organic piece that subsequently became the cover for the edited collection by Masters and Houston. It underscored the importance of the connection with nature because for him the psychedelic experience "was the real reawakening of our contact with the natural world." He then painted *Flying Leap* in 1966, for which he used dots in a way similar to Australian aboriginal art. But as he contends, those Australian artists were not yet known in the Western world, and for him the most obvious explanation is that he must have encountered aboriginal Australians during a DMT experience and learned about dot painting then.[31]

In spite of their explicit connection with psychedelic drugs, the aesthetic qualities of both paintings greatly appealed to highly influential New Yorkers. *All Things Are One Thing* was purchased by Reed Erickson, who by then had become a man as a result of a sex change. Erickson was a tremendously wealthy person who had founded the Erickson Educational Foundation in 1964 to support the study of transgender issues as well as Masters and Houston's research.[32] *Flying Leap*, meanwhile, was bought by economist Stanley Scheinbaum, famous for organizing the defence of whistleblower Daniel Ellsberg and for founding People for the American Way.

As Abrams was reaping the success of his art, others were likewise drawing inspiration from LSD. A thirty-three-year-old painter, who had taken the drug some thirty or forty times, claimed in 1966 that "almost all the people I know who are in any way connected with art or writing have tried it,"[33] and a year later, Stanley Krippner conducted the first major study on psychedelic artists. Most of them came from the New York area, though some came from other parts of the US and from Europe, and a sizeable majority claimed that the psychedelic experience had led them to revisit their work in some way or another.[34]

Meanwhile, the Abrams' Brooklyn apartment had become a rallying point to trip surrounded by Isaac's art, and Nina Graboi, who had since become friends with them, had one of her most memorable psychedelic experiences there. In 1966, Isaac had painted the two pillars flanking the main entrance of the Center for the League for Spiritual Discovery, and one of his paintings had also found a way into her Third Force office.[35] Abrams's psychedelic art greatly appealed to her because it had the ability to recall part of the psychedelic states of awareness and it "reflected dimensions accessible only to the turned-on eye." In the Abrams' apartment, her trip was a strong aesthetic experience in which she saw herself and her companions fathoming the heavens on a spaceship. From above she saw the earth "full of Adams and Eves who gradually evolve and master technology throughout the ages. They went through a scene of war that soon made way for the prosperity and consumerist frenzy of the previous decade. Then, they moved back into the Sixties with its music, love and innocence."[36]

While Abrams continued his ground-breaking painting, Leary and his associates went on to create what was perhaps the most ambitious attempt to translate the psychedelic experience into a form of multimedia theatre dramatizing the life and times of mystics and religious figures. In doing so, they allowed psychedelic art to reach new heights of visibility, leading the world of film to take notice.

Psychedelic Celebrations

A noteworthy but understandable aspect of Leary's involvement with theatre and light shows[37] is that their content changed markedly after his sentencing. In 1965, the psychedelic movement's shows were certainly eclectic, but they lacked a salient religious message that became far more explicit the next year when the High Priest decided that the best way to gather popular support was to present LSD as a sacrament.

In April, a group of Millbrook residents organized an Experiential Theater Evening at the Village Vanguard. The event boasted an impressive cast: Metzner, Alpert, Hollingshead, Watts, jazz figures like Steve Swallow, Peter Larocca, and Charles Mingus, but not Leary, who was in India at the time.[38] The purpose of the event was to replicate the sensory bombardment of the psychedelic experience without drugs, but the reception was lukewarm. As one reporter wrote, "A hundred would-be experiencers were turned away, business at the bar was slow, and the audience was rapt and curiously split."[39]

That same year, Leary collaborated with Gerd Stern and USCO, a group of multimedia artists with interdisciplinary backgrounds who were strongly influenced by Marshall McLuhan. In order to create total environments through audio and visual techniques, they developed a sensory overload model. As Stern described it, "when you walk down the street you take in, say, 50-million inputs – sights, smells and so forth. You process and cope with them on many levels. Here, we create an overload situation where you can't bring in all of your critical baggage. [It] allows the information to get straight through as emotional input."[40] The purpose of that experience "was to break through that linear time and space dimension so that you could go someplace else."[41]

USCO created a total environment at the Riverside Museum, where spectators enjoyed their multimedia light shows with audio collages and incense smells. In the first of the three rooms, they created a "light garden" in which spectators could "activate flowers made of lights by walking on floor switches." In the second room ("the cave"), they "lay down on a rotating couch, and contemplated the pictures of demons, gods, and humans painted on the ceiling and the walls around them." The third room, dubbed "Creation," was a meditation space full of spiritual imagery. "In it were five nine-foot high paintings representing the planets in their orbits, the seven spheres, the Tree of Life, a male figure of Shiva, Hindu god of energy. His outflowing energy was symbolized by a central, pulsating light from which painted lines radiated."[42] They called the performance a "be-in"[43] because rather than simply looking at the show passively, the audience was supposed "to exist in the show" and fully experience the disorientation and – potential – transcendence through external stimuli.[44]

With Stern and USCO, Leary created a series of happenings intended "to carry the message of consciousness expansion to larger audiences and to bring much-needed financial income to the ever-changing Millbrook community."[45] They ran shows once a week at the New Theater in midtown for about eight weeks and gave the proceeds to support Leary's psychedelic movement. To help create the perfect atmosphere, the Abrams moved all the paintings from the psychedelic gallery to the theatre.[46] During the event, Leary gave lectures on the "theoretical background necessary for an understanding of the new techniques of audio-olfactory-visual alteration of consciousness."[47]

Isaac remembers how the place was absolutely packed with psychedelic fans and further illustrates the momentum his own exhibition had generated. At one point, Leary asked, "'Well how many people here have had the psychedelic experience? Gotten high?' Suddenly, everybody raised their hand [laughs]."[48] Much to the dismay of Stern and his colleagues, however, "Timothy was kind of a dry, boring lecturer in those days … it was the middle of this really turned-on show, and here was this professor standing up in the front going on and on." Fortunately, Beat poet Michael McLure had given USCO tapes of people screaming to interrupt Leary and create confusion.[49] Others in the audience were unimpressed. Though she managed to get an invitation, psychedelic activist Lisa Bieberman did not fail to notice the staggering $40 cover charge (more than $300 as of 2020) for one of the shows.[50] For USCO, the show nevertheless enabled them to meet other psychedelic artists like Isaac Abrams, Rudi Stern, Jackie Cassen, and Richard Aldcroft.[51]

After 1965, Leary became much more intent on presenting the LSD experience along spiritual lines. It is unclear how this idea originated, however. Back in September 1961 and immediately after Wasson's dismissal, Leary had wondered about the best way to promote the drug over drinks at the Friedmans. Eventually, he had decided that a religious organization was the way forward and that it would help to frame the psychedelic experience under a legitimate light: "It's hard to attack a religion. Consider the Native American Church. It uses peyote. Active ingredient: mescaline. About 200,000 members. Nobody bothers them and they don't bother anyone else."[52] This might have been an overstatement, but in any event, it was a clear indication that Leary was open to strategically presenting psychedelics as adjuncts for spiritual practices.

Five years later, Isaac Abrams visited Leary at Millbrook, and it seemed that he had forgotten his idea:

> I know that he was talking to his lawyer from Texas and I was visiting at Millbrook and I came along and Tim said: "Isaac, come on in and sit down!" And they were talking about this court concerning smuggling marijuana, for which he went to jail. And I said "well maybe, American Indians take peyote as a sacrament. Maybe this is a similar thing." And this lawyer said "that's a hell of an idea, Tim!" And the next thing you know, they were calling it a sacrament. And all I did was say the obvious. I thought it was quite obvious.[53]

Soon after, Leary created the league to underscore this connection, and to fund it he ran a series of psychedelic plays in the East Village to make a similar case while highlighting the talents of multimedia artists.

The light shows of Leary's Psychedelic Celebrations were masterminded by Jackie Cassen and her partner Rudi Stern. Cassen was an early light artist who had pioneered the use of slides and had exhibited some of her work at the Abrams' gallery. Stern was an admirer of Thomas Wilfried and a painter by trade who had studied in Europe. In 1964, he went to the Bridge Theater on St Mark's Place, and there he saw awe-inspiring "projections of circles, handmade circles, from two slide projectors with somebody's fingers alternating between the lenses. You changed the slides with your palm, and you covered the lens and you created an animated rhythm." That same evening, he met Cassen, who became his close collaborator for several years. Back at Stern's place, they took some acid and spent most of the night looking at a candle on the other side of a bombsight lens, which turned the room into an M.C. Escher painting.

Stern and Cassen were already showcasing their talents at the Polish National Home on St Mark's Place[54] when they were invited to do a light show based on Herman Hesse's *Steppenwolf* at Millbrook during the summer of 1966.[55] Among the attendees was an ambitious young producer and an acquaintance of Billy Hitchcock, David Balding, who approached Leary to organize a series of plays in the city. Nina Graboi made use of her apartment as a base camp for the cast and crew, which featured Leary, his new wife Rosemary, and Metzner. From Stern's perspective, this multimedia art was a way of returning to a very basic form of theatre: "[Antonin] Artaud first envisioned a theater taking the form of mythic structure – light, sound, and shadow replacing narrative, pantomime replacing acting."[56]

The first show was called *The Death of the Mind*, and it was meant to dramatize Hesse's novel. It opened on 20 September 1966 at the Village Theater, in the same building that now housed the *East Village Other*. Scores of New Yorkers flocked to see the play, and "the crowds … stopped traffic on Second Avenue." The show was a sell-out for six weeks.[57] Among the 2,400 attendees were prominent intellectuals, artists, and celebrities like the great conductor Leonard Bernstein, *Partisan Review* editor Lionel Trilling and his wife and literary critic Diana, and Academy Award–wining choreographer and dancer Jerome Robbins.[58]

According to Rudi Stern, most of the people who attended were under the influence of psychedelics. Upon entering the theatre, they could listen to Peter Walker (a key figure in the Greenwich Village folk revival) playing ragas on his guitar to help create a meditative atmosphere. For the actual show, they had set up complex light-show equipment with three screens. One sequence used red paintings and was designed to simulate "a trip in the bloodstream of Harry Heller and … to visit the Magic Theater of Steppenwolf." Throughout the show, Stern gave his orders to assistants through a walkie-talkie that the whole theatre heard very clearly, blurring the boundaries separating the audience from the crew in the process.[59]

Even though the Celebrations were part of the larger tradition of New York's artistic avant-garde, it explicitly extended into the realm of spirituality. *Death of the Mind* began with Leary reciting a prayer,[60] and Graboi remembered that "The aroma of incense filled the theater, bells tingled, beads shone."[61] Several attendees wore buttons that read "Psychedelize Suburbia," and one reporter noted that these buttons, along with paperweights, peacock feathers, and diffraction disks, were all considered to have in common the shape of a mandala.[62] As Krippner sums it up, "It took on the trappings of a church service."[63]

148 | PSYCHEDELIC NEW YORK

The success of the first celebration prompted Leary to organize a second show on 23 October, *The Reincarnation of Jesus Christ*. Cassen and Stern shot a misty reversed-negative film of a man walking in Harlem and superimposed slides narrating the life of Christ and the history of the Roman Catholic Church, with its saints, virgins, and martyrs. To accompany the play was a samba version of *Missa solemnis*.[64]

Although *Reincarnation* carried explicitly religious themes, it also illustrates Leary's iconoclastic suspicion of monotheistic religions. During the play, the audience could see Jesus climb on a cross behind a screen. Leary then walked to him on stage and cautioned him against his suicidal tendencies and the impact it might have on Western culture: "Hey, Jesus, if you go through with this you'll leave a 2,000-year-old tradition of pain and guilt. Centuries of Christian soldiers marching with bloody swords to avenge you." Instead, he suggested that Jesus accompany him for some beers and "sassy girls" and that they "start a religion that laughs and sings to the love of life." He then went behind the screen and appeared to pull out the nails from the cross.[65]

This irreverent approach to the central myth of Christianity did not sit well with Michael Itkin, however, who had joined the league and closely followed Leary's psychedelic journey. Itkin himself had incorporated the Psychedelic Peace Fellowship as a church, and the fellowship had just held its first meeting in an East Village restaurant.[66] He had collaborated with the Millbrook crew for *Reincarnation*, but in a subsequent open letter to Leary he told him that he was officially disaffiliating from the league because Leary had failed to portray the mystical transformation Jesus underwent to become a holy man. For Itkin, this inward metamorphosis was "a revolutionary Gospel of love which requires a life of active service to the poor, the hungry, the downtrodden, the oppressed, the imprisoned, the sick, the homeless, the beggar." By omitting this aspect of Christianity and its social import from his show, Leary had turned it "into a mockery of Christianity."[67]

Unitarian preacher Walter Kring was another clergyman to see *Reincarnation* and to find it offensive. While he admitted that "the evening was an aesthetic experience, and I think a good one," it was hard for him to see Leary as anything but a charlatan offering a good show. Leary's religion lacked the discipline of the Native American Church members and ran the risk of fostering withdrawal from the real world. Though Kring agreed that under the right circumstances psychedelics had a genuine religious import, he strongly suspected that Leary's attempt to clothe the acid experience in religious meaning was a calculated ploy to find support for his upcoming marijuana trial.[68]

The way Leary liked to wind down after his performances would lend credence to Kring's suspicions. He routinely removed his white garments and donned a suit and tie to hang out with the Madison Avenue crowd at the Playboy Club at 59th Street and 5th Avenue. There, the waitresses dressed as bunnies frequently complained about a middle-aged drunk pinching their backsides.[69]

From Light Shows to Film

Itkin and Kring's disavowals did not stop Leary from carrying on with the Celebrations. *The Illumination of the Buddha*[70] was produced by Metzner, who had been studying the Buddha's life story. On that occasion, he worked with a group of filmmakers called The Third World, which included Bob Lowe, a Columbia academic from the film department. Together, they projected hundreds of slides on a screen using a dissolving unit that enabled the images to merge and create a strong psychedelic effect with "much more mythic and archetypal content – rather than just abstract color patterns." The show was such a success that the group toured the country, with performances in Chicago, San Francisco, and Santa Monica.[71]

Third World artist Gray Henry was part of the crew that worked on *Illumination*. After the show, she became actively involved in producing film at their Lower East Side studio. They organized a light show for a Janis Joplin gig, and soon after a film company offered to finance a production of their choice. The movie, which was shot at Millbrook and involved Leary and Charles Mingus, was a psychedelic standoff opposing Indians, whose clothing and tepees were covered in DayGlo paint, and cowboys, who represented the younger generations and their parents, respectively.[72]

Leary's involvement in film took on an unexpected turn around that time. In 1967, a Hollywood producer approached him to adapt *Death of the Mind*, but the prospect of money immediately created a rift between him and Cassen and Stern. According to them, Leary had negotiated the contract behind their backs, and as a result the producer had made them feel as though they were mere technicians when they had actually designed the first Celebration. Leary, on the other hand, believed that Stern and Cassen simply "wanted big money, a contract, and control over the movie," and he pointed out that no league member could "accept profit from LSD activities, films, or lectures." Given that Cassen and Stern threatened to sue the producer and Leary for $1 million, it is unsurprising that the movie did not materialize.[73]

Leary had other entries into the world of cinema. Around the same time, he connected with filmmaker Otto Preminger, who had attended the Celebrations. Preminger was looking for information on acid for his film *Skidoo* (with Groucho Marx's final appearance on screen), and Leary organized an LSD session in Preminger's luxurious apartment in Manhattan. Even for a veteran of hundreds of trips, it was a fascinating aesthetic experience, as he entered "Otto's plastic-fantastic white-and-chrome, futuristic projection room, which bristled with dials, lights, levers, and other control-panel paraphernalia."

After the acid kicked in, Preminger became hyperactive and decided to turn on the television, changing channels but also the colours and focus. At first, Leary saw this as counterproductive because it favoured escapism rather than introspection or profound interaction with the environment. He looked for some Ravi Shankar records to try and channel the trip into something more manageable, but he could only find film scores in Preminger's collection. Preminger switched on two other television sets, and Leary wondered how he could stare "with gleeful satisfaction at a screen flickering with random patterns and dots," until he had an epiphany: as a director, Preminger "took on the godly task of inventing a reality – he selected plot, location, actors. He then externalized his vision on film and marketed it so that millions of human beings could inhabit his creation." Following this session, he concluded that advanced information and communication technology had the power of extending the brain and could ultimately lead humanity to the next stage of evolution.[74]

Preminger's *Skidoo* was not the only movie to be affected by the psychedelic movement, according to Leary. The former Harvard professor was a consultant for Hy Averback's *I Love You, Alice B. Toklas*, which features Peter Sellers and was written by friends of his. He also claimed that Stanley Kubrick's *2001* was inspired by their Psychedelic Celebrations and that the Broadway musical hit *Hair*, which focuses on a group of

Bohemian activists in the city and depicts drug use, was supposed to be partly based on their communal experience at Millbrook – many of the actors were acquaintances.[75]

Others, like Krippner, came to appreciate how psychedelics could influence the appreciation of film. On one occasion, he took LSD in Brooklyn with some friends and then proceeded to paint a Volkswagen bus. After that, he took them to the pictures to see *Freaks*, which featured characters with pointed heads. Some of those who attended began to feel their heads stretch out and point, just as in the film. Krippner, though, is quick to point out that it was an "artistic experience" rather than some amusing activity to do while high.[76]

Soon psychedelics were reaching artists using a major technological innovation: the portable camera. Before this mini-revolution, cameras had remained in studios, but by the late 1960s, artists, scientists, and political activists alike were experimenting with it. Some of those artists were so influenced by LSD that they believed that "drugs were an essential model for what video could be as a technology of consciousness."[77] Among them was Eric Siegel, who was then working on visual feedback and who found a way of creating kaleidoscopic effects by pointing a camera at its monitor. In May and June 1969, Siegel's work was exhibited at the Howard Wise gallery and made a great impression on Nam June Paik. Paik began working on video synthesis, which he saw as an eminently psychedelic process. For him, drugs allowed a unique participatory experience that enabled users to be simultaneously artists, art consumers, and critics.[78]

This approach was reminiscent of some of USCO's total environments, and it is no surprise that the collective collaborated with filmmaker Jud Yalkut, who produced disorienting films in an attempt to "find another way to hit people, to dislocate them, and then re-center them at the end – very much a trip analogy."[79] Masters and Houston described his art as "a torrent of hurtling colors and lights, forms blinking, whirling, and surging. Image follows image in rapid-fire succession, distorting awareness of time and space as the sensory bombardment continues."[80] For Gerd Stern, a testimony of Yalkut's use of psychedelics is apparent in his heavy use of the in and out zoom.[81]

This could be seen in Yalkut's collaborations with Yayoi Kusama, a Japanese polka-dot artist who had been suffering from hallucinations since she was a child.[82] In March 1968, Kusama presented her "Self Obliteration"[83] at the Cooper Square Arts Theater in front of a crowded audience. To accompany the happening, a band of late-teenagers called "The Dayz Beyond" played psychedelic rock. Kusama entered from behind the stage, "dressed in red leotards with white dots sporadically covering her outfit and wears a long-furred black coat." She was soon followed by three semi-nude men who wore US flags around their waists. As she began to paint dots on their skin, more naked or near-naked participants joined in. Then a fake policeman arrived on stage, swinging his club and shouting that everyone was under arrest. He was wrestled down to the floor and stripped. Kusama then produced a print of the *Mona Lisa* and began painting dots on it, while a film partly made and edited by Yalkut appeared on a screen just above the band. The whole event was intensified by flashing strobes.[84]

Cerebrum

By the end of the Sixties, multimedia art was conquering new audiences. It had already found its way into rock concerts and psychedelic night-clubs like the Electric Circus, but the venue that best embodied these ground-breaking total environments was Cerebrum, which hardly qualified as a discotheque or a traditional entertainment venue. Cerebrum, which had no nightclub, dance hall, or liquor licence and did not allow smoking, challenged the conventional patterns of entertainment by offering a deeply experiential setting designed to stimulate all the senses. All this was achieved by expanding the output of the multimedia light shows and by offering a new vision of night life that blurred the boundaries between adulthood and childhood and between socializing and play.

Cerebrum was located on Broome Street close to Broadway, and its architecture was masterminded by John Storyk, who designed Jimi Hendrix's Electric Lady Studio. It was founded by Ruffin Cooper and some friends in 1968. Cooper was the gay son of a Texas banker who lent him the money for the venture, and he believed that conventional entertainment was dull and longed to offer "freedom – to do anything you want or play at being anyone you want."[85] Larry Vigus, who guided patrons through the experience, remembers how Cooper first came up with the idea of the venue. Cooper had been a theatre student with interests in performance arts. He and some friends enjoyed smoking grass and playing games under the influence. They would play with light, sounds, fabrics, balloons, feathers, or plastic. They thought this should be shared and decided to create "a place where people could go and be among other people who were stoned."[86]

Upon entering the venue, patrons were invited to pull on a translucent toga and remove their clothes from underneath. Then they arrived in a large room with a floor of more than a dozen white carpeted platforms and with flashing lights bouncing off mirrored globes and pictures of eyes, the Buddha, and a waterfall projected on the walls and ceiling, among many other commonly used images. The participants were given items such as stereo headphones, glowing orbs and prisms, light boxes, and plastic pillows, and they were invited to take part in games, like building a tower with blocks of glass, playing with a big weather balloon and a giant parachute, or just pretending to be an angel.[87]

In this way, Cerebrum was not a place for socializing but for art and for highly experiential activities meant to echo the psychedelic experience and its ability to undermine boundaries. The idea was to "disorient, obliterate the body-to-ground relationship, and open the door to sensation,"[88] with or without the help of psychedelic drugs. Art critic Gene Youngblood, who took part in the Cerebrum experience, felt that "one is voyeur, exhibitionist, and participant. One is both male and female."[89] Vigus also contends that because everyone wore white togas, "the uniformity removed the costumes of 'class' and status."[90]

Yet for all its innovations, Cerebrum was a short-lived venture that lasted only nine months. One reporter criticized the club because the translucent togas favoured voyeurism, whereas organizers and staff (such as Vigus) claimed that they increased freedom and communal bonding. "Several men said they couldn't stop looking at the just-perceptible nude bodies all around them. They were turned on by the looking and not by the joining-in possibilities Cerebrum offers."[91]

That did not stop patrons from turning up under the influence of LSD, while the eighteen revolving people on staff were equally fond of drug use. Vigus, however, makes it clear that the staff discriminated between lay and spiritual drug use. "Grass and hash were used daily but LSD and psilocybin was saved for special occasions and often treated in sacramental fashion rather than as a PARTY DRUG or just to highlight routine activities."[92] He also points out that his group discriminated between "good" and "bad" drugs, at least during their time at Cerebrum. "In general, we looked down on speed. We also looked down on people who used downers like heroin … A lot of us (most of us) didn't use beer or hard liquor at all." Yet Vigus occasionally snorted cocaine and smoked opium.[93]

A psychedelic drug like LSD could trigger profound visions of swirling patterns, iridescent light, and otherworldly encounters and cause profound alteration of the ordinary waking states of consciousness. This not only led to the production of a new type of visionary art but to new aesthetic sensibilities resulting from acid use rather than just the exposure to psychedelic culture. Psychedelics were instrumental in the popularization of this new form of art that extended beyond painting: psychedelia permeated theatre and cinema and spurred the development of sophisticated multimedia and interactive installations.

Psychedelic art was a major component of the broader psychedelic culture and a fitting illustration of its complexity. It created a new way of making, understanding, and revisiting art, as well as new forms of socializing centred on transcendental experiences that could be simultaneously entertaining and aesthetic. It found itself at the crossroads of technological innovations, a desire to probe the mind in a near-scientific way, and an expression of a new form of spirituality, usually removed from dogmatic imperatives.

Among the many artists who had their careers influenced by LSD and psychedelics, Isaac Abrams certainly stands out for his endurance, but in the larger history of psychedelic New York, the first psychedelic art exhibition was arguably his and Rachel's greatest contribution. One reason that both Isaac and psychedelic art have remained on the periphery of art history is that they were obscured by pop art and Andy Warhol. "I couldn't possibly compete with the whole pop art movement of the cultural establishment," laments Abrams, "which was much more comfortable with the pop art movement. Because essentially it enthroned American commercialism and my vision was somewhat different than that."[94] While it might be unsurprising that an art that had explicit connections with mind-altering drugs enjoyed a more limited success, psychedelic art showed important staying power, as evidenced by all the artists who followed in Abrams's footsteps.

7
Changing Scenes
Prohibition and the Demise of Psychedelic Idealism

As the Sixties were coming to a close, New York psychedelia included a vibrant art scene and even a handful of scientific investigations into LSD. However, reports of adverse reactions to psychedelics were fast becoming a source of concern for medical authorities. At Bellevue Hospital, psychiatrist William Frosch noticed a sharp increase in psychotic episodes resulting from acid use. Extreme forms of panic were particularly commonplace among dropouts in their late teens and early twenties, like a young man who was admitted after hearing "God's voice" and almost stabbing a friend in the back.[1] Soon Brooklyn District Attorney Aaron Koota became the most vocal opponent of non-medical LSD use and launched a campaign to raise awareness about the dangers of psychedelic experimentation among the young.

The equation of youth and drugs received an untimely boost from Timothy Leary, who was now aggressively courting the baby-boomers. During a Town Hall lecture on 5 April 966, a couple of weeks before Koota's campaign, Leary was adamant "that the present generation, under the age of 25, is the most sophisticated, intelligent, wise, the holiest generation in our history." Unfortunately, the young were being persecuted by the "middle-age, middle-class, middle-brow, whiskey-drinking persons who pass our law."[2] Pitting the young against their elders in such an explicit way, however, played into the hands of the prohibitionists and gave LSD more publicity than it needed.

Runaway children[3] who were drawn to the excitement of living in East Village crash pads exacerbated the feeling that the young were out of control and drew the ire of the local working class. While the *East Village Other* carried on its psychedelic mission, its neighbourhood was overwhelmed by indiscriminate drug use, and soon the paper's offices "served as an information clearinghouse to assist runaways with shelter, food, transportation, or a telephone call home."[4] But the locals, who had very few prospects of leaving this rundown area, were furious to see the carefree youth flock to the Village, and they were dismayed by all the panhandling, the illicit drugs, and the increase in rents that came along with them.

In fact, real estate investors and landlords briefly tried to cash in on the Village's trendy aura, hoping to ultimately attract "a broader and more equivocal category of upscale middle-class residents."[5] While some activists at least tried to help the Villagers by organizing street patrols and by provocatively transferring part of the local garbage excess to the recently opened Lincoln Center,[6] it soon transpired that the quarter was not the countercultural bastion some thought it would become.

Notions of psychedelic exceptionalism were soon lost in a terrifying surge of narcotics. At the turn of the Sixties, New York was still surprisingly prosperous compared to other US cities,[7] but it had "more addicts, more crime, and more disorder than any other major American city," even if this was merely an acute symptom of nationwide urban decay.[8] The broader political climate further exacerbated the feeling of impeding downfall. As the anti-war and civil rights movements were splintering as a result of internal radicalism, New York City went through significant strikes coming from teachers, the police, firefighters, and the sanitation sector, followed by the Stonewall Riots of 1969. "1968 and 1969 were the two angriest years I ever lived in America," filmmaker David Hoffman sums up. "People yelling all over the place, screaming on the streets, screaming at each other."[9]

In this charged atmosphere, many weary acid heads moved away from drugs, thanks to Indian teachers promising to heal the ontological wounds resulting from consciousness-exploration. By turning to alternative religions, former users joined the tired political activists who had grown disillusioned with protest and saw spirituality as a panacea.[10]

Hence, these new gurus managed to reconcile the overarching tension between New Left politics and the psychedelic counterculture.

But all the changes that occurred in the East Village were not enough to effectively end New York psychedelia, which continued to receive favourable coverage in the above-ground media. Just before the Koota campaign, *Life* published a balanced assessment of LSD that discussed the new problems associated with non-medical use while suggesting that prohibition would have disastrous consequences. It was only after Henry Luce's death in February 1967 that *Time* and *Life* lost interest in the topic.[11] A year later, the Hearst corporation formally relinquished its anti-drug agenda by launching *Eye*, a hip magazine featuring sympathetic articles on the acid culture, which lasted until 1969.[12] And in midtown, the New York jet set continued to indulge in LSD and other drugs, oblivious to the plight of working-class locals and Long Island runaways, while the rhetoric and imagery of psychedelia made inroads into the area's business, advertising, and entertainment sectors.

The Backlash against LSD

Soon after the Drug Abuse Amendments of 1965, Aaron Koota began his high-profile campaign against LSD. Koota was born in Brooklyn to Russian immigrants in 1906, and in 1950 he joined the rackets bureau of the Kings County District Attorney's office, which was then working on a gambling case that led to a massive purge of the local Police Department. In 1964, he was elected district attorney of Brooklyn,[13] and in April 1966 he told the media that acid was endemic in the country's high schools and proposed to make the distribution of the drug a felony punishable by a seven- to twenty-year jail sentence.[14] A few days later, he claimed that high school and college students were manufacturing LSD in the chemistry classrooms, and he set up a special phone line for the narcotics squad to receive information about the drug.

Crucially, though, Koota "refused to divulge how many schools, how many youngsters or which schools were involved."[15] Several officials highlighted this lack of evidence, and the director of health education for the Board of Education contended that "so far not a single case of the use of LSD by students has been reported to [his] office."[16] Over in the Bronx, the James Monroe High School principal wrote Koota a strong letter demanding apologies for tarnishing the reputation of several schools.[17]

Koota also suggested that the underworld had moved in to take control of the acid trade and claimed that "The profits from the sale of (LSD) are obviously tremendous,"[18] when a drug like LSD, which rarely sold for more than $2 a hit at the time,[19] presented a weaker value-for-money than physically addictive drugs. "This business about making LSD in school laboratories is preposterous," charged a Columbia student. "I know the formula and I've had enough chemistry courses to follow it; but I couldn't make LSD if I spent a year in a lab."[20] At the FDA's offices in Brooklyn, the acting director of the New York field station of the Bureau of Drug Abuse Control admitted that they got "more actual LSD cases that were developed in New York than in any other section of the country" but they had no hard evidence of connections with the Mafia.[21]

It is hard to see Koota as anything other than a "headline-hunter," as the *New York Times Magazine* subsequently portrayed him. A year later, he claimed that he had formulated his accusations based on letters from parents forwarded by the Board of Education. But although the board dismissed these claims as unfounded, Koota "did not withdraw his accusations, explaining that he used LSD as a 'generic' term for all kinds of hallucinatory drugs, some of which can be manufactured – or at least distributed – in the schools." He justified this equation by arguing that he had a moral duty to warn parents about the drug peril.[22] Regardless, two separate bills to make the distribution of psychedelics a felony were introduced in April 1966 by Anthony Travia, Democrat of Brooklyn, and Norman Lent, Republican of Nassau.[23]

A few days earlier, New York had been rocked by a gruesome killing attributed to LSD, and in retrospect it mattered little that suspect Stephen Kessler was subsequently acquitted on the grounds of mental insanity and that the drug he had ingested before the murder was not acid.[24] This was enough to equate the distribution of LSD with the peddling of addictive narcotics. On 28 April, the State Senate in Albany officially banned the sale, possession, and use of psychedelic drugs.[25]

With policy-makers successfully implementing tighter measures, law enforcement agents could now challenge acid users in a much more aggressive way. On 15 July 1966, Nelson Barr was arrested for selling LSD to an undercover FDA agent and received a one-year prison sentence and a $500 fine. While his lawyer prepared an appeal, Barr was sent to Rikers' Island prison and was immediately placed in isolation. The reason, he believed, was that the inmates and the prison guards were so curious to hear about the effects of LSD.[26]

Howard Lotsof was another to be convicted under the new law. Back in 1963, two FDA agents had raided his Brooklyn laboratory through which he had been ordering large quantities of mescaline, but Lotsof had calmly told them that he was testing the drug on rats. The new legislation, however, changed everything. When one former user was arrested for possession, he gave away Lotsof. The judge dismissed his claims that he was successfully treating addiction with ibogaine and sentenced him to fourteen months in prison after finding him guilty on four misdemeanour charges.[27]

Predictably, the change in legislation was a blessing for drug dealers. Before the new law, investigations on New York campuses suggested that drugs were far from prevalent and the few colleges that reported occurrences indicated that students tended to experiment with grass, speed, and barbiturates rather than LSD.[28] But months later, New Yorkers discovered that psychedelics were now being manufactured in clandestine labs. In the process, these new networks began selling acid like any other psychoactive commodity and watered down the drug's aura of wonder chemical.

In September 1966, one magazine reported on a Harvard dropout who had moved to New York to work as a chemist for organized crime, manufacturing between 50,000 and 100,000 LSD doses a year, while his employers sold other drugs like hashish, cannabis, cocaine, and heroin.[29] The following year, the BDAC stated that its New York regional office had seized 111,631 doses of LSD, nearly 4,000 doses of DMT, and 44,000 doses of MDA for a combined street value of more than $800,000 (more than $6.5 million in 2021).[30] The MDA was seized in a Chambers Street laboratory that had the capacity to produce some 15,000 doses of the drug as well as 50,000 doses of LSD.[31]

Bathtub acid was becoming a reality, and there is good reason to believe that the chemists were highly skilled and in possession of state-of-the-art equipment rather than undergraduates sneaking into university labs. An expert toxicologist from Suffolk County contended that "It requires time, skill and special chemicals. A graduate student,

160 | PSYCHEDELIC NEW YORK

who may be alone in a lab at night, could make LSD, especially if he had access to lysergic acid, but I do not believe an undergraduate could, and certainly not a high school student."[32]

Soon there were even clearer signs that the Mafia was taking control of the acid trade. Over in Washington, DC, the chief of Drug Abuse Control for the FDA claimed that the Cosa Nostra had become interested in LSD.[33] This was backed by a New York chemist who once told Leary that he was looking to start his own lab because he did not want to enrich the mob figures operating an acid business in Queens.[34] One dealer claimed to sell the drug to clients aged between eighteen and twenty-five years of age who usually came "from rich bourgeois families." Mostly, he dealt thousands of doses, and the transactions involved sums of money between $300 and $1,500, whereas a $200 deal was considered important during the previous year. When asked if the underworld had effectively taken over the LSD trade, he answered that one of his business partners was allegedly "assaulted by supposed Mafia people and his personal property was destroyed. Supposedly it was for underselling."[35]

With organized crime now involved in the acid trade, addictive narcotics posed a greater challenge to psychedelics. In 1969, an eighteen-year-old LSD user begged Leary for help because he was trapped somewhere between the awe of the psychedelic experience and the enslavement of heroin, speed, and barbiturates: "When I trip I reach illumination … but when I return to my ego, I find myself taking the same narcotics."[36] EVO journalist David Walley once met a struggling Black teenager who forced him to give him five dollars with a piece of broken glass, but in spite of this mishap, Walley sat down to learn about his life and his drug habits. The young lad had first tried LSD sometime in 1966 when he was merely twelve years of age, and during a subsequent trip he saw the faces of two people he had allegedly killed infested with snakes. He was now living on the streets and shooting up smack.[37]

Whereas a drug like LSD heightens awareness, heroin does the opposite by numbing the senses, and it is understandable that a teenager coming from a harsh socio-economic background should find more comfort in opiates than in acid. By contrast, it is more likely that a better-educated journalist would be more interested in using the vision-inducing LSD and in building on the experience for his own betterment. As activist David McReynolds summed up, "People in Harlem did not want their consciousness expanded. They wanted it closed down. They didn't want to see more things, they wanted to go to sleep, to pass out, and heroin could do that and LSD could not."[38]

Black New Yorkers had such a long history of drug problems that there was little chance they would be impressed by claims of chemical enlightenment. 1967 might have been the year the Beatles released their seminal "Sgt. Pepper's Lonely Hearts Club Band," a mind-blowing album with explicit references to the psychedelic world, but it was also the year the less-known soul singer and songwriter Rex Garvin released "Believe It or Not," which openly cautioned about the perils of LSD. Garvin had grown up in Harlem in the previous decades, a few blocks away from the Apollo Theater on 125th Street, and by the time he was sixteen, he was already touring with famous Black musicians. There he saw his older peers drink heavily and smoke pot, which he took on moderately much later in his life. But when acid became commonplace, he found it downright frightening. "LSD was popular in the white community," remembers Garvin. "You see, a lot of people when you're on tour want you to try things. I was scared to try it. I remember a guy who told me he tried that shit and woke up in a gigantic vagina. I didn't want to feel that shit."[39]

For light-show designer Joshua White, it was cocaine that spelt the end of psychedelic innocence. After the 1969 Woodstock festival and the comeback of cocaine,[40] his coworkers began to overindulge. "It was very cheap," White recalls, "everybody took it, and suddenly everything got much meaner. When people on cocaine are threatening to kill you, even though I wasn't afraid, I just felt it was time to move on."[41] And for someone like Leary touting psychedelics as catalysts for social change, amphetamines had also become nothing short of a counter-revolutionary chemical, which had dented his hopes of a swift psychedelic revolution.[42] To make things even worse, the quality of LSD was changing quite dramatically. Jean Houston was one of many who cautioned against fake acid, which was "as bad as bathtub gin."[43]

In the late Sixties, a new brand of "Orange Sunshine" LSD became a minor sensation on account of its incredible potency and because it was supplied by an idealistic network known as the Brotherhood of Eternal Love.[44] One dealer was enamoured by Sunshine, but he dismissed "new" drugs like MDA because they had no spiritual quality. And other kinds of acid now contained so many additives that he discriminated between pure LSD and mediocre street acid. "Beware of 'Orange Wedge,'" he cautioned the EVO readers, "which started out as a relatively good product, but has been messed with since. They have Strychnine and Belladonna and god knows what other weird, fucked-up, bad Karma drugs into it."[45] More specifically, a study of black market acid claimed that less than 10 per cent was pure and not altered with methedrine, heroin, atropine, and strychnine.[46]

Methedrine (a powerful methamphetamine), in particular, was another narcotic that typified drug use in the late Sixties. As Abbie Hoffman cautioned, "There's a notable absence of LSD, and a very high increase in the use of meth. It's a very self-destructive drug, and so there's a lot of violence."[47] Other radical leftists claimed that the drug had become popular among some acid heads because it was close enough to the psychedelic high, and they connected the rise of methedrine-laced LSD with the Mafia's involvement in the trade. Whereas an acid user would perhaps take the drug once or twice a week, a methedrine user might take it four or five times a day to satisfy the craving. So it made economic sense to mix the drug with psychedelics to gradually lure LSD users into using methedrine on a daily basis.[48]

Around that time, the new drug STP was initially mistaken for LSD, despite its much longer and more powerful effects. The *Village Voice*, which was still keeping track of the latest psychoactive trends, soon published vivid accounts of STP trips to warn against the super-hallucinogen,[49] which could turn a user's body into "a conductor for tens of thousands of volts."[50] Amelie Edwards, who once took the drug and saw the walls crawling with insects, remembers the confusion and paranoia it created among the Village acid heads. "So people would start to be afraid of taking acid because – you'd always ask: 'does it have STP in it?' 'Is it STP?'"[51]

As one of the few shining lights of the end of the decade, the *East Village Other* likewise became concerned about the changing drug scene and cautioned its readers about dangerous substances while pointing to unregulated alternatives. A few months after the banana hoax, the paper published an anonymous letter describing how to get high with an "Instant Icer." This involved spraying some of the icer into a leak-proof plastic bag and letting it warm at room temperature. Then, you only needed to inhale the contents deeply and hold your breath for a sixty-second high.[52] On the other hand, the paper warned against anesthetic cyclopropane (Trimethylene), which was mistaken for nitrous oxide and could cause arrhythmia and respiratory failure,[53] and against smoking hydrangea because it could lead to a carbon dioxide overload in the bloodstream. Instead, the paper recommended licking "magic toads" that contain bufotenine.[54]

Once There Was a Village

In spite of the *EVO*'s best intentions, the East Village did not become the psychedelic haven many hoped it would. In 1967, the Ninth Precinct reported a 28 per cent increase in narcotics arrests and a 51 per cent jump in felony narcotics arrests.[55] For the locals, it was a veritable epidemic. During that summer, Yuri Kapralov and his family were living in a four-room apartment close to Tompkins Square Park, and Kapralov might be sitting on his stoop around eight or nine in the evening when the open peddling would begin:

> and a well-dressed guy would walk by and he'd be singing, "Acid, acid, get your beautiful acid ... only ten tabs left, beautiful acid ..." Two minutes later, another dude, singing in a low baritone, "horse, horse ... ride a pony, two bills, sweet smack ..." Another five minutes, a small freckled chick about twelve would be dancing around, playing with her dog: "Jamaican, Jamaican, anyone for grass? Ten an ounce, thirty cents a joint, California joint ..." ... And you could simply buy whatever your heart desired, heroin to mescaline, from seven- or eight-year-old kids riding on their bikes around Tompkins Square Park.[56]

In the park, LSD remained a feature, but Richard Goldstein, for one, "probably saw more heroin than anything."[57] The local smack trade was controlled by Puerto Rican gangs who saw psychedelics as a threat to their business, and many acid heads were beaten up and robbed in the park as a result.[58] Contrary to the prevailing notion of the time, street gangs had remained a presence in the East Village even before their re-emergence in the 1970s when New York's stalling economy led struggling working-class youth to turn to gangs as they had done after the war.[59]

164 | PSYCHEDELIC NEW YORK

Violence in the Village made the headlines in October when the naked bodies of two well-known acid heads, twenty-one-year-old James Hutchinson (better known locally as "Groovy") and eighteen-year-old runaway Linda Fitzpatrick were found horribly mutilated in an East Village basement. A young commune-dweller known locally as Galahad blamed the killings on greedy "Pushers from uptown" who did not like the idea that Hutchinson was dealing drugs "at cost price."[60] Beat poet Ed Sanders remembers Hutchinson, who briefly turned his Peace Eye Bookstore into "a mattress meadow" for the runaways,[61] as someone who "preached the message that a person could both serve AND stay high and party while doing good."[62]

Amelie Edwards painfully discovered how crash pads were being affected by addictive drugs when she ended up in a commune made up of speed and junk users. "They were thieves, they were heroin addicts," she recalls. "They did everything bad. I mean, they had me go to the department store with a phony credit card and charge things." There was precious little LSD available, and the people there soon grew tired of her because they had to prepare the needles for her.[63]

By then, the Villagers could no longer count on the Psychedelicatessen for supplies. While the iconic head shop was freely dispensing acid to local users, it also had its share of problems. Soon after it had opened, a man had approached Susun Weed and suggested that she pay him to "protect" the shop. Not realizing he represented the Mafia, she had refused, and as a result, the store was vandalized and robbed over and over. On the one occasion that a thief was caught in the act, however, he claimed that the drugs he was arrested with were stolen goods from the Psychedelicatessen.[64] This marked the beginning of a police investigation that culminated in a June 1968 raid during which the "house stash" (magic mushrooms, pot, and hash) were seized.[65] The commune, which dispersed but stayed in touch, had to close the store and give up their brownstone.[66]

Outside the communes and crash pads, the continued arrival of suburban teenagers had become a nuisance for the locals. "We have to live in this shit," an incensed taxi driver complained. "They don't. I don't understand these young punks."[67] Another resident, who had long been trying to move out of the area, was just as livid: "Let me tell you, one day I saw two of these hippie animals screwing in the park – right out in the open! Is this any place to bring up my kids?"[68] Beyond the moral outrage, promiscuous sex contributed to the spread of venereal diseases, and soon some Villagers set up Contact, an emergency shelter where street kids with VD and hepatitis could get treatment. A psychiatrist and a psychologist also came over once a week to talk them out of drugs and suicide attempts.[69]

But more and more drugs kept coming their way. At the turn of the 1960s, the Village went through a gigantic wave of heroin, and on Kapralov's block, Slavic and Puerto Rican kids, who had hitherto stayed clear of smack, started shooting up. The situation had become desperate:

> I knew only one old woman on our block who had *not* been mugged. That was the Carpatho-Russian lady who was now our [building superintendent]. She always carried a big club. Fewer than 20 percent of all apartments were NOT ripped off. I'd also make a conservative estimate that approximately one hundred people on our block felt the knife or looked at the gun, or both, in '69 and '70. At least twenty people were stabbed. At least five were shot. Three were killed, as far as I know. I don't know how many died in the hospitals later. Needless to say, the cops did nothing.[70]

Along with all the damage to people and property, several smack users died of overdose during the heroin peak. In the winter of 1970, Kapralov moved to an apartment on 11th Street where the entire basement was full of heroin users. After a lock was added to the front door, the building lived on in relative peace,[71] but on 22 March, the entire neighbourhood heard a bomb detonate at the Electric Circus, which injured seventeen people. On 7 August 1971, the club closed for good, less than two months after the Fillmore East had likewise ceased to exist.[72]

The local drug world took on a far more sinister turn the next year. Kapralov had befriended a seventeen-year-old female runaway from Wisconsin, but when he finally found an apartment for her to move into, she unexpectedly disappeared. After asking around and finally confronting a smack addict named Jack, he learnt that he had sold her to some gang over in the Bronx for two hundred dollars. Kapralov pulled his knife out and threatened to kill him if he didn't bring her back. When he did, the teenager looked like she had aged several decades.

166 | PSYCHEDELIC NEW YORK

Jack had given her some Sunshine acid that was far more powerful than anything she'd ever tried. She was then raped by two of Jack's friends, including one who hit her with his belt. Later, Jack gave her a drug that knocked her out, and he then drove her off to a vacant storefront where he sold her to a Dominican slave ring that offered runaways to their clients. For the next four days and nights, she was raped multiple times by several men, but then she was resold to a sadist who kept her in a pitch-black, soundproof room. That man fed her a combination of acid and speed and beat her up regularly for hours at a time. When Jack finally "bought" her back, she was blindfolded until she arrived on 10th Street. A friend of hers called Kapralov, who then took her to the psychiatric ward at NYU hospital. Over the next few months, Jack continued to be involved in the local slave trade to support his heroin habit until he was killed by a mugger he tried to resist.[73]

My Sweet Lord

As the East Village was wrestling with drugs and crime, the quarter witnessed the arrival of Indian gurus who lured tired acid heads into their drug-free religions while promising them enlightenment. These spiritual teachers were able to travel to the US following the Immigration and Nationality Act of 1965 that lifted the restrictions on immigrants from Africa and Asia. Invariably, they dismissed psychedelics as an ersatz of spirituality. With so many acid users going through existential anxiety after experimenting with drugs, these charismatic leaders found a fertile breeding ground.

Part of the counterculture first heard about these gurus in the pages of the *East Village Other* soon after the paper's creation. Peter Leggieri remembers the day Walter Bowart encountered Hare Krishna leader Bhaktivedanta Swami Prabhupada in Tompkins Square Park. That day, Bowart had dropped some acid and strolled to the park where he saw Prabhupada, "dressed in golden robes and sitting in a lotus position under the giant tree that now bears his name." He rushed back to the offices immediately, ordered his coworkers to stop the presses, and begin drafting a story about the "holy man." John Wilcock turned to Leggieri, who was their only colleague with a smattering of theology. His article went to press, and decades later Leggieri learnt that the original article had been reproduced in Hare Krishna's main temple in India.[74]

Prabhupada had arrived penniless as early as 1965 and started chanting Hare Krishna in the park. Allen Ginsberg soon became a disciple, and as he recalled, "Immediately dozens of young LSD freak-outs flocked to sing the Harekrishna Maha-mantra with him – chant for the preservation of the planet."[75] Buoyed by this initial success, Prabhupada founded the International Society for Krishna Consciousness in a Lower East Side storefront in 1966.[76] The guru insisted that the effects of LSD were temporary and that users always had to come down at some point. Instead, with "Krsna [sic] consciousness, you stay high. Because you go to Krsna, you don't have to come down. You stay high forever."[77] To achieve this, one had to relinquish drugs, alcohol, and extramarital sex and take on chanting, which was accompanied with cymbals, tambourines, sticks, drums, bells, and a small reed organ.[78]

The American Hare Krishna movement soon became one of the major forms of post-psychedelic spirituality. In 1966, a Columbia dropout and LSD user named Keith Ham met Prabhupada on the Lower East Side. The next year, he became Swami Bhaktipada, and in 1968 went on to form what would become the largest Hare Krishna community in the country.[79] By the end the decade, it was a nationwide movement drawing former acid heads as well as scores of former protesters who had likewise gotten tired of activism.[80]

For the Village Ukrainians, however, Hare Krishna was just another source of trouble coming from the middle-class young, and they had to complain about the chanting in Tompkins Square Park. When the police showed up, the argument descended into a riot, and the officers made dozens of arrests while occasionally resorting to violence. As the prisoners were being taken to court, the protesters organized through the underground media channels, and the entrance to the court room was soon blocked by a human chain of protesters singing Hare Krishna.[81] Subsequently, Krishna followers found sanctuary at the Electric Lotus head shop and could meditate in a backroom chamber clouded in aromatic incense.[82]

Perhaps the most famous convert to Eastern spirituality was Richard Alpert, who travelled to India in 1968 and returned as Baba Ram Dass, freed from psychedelics. In December, the former Harvard psychologist gave a talk at the Universalist Church on 76th Street, "wearing meticulous Indian white." Ram Dass claimed that his drug-free religious conversion to yoga made him feel as though he was under the mild but constant influence of hashish, a state he could never maintain with psychedelic drugs.[83] His influence quickly reached the East Village, where Nina Graboi bumped into a former regular of the Center for the League for Spiritual Discovery. Since those days, he had been ordained Surya Das ("Servant of the Sun") by Ram Dass and had delved deep into Eastern spirituality.[84]

On 12th Street, the Yoga Head Program was run by Guruprem, who had once been an LSD dealer in the Village but had since given up drugs after contemplating suicide.[85] Guruprem had learned his trade from Swami Satchidananda, who saw psychedelics as enslaving but was always patient with his students, confident that they would naturally embrace his "true" consciousness expansion. "Kids have been spoiled by acid," claimed one of his disciples. "They won't accept anything unless they can feel it." His followers set up a "tribal store" on East 6th Street that was meant to give the group more visibility. It had its fair share of DayGlo paint, tie-dye bunting, and strobe lights, as in typical head shops, but it also featured a life-size photograph of the Swami, clearly indicating that this was to be a spiritual place as opposed to a beacon for psychedelia.[86]

The End of the Psychedelic Movement

Gurus easily tapped into the new spiritual marketplace because by then Leary's psychedelic movement was crumbling. In the final part of the Sixties, the High Priest was spending most of his time in California, and his mounting legal issues finally caught up with him in 1970 when he began serving his jail sentence. His relatives and friends scrambled to assist him, but this was a far cry from the support the Leary Defense Fund had received in 1966. In such a charged political climate and amid rampant narcotic abuse, psychedelic idealism had become a relic of the Sixties.

In May 1970, Rosemary Woodruff Leary put on a benefit, and it was telling that the event was organized back in Greenwich Village where it had all started. But the atmosphere was just as bad as in the East Village. On 6 March, a detonation in a West 11th Street apartment killed three people and injured two others. The bomb, which exploded prematurely, was assembled by the Weather Underground, a radical leftist group that had turned to violence at a time when their leaders were experimenting with strong doses of LSD.[87] Acid reinforced their political views and kept them aware of their revolutionary objectives,[88] and from this perspective, LSD was a tool for destroying the state rather than a catalyst for global peace.

In spite of the shocking news, Woodruff went ahead with the fund-raiser at the Village Gate, a nightclub located at the corner of Thompson and Bleecker streets that had been providing jazz, folk music, and avant-garde entertainment to the local Bohemians for more than a decade.[89] The nightclub had also helped activists by hosting a benefit for the Congress of Racial Equality in 1961[90] and for a jailed protester in 1968.[91] That same year, Norman Mailer gathered enough signatures to run for New York City mayor, and his campaign manager organized a rally there, "amid the pulsing music and lights of an acid-rock band." The event, however, was a public relations disaster for Mailer, who overindulged in whiskey and hurled profanities at a group of feminists.[92]

The Leary fundraiser somehow managed to fare even worse. Graboi was among the attendees that night, and she had swallowed a tab beforehand, "In honor of Tim." As she walked through Bleecker Street, she realized how inhospitable the city had become, and inside it was a very different crowd compared to the peaceful days of the Center for the League for Spiritual Discovery. Prominent figures like Allen Ginsberg and Alan Watts were attending, but so were political radicals like Abbie and Anita Hoffman and Jerry Rubin. Thrown into the mix were "a sprinkling of jet-setters, and some secret service men with hard faces and guarded eyes."[93]

The one thing these New Yorkers did share was a ravenous appetite for LSD. As Anita Hoffman recalled, "The punch was spiked and everyone was on acid."[94] Woodruff had invited some former Millbrook light-show artists, but by the time they were supposed to perform they were lying under the tables, completely incapacitated.[95] Abbie Hoffman was another who had overindulged, and he was in no mood for a peaceful party. Earlier that month, the National Guard had shot at some protesters during an anti-war rally at Kent State University, killing four, and earlier that day some New York longshoremen had beaten up anti-war activists while the police looked the other way.[96]

The furious Hoffman soon pushed a speaker off the stage. "If you want Tim Leary out of jail by July 4th," he frantically lectured the crowd, "then let's tear down the walls of his prison – because that's the only way he's going to get out."[97] Graboi's acid tab was still coming on as she saw Hoffman stare directly at her, his face red with anger. Soon after, her consciousness began to disintegrate, and in the heavy atmosphere of the Village Gate basement, the LSD became overwhelming. She spent the night half-conscious on a thick coil of rope while her friends pondered calling an ambulance.[98]

Meanwhile, Woodruff saw all the wealthy donors leave the nightclub one by one as Hoffman raged on. To make things worse, he attacked and destroyed an expensive loudspeaker. By the end of the evening, the fundraiser had cost her $3,000.[99]

Meanwhile, Midtown ...

As the Village Gate fiasco revealed, psychedelia did not have a viable future in downtown Manhattan, but the presence of jet setters, on the other hand, suggests that wealthy New Yorkers were still interested both in LSD and its concomitant psychedelic culture. While the East Village was mired in drug abuse, psychedelia found a home midtown where the upper class continued to experiment in their bubble of wealth and power, while the corporate and advertising sectors saw a unique opportunity to recycle its codes for commercial purposes. This was a testimony of how far LSD and psychedelics had gone since Leary had introduced the local jet set to psilocybin back in 1961.

In 1967, Millbrook resident Art Kleps assumed a greater presence among the New York upper class, while Leary was looking for support all over the country and making occasional appearances in the city. Around that time, Kleps met Joe Gross, a late-thirties psychiatrist practising in a penthouse overlooking Central Park and the Guggenheim Museum. Gross loved the Millbrook scene and regularly visited Kleps there. He smoked a little grass now and then and ended up trying LSD at the commune.[100]

But most of these well-to-do New Yorkers gravitated around Peggy Hitchcock, who regularly offered carefree entertainment in her five-storey house off Fifth Avenue. That same year, Hitchcock hosted an LSD party. "A bar had been set up in the second-floor hall, at the top of a curving, marble staircase," recalled Kleps. "Peggy's butler poured and stirred, and a dozen people, drinks in hand, were milling around in a large sitting room to the right of the stairs." She then led Kleps and Bill Haines, another Millbrook resident, to prepare a punch for the guests on the third floor. Kleps and Haines began adding acid drops from a vial so that it worked out to approximately 40µgr per cup. This would make the experience manageable for novices, and experienced acid heads could always go for more.

When they came back down with the punch, they bumped into a nervous Leary who could not wait to try it and was having an animated conversation with a young Episcopalian priest. As the drug hit the party, however, the priest was appalled by the scene. At one point in the evening, Haines retreated to the library to meditate in a dark corner, and the distraught priest came in, unaware of his presence. He telephoned his bishop and told him that everybody was flying on acid and behaving insanely. Haines found it outrageous that one of Hitchcock's guests would report this and thought of "bombing" him by giving him acid without his knowledge or consent.

Haines had a brief discussion with Kleps and Leary about the ethics of bombing, but all three came to the conclusion that the case warranted an exception. "With great aplomb," Kleps recalled, "Haines walked around behind his target's table and deftly demonstrated that the hand is quicker than the eye. It became evident, an hour later, that the priest loved the stuff. The transformation was abrupt. One moment he was grimly sitting in a corner sipping his gin and the next moment he was on the dance floor with Peggy, putting on an exhibition of pelvic-thrust, head-jerk dancing worthy of the most primitive teenager.[101] The priest went apparently unharmed, yet this anecdote illustrates how flawed the ethics of the psychedelic movement had become. Isaac Abrams, for one, would have been shocked: "I always thought dosing people, meaning giving them LSD without their voluntary participation, was really bad manners. In the worse sense of bad manners."[102]

Meanwhile, Van Wolf's place continued to draw wealthy New Yorkers intent on psychoactive licence. On Christmas Eve, he threw a party, and Kleps was struck by the casual use of cocaine and marijuana among the jet setters: "Little cut glass salt dishes filled with cocaine sat on every table, complete with tiny salt spoons to lift the stuff up to your nose with for inhalation. A huge Black man, dressed in full livery, sat behind another table rolling perfectly cylindrical double-length joints out of four standard-sized papers for the guests." Not every guest indulged in coke and grass, but even then they were totally indifferent to the scene.

After Christmas, Kleps spent a few days in a state of drunken stupor at Billy Hitchcock's apartment. When he finally sobered up, Billy took his family and Kleps out for dinner. On the way to the limousine, he casually told him that his son had ingested an LSD tablet, which had "probably looked like candy to him." Hitchcock's wife Aurora did not seem happy about it, but then she believed that "all children were 'naturally stoned' anyway." Nevertheless, Kleps became anxious after doing the maths: "before we got to the restaurant it struck me that 300 micrograms for Little Billy was the equivalent of about 2,000 for me in terms of body weight." Kleps and Hitchcock worked through a few bottles of Beaujolais when it dawned on them that Hitchcock's son might be on his way to permanent brain damage. Back at his apartment, Billy Jr kept his mother up all night long while Kleps slept heavily under the influence of a downer.[103]

The way the Hitchcocks treated this episode speaks volumes about their status and reveals how unconcerned they were about the controversies surrounding LSD. It also suggests that they had not been reading the papers. Back in April 1966, the media had widely covered a similar accidental ingestion of LSD by a five-year-old girl in Brooklyn – her uncle had left a saturated sugar cube in the refrigerator.[104] The incident was related in popular magazines, and the *New York Times* published three articles about it,[105] but it appears that the news did not reach the Hitchcocks and the New York upper class that carried on using LSD casually.

And there is a very simple reason for their continued use of the drug: Billy Hitchcock was now involved in a large-scale acid trafficking conspiracy. In 1966, Nick Sand visited Hitchcock in his apartment, and together they smoked some DET, by which time Hitchcock was already the veteran of approximately twenty-five LSD trips. A year later, Augustus Owsley Stanley III, another idealistic chemist otherwise-known as "Bear" in the psychedelic underground, also paid him a visit from California. Along with Sand and another brilliant chemist by the name of Tim

CHANGING SCENES | 173

Scully, they began a multimillion-dollar LSD distribution scheme, and Hitchcock made use of his wealth and connections to fund the chemists, launder profits, and assist with legal matters.[106] By then, Hitchcock had already teamed up with his old friend Charlie Rumsey, another wealthy New Yorker who was the nephew of businessman and politician Averell Harriman. Rumsey was actively involved in the Millbrook scene, but in midtown he was better known for supplying the local jet set with LSD.[107]

That Hitchcock ever chose to get involved in such a risky operation is quite perplexing, given that he was drawing between $5 and $7 million a year in interest from the Hitchcock family trust fund.[108] For all his attention to the psychedelic experience, maybe Hitchcock was just another member of the New York upper class attempting to increase his wealth.[109] In any event, the rich did not have to worry about the purity of the LSD they were using, while teenagers poisoned their bodies with fake acid in the East Village.

While well-to-do New Yorkers like the Hitchcocks and Van Wolf were using drugs by way of entertainment, others realized that there was money to be made with psychedelia. The upper class certainly allowed people working in the business, entertainment, and advertising sectors to discover psychedelics, which probably influenced their trades. By the time Leary had announced the creation of the league at the Advertising Club on Park Avenue, a thirty-six-year-old account executive for one of the biggest advertising agencies in the city had already taken LSD twice because he was looking for a strong emotional experience and he feared that he might lose his sensitivity toward his job.[110]

However, it is more likely that the commercial opportunities that arose in the second half of the Sixties came about as a result of psychedelia's own visibility rather than by entrepreneurs undergoing life-changing experiences with LSD. A testimony of the ever-growing popularity of psychedelic aesthetics is their seamless transition into Madison Avenue when advertisers realized that psychedelia could "provide maximum dramatization of an otherwise mundane product."[111]

This occurred at a time when the industry was undergoing deep changes. Back in the 1940s and 1950s, "Admen were hopeless yes-men, dedicated to affirming their clients' every whim." Thinking outside the box was virtually unheard of, and the most rewarding position they could hope for was the account man, "whose job was simply to entertain clients with stiff drinks and a smooth line – advertisements themselves ... were secondary."[112] The first agency to depart from the robotic advertising of the time was Doyle Dane Bernbach with a landmark 1959 commercial for Volkswagen. Bill Bernbach had skilfully tapped into the growing skepticism toward advertising while inserting critiques of consumerism through "what we might call anti-advertising: a style which harnessed public mistrust of consumerism ... to consumerism itself." The entire industry was stunned by this radical turn, but it quickly followed Bernbach's lead.[113]

After the birth of hip advertising, there was nothing particularly controversial about Leary's fantasies of chemical revolution and individual liberation through LSD, a drug known in some scientific circles for its ability to stimulate creativity.[114] Rather than posing an existential threat to the sector, psychedelia was a reinvigorating cultural force that helped advertising move away from the tedium of the previous decades.

Madison Avenue, which had already hosted the psychedelic showcase in February 1967, formalized the connection that same year when Ernest Dichter of the Institute for Motivational Research suggested that the sector pay attention to the acid culture and use "animation with psychedelic colors and motion" to convey new and exciting meanings to products. In September, an article in *Madison Avenue* likewise instructed admen to take this culture seriously. While it stopped short of telling them to turn on, it stressed that many LSD users were able to transgress ordinary states of consciousness.[115]

Perhaps the most fitting example of this transition into Madison Avenue was the art of Peter Max, who is best remembered for working with the Beatles on *Yellow Submarine*. Max made a fortune in advertising by recycling psychedelic codes, which formed the basis of his "Transit Art" produced on behalf of the Metro Transit Advertising that owned a franchise on about 20,000 vehicles. By 1969, his company had printed 2.5 million posters, and his designs had appeared on more than forty products and in boutiques and restaurants. As one of his clients summed it up, he "has serious interest in making money ... He's made everyone realize that there's a demand from the youth market."[116]

But even if Max can be remembered as a hard-nosed businessman who had enough flair to see the commercial potential of psychedelic art, the psychedelic experience had nonetheless made a genuine impression on him. For all the talk of shallow commercialism, Max was drawn to the spiritual import of psychedelic drugs: "They bring peace to the nervous system … so you can receive all the transmissions of the cosmos." In fact, it was Max who had persuaded Swami Satchidananda to move to New York after meeting him in Paris and telling him about the fledging psychedelic scenes in the United States.[117]

Around that time, advertisers were likewise using psychedelic jargon to sell their products. For example, one shoe brand suggested that you "take a trip down and get the shoes that will really turn you on," and a vodka brand also advertised "Turn on a White Christmas."[118] Light shows followed the same path when the Best & Co. department store hired Jackie Cassen and Rudi Stern for a window promotion using multimedia techniques.[119] In 1966, another advertising company designed an ad to help its clients appreciate the numbers and wealth of the baby boomers,[120] and a year later, the firm realized they could also tap into the growing psychedelic culture. They did a presentation at the Village Gate called "What Turns Alice On" using "dance, music, film and exotic lightning effects" in front of a group of 110 executives of a food manufacturing company. One company spokesman made it clear that they had no interest in taking drugs but that they took psychedelia very seriously: "We're telling the industry that if you're looking for a new form, choose one they understand and dig, that they will groove to. It's not based on the fact that your audience is taking drugs and will turn on when they look at a TV set."[121]

In 1967, the *New York Times* reported that "the multimedia technique is helping to convey information, provide entertainment, create aesthetic experience, sell products and even further medical research." The paper claimed that one firm had increased its sales by 11 per cent "with the aid of rock 'n' roll music, slide and movie projections and a battery of pulsing strobe lights." Another company, Sensefex, even began offering advice on multimedia environments for corporations looking to improve their marketing strategies. Tellingly, the directors of Sensefex revealed that "our three muses are Tim Leary, the Beatles and McLuhan."[122]

Locally, psychedelia was also influencing off-Broadway theatre. In September 1967, Robert Joffrey's *Astarte* premiered at the City Center Theater on 55th Street. This "psychedelic rock ballet" interpreted the myth of the love goddess and featured two dancers who coordinated with the music, as well as kinetic scenery displaying psychedelic images that were sometimes superimposed on the dancers. As one journalist noted, "The film images dwarf the dancers, and they try out their puny love on a naked forestage, while behind is a wall of giants, images of themselves embracing, moving together, challenging, one image cutting across another, and yet another as the screams on." Although he acknowledged the borrowing of "psychedelic techniques," he contended that this piece had taken multimedia art to a new stage by moving away from the avant-garde.[123]

Multimedia installations likewise gave a new aesthetic direction to discotheques, as they had done at the Electric Circus. All over the city, club owners became interested in these experiential techniques, and they hired light-show artists to create uniquely interactive environments that departed from the typical ways of socializing by "turning on their patrons with high-decibel rock n' roll combined with pulsing lights, flashing slide images and electronically tinted 'color mists.'"[124] Their commercial success was based on a tangible acid substrate: "Associating the psychedelic experience with the discotheque has the same function as the posters, insofar as it announces that this is a place to which people with certain already formed tastes, interests, and curiosities will want to come."[125]

Naturally, these novel forms of entertainment attracted acid users who sought to enhance the drug experience or simply to enjoy it with their own psychedelic sensibility. As a result, these crowded environments made for excellent hangouts for dealers. One twenty-three-year-old LSD seller claimed that most of his clients were "kids with plenty of money in their pockets" who did not need to work and added that they were "the kind of kids who've got the money to make the discotheque scene."[126] Indeed, one acid user revealed that "You can walk into half the discotheques in the city and make a contact in five minutes."[127]

The son of Adlai Stevenson, Borden, realized the commercial potential of such ventures when he opened Cheetah on Broadway and 53rd Street with the help of Olivier Coquelin, the mastermind of the postwar discotheque scene. During occupation, the Nazis indulged in the Parisian cabarets, but jazz clubs were banned because of their connections with America, Blacks, and Jews. As a result, "illicit clubs adopted the low-key approach of playing records over crude public-address systems, since live performances, for so many reasons, were impractical." Jazz quickly became the music of the resistance, and the discotheques that blossomed in Paris after the war were a tribute to America and jazz culture while keeping their subversive and underground edges.

It was fitting, then, that Coquelin, who was granted American citizenship after serving in the Korean War, completed this transnational exchange by successfully importing this virtually unchanged discotheque template. On 31 December 1960, America had its first disco on Sutton Place, which was explicit about the French connection – Le Club. The Parisian discotheque, however, had an elitist dimension that also crossed the Atlantic, and a venue like Le Club and the discotheques that followed in the early Sixties typically charged astronomical fees at the doors and sometimes required patrons to pay annual dues. The democratization of discotheques happened as the British Invasion was sweeping America, courtesy of Sybil Burton, who opened Arthur, close to Le Club. Burton was a Welsh actor and the daughter of a miner, and she believed that the discotheque should be available to people of all classes who wanted to dance the Jerk, the Watusi, and the Boogaloo.

With Cheetah, Coquelin took the popular discotheque to another level by opening "an arena-style club with an eight-thousand-square-foot dance floor, sound provided by three alternating rock bands (as opposed to recorded music), a library (!), a TV room, and a movie theater, not to mention a boutique where disco-goers could buy clothes for the evening (and put aside whatever they came in wearing)."[128] By then, Coquelin had identified psychedelia as the next big thing, and he gave his latest invention the psychedelic edge necessary to attract New Yorkers looking for a mind-blowing total environment.

Like the other psychedelic nightclubs that were sprouting all over the city,[129] Cheetah offered a total environment with "sound, lights, textures and movement all fused together in a total assault on the senses and emotions."[130] The visuals were designed by Cassen and Stern,[131] and the club featured a sophisticated light installation programmed to change colour and intensity according to the music. The light would bounce off the walls lined with mirrors and aluminum sheets, while thousands of rainbow-coloured light bulbs went on and off.[132]

As at Cerebrum, the club did not sell hard liquor in an attempt to turn away the older generations. Instead, many showed up under the influence of LSD to enjoy the experience.[133] But even those who did not turn on found their habitual consciousness altered. One female partygoer claimed that "It was taking an LSD trip without the LSD," and a young man, clearly affected by the disorientation, said that "It was like being inside a giant combination jukebox and pinball machine."[134]

Though Cheetah built its base on the younger New Yorkers who were acquainted with the psychedelic culture, some of the patrons included celebrities like Peter Fonda, George Hamilton, and Catherine Deneuve, and the club also held a gala to support Eugene McCarthy's run for president. In the summer of 1967, it became a meeting ground to ease the tensions in the East Village[135] by hosting the Grateful Dead and the Group Image for the first in a series of "Inter-Tribal Community Benefits."[136]

Yet club owner Stevenson had no time for psychedelia. "I'm not a nightclub man," he freely confessed, "and the [new sound] drives me out of my mind." Indeed, his venture was solely a way of reaping the benefits of the current fads, even when they included elements of psychedelia. Stevenson openly admitted that "it's kind of ridiculous ... to talk about the 'need' for a new nightclub, but I do believe that Olivier has a remarkable grasp of what young people are looking for in entertainment today."[137]

Combined with the rise of psychedelic advertising on Madison Avenue and the continued drug parties among the upper class, a discotheque like Cheetah confirmed that midtown Manhattan was becoming a new focal point for New York psychedelia. While this did not hold in the following decade, another transition to nearby Central Park occurred soon after and allowed the green sanctuary to become the city's new psychedelic hotspot.

As New York City entered recession, the psychedelic counterculture basically disintegrated. Prohibitionists ramped up the anti-drug rhetoric by tying drugs to youth, which by then had certainly become a visible category of acid users. In the East Village, rampant drug use combined with sexual promiscuity and violence was a fitting counterpoint to San Francisco's Summer of Love, leading the working-class locals to occasionally take action against the newcomers. Some acid heads soon turned to Eastern gurus for counselling and ended up moving away from LSD. And as the new decade began, Leary was behind bars, and a few years later his psychedelic career was formally over when he collaborated with the FBI in return for freedom.

The few Village restaurants and shops that had been there before the newcomers certainly welcomed the minor economic boom resulting from the changing demographics,[138] but by 1968, only 6.3 per cent of the Lower East Side's housing stock was occupied by middle-income tenants, and those upwardly mobile New Yorkers were concentrated in specific areas.[139] While the western part of the Village did experience a wave of real estate speculation that caused the rents for apartments close to St Mark's Place to double between 1966 and 1967, this brief interest was not enough to attract "the levels of capital investment required to sustain a major rehabilitation of the area's aged housing units."[140] Because real estate interest was closely linked to the Village's hip image, it soon had to look elsewhere.

And yet, psychedelia was a now such a cultural force that it found a place in the city's advertising and entertainment sectors. Madison Avenue and Cheetah undoubtedly exploited psychedelia for commercial purposes, and it would be easy to dismiss this as cynical commodification. But this would imply that there existed a monolithic and fundamentally anti-capitalist psychedelic culture, when New York psychedelia was largely the reflection of the city's pluralism. In spite of the mounting controversies, advertisers allowed this culture to reach unprecedented levels of visibility. All this, however, would not have been possible without the initial success of psychedelic art and light shows, as well as the gradual popularization of psychedelic slang and codes resulting from acid use all over the city. As the final chapter will further illustrate, psychedelia was not going to disappear with the Sixties.

The Sixties Happened in the Seventies

In the 1970s, it seemed as though psychedelics had vanished from the psychoactive landscape, which was dominated by narcotics. While amphetamine abuse did not disappear completely, Americans no longer viewed speed as a harmless thrill, and the federal government took significant measures to curb pharmaceutical production.[1] But in 1970, New York's heroin wave reached its peak. Blacks and Hispanics were disproportionately affected, and several Harlem community leaders vocally supported stricter laws to curb narcotics use. Early in 1973, the Rockefeller Drug Laws introduced tougher penalties for drug offences (including cannabis) and mandatory prison sentences. The consequence was a strong increase in incarceration rates, particularly for ethnic minorities.[2]

At the same time, the city's looming bankruptcy caused bankers and politicians to exploit New York's economic crisis by slashing services and firing thousands of municipal workers, which ushered in a new era of fiscal conservatism.[3] The city's Department of Health had to cut $1 million from its methadone substitution program between 1974 and 1977, and the city's narcotics squad and the special narcotics prosecutor saw their respective budgets shrink as a result of the cuts. By 1985, 30,000 registered drug addicts were in treatment, but that figure paled in comparison with a staggering grand total of 250,000 known addicts in the city, many of whom became infected by HIV/AIDS by sharing their needles.[4]

But psychedelia lived on. In the late Sixties, Central Park assumed the quality of a green haven for acid heads who had realized that concrete and steel made for an inhospitable setting and that areas featuring natural landscapes were far more supportive. Young people could spend hours under the influence by the Bethesda Fountain, and a few years later it was a popular place for dealers and for graffiti artists. Other acid heads preferred to leave the city in order to live in the peace and quiet of the country, but at least some of them maintained ties with the metropolis.

In the following years, the police continued to seize large quantities of LSD in the city in spite of widespread cocaine and crack consumption, while the more knowledgeable New Yorkers like Ed Rosenfeld got their hands on obscure psychedelic chemicals that were then unknown to authorities. Psychedelic art continued to find space in the Manhattan galleries, and the first generation of psychedelic artists were joined by painter Alex Grey, whose work was a fitting embodiment of the intertwining of the scientific and spiritual components of the LSD experience.

But one of psychedelia's most obvious signs of longevity lay in Howard Lotsof's investigations into ibogaine's anti-addictive properties. His movement found the support of the radical left, marijuana activists, and later the Black Panthers, who all saw ibogaine as a promising way of helping some of the city's blighted neighbourhoods where addiction was rife. Since the beginning of this therapeutic movement, several clinics offering ibogaine-based therapy have opened around the world, and they now offer one of the most innovative treatments for substance abuse disorders.

In this way, Lotsof's movement fundamentally disrupts the notion of a contemporary psychedelic "renaissance." While Charles Dahlberg's research shows that all the non-medical controversies of the Sixties were not enough to effectively terminate LSD science then,[5] Lotsof's efforts to promote ibogaine-based medicine hints at even greater historical continuity and suggests that psychedelic science never really ended in New York City. That it operated at the crossroads of medicine and political activism further illustrates that psychedelics rarely remained tightly confined to one particular realm and allowed his movement to easily find supportive audiences around the city.

Central Park in the Seventies

At a time when many Americans were rekindling their interest in old traditions of pastoralism and anti-urbanism,[6] many acid heads chose to leave New York City in order to get closer to nature. In particular, the baby boomers, who had grown up in suburbia close to fields and forests, and those who often vacationed outdoors, came to develop a stronger environmental awareness than their elders. Some members of the radical left and the counterculture likewise criticized the increasingly visible consequences of pollution and joined the chorus of environmental protectors.[7] With their ability to trigger feelings of intimate connection with nature,[8] LSD and psychedelics played a part in fermenting a greater appreciation for natural settings.

In fact, some LSD users had already concluded that the metropolis was not the best setting for intense psychedelic experiences. "The city is a very bad place to take LSD," claimed Eve Babitz, "because you suddenly become aware of all this steel and concrete and hostile faces and impossible chores that you cannot do when you are on LSD."[9] Yablonsky's interviewee Sonny concurred: "Cities as a human environment are architecturally negative." As a result, many of his acquaintances "decided to get out into small tribes, find an open area of open land or woods somewhere, do their thing, and live in the country."[10] Another user had suffered an existential crisis following his experimentation and realized that he had "become intensely aware of the spiritual suffocation of the city life." This separated father of two was now looking for a community "composed of really tuned-on people who would have a sense of responsibility towards the community and its members."[11]

The Third World studio also grew tired of the city. After spending time in Millbrook, "Most of us on the crew felt we could not return to the Lower East Side, the dirty pavements, and the Bowery bums," Gray Henry recalls. Bob Lowe moved to California and became a healer. Others went to Chicago to join the anti-war movement, while Henry married a Venezuelan and ended up living in Cairo.[12]

Around that time, the Abrams gave birth to their first child, and they moved to Woodstock, New York, at the turn of the decade because Rachel wanted to raise her daughter in a better environment. "We were going to the park," she remembers, "and she was crawling around picking up cigarette butts and empty beer cans. And I was just disgusted with it."[13]

THE SIXTIES HAPPENED IN THE SEVENTIES | 183

Nina Graboi likewise moved to Woodstock in 1969 after realizing that the "decaying city" was no longer a suitable place to take acid in.[14] In this "New Age community bursting with creativity and vitality," she opened a shop selling Indian products and artefacts, which was followed by a personal development centre and various other occupations.[15] For psychedelic artist Martin Carey, settling in Woodstock also made sense because of the town's acceptance of eccentric lifestyles and the proximity to the New York marketplace.[16]

But some New Yorkers continued to take acid in the city. One LSD dealer admitted that he preferred to enjoy the experience at home but that he forced himself to do it on the streets, "Otherwise I would be living in my own little world and wouldn't be aware of what's happening around me. I wouldn't be aware of other people's ideas and the trips they are on." Yet he also liked to be in contact with nature, and he saw the country as a safety valve: "If I become deranged from the pressure I shall split the scene, go out into the country and recover my head."[17] Others realized that parks made for good spots to enjoy their experiences amid the overcrowded urban spaces. "Mostly I turn on with Jim and Rick," one of them told Graboi. "We go to the park in Brooklyn [likely Prospect Park]. We have a ball." During their trips, they could see "the trees dance and everything is, like, alive!"[18]

Central Park soon became a well-known sanctuary for such users, perhaps because it was also an important public space for social movements. In April 1967, Martin Luther King attracted more than 100,000 civil rights demonstrators, and in 1969 "lesbians and gays marched from Greenwich Village to Central Park to hold a 'gay–in' on the Sheep Meadow."[19] In part, this expression of pluralism was the result of mayoral policies designed to encourage meetings locally. Indeed, the Lindsay administration "shut down Central Park to street traffic on weekends to encourage people to walk, bike, run, skate, and stroll through it more freely" during the summer of 1966.[20] This led to the gradual desegregation of the park, which allowed white New Yorkers to ride through areas that had been previously confined to Blacks and other minorities. It was hardly surprising, then, that psychedelic drug users saw it as a safe spot in which to turn on.

Amelie Edwards, for one, enjoyed dropping acid by the Bethesda Fountain, where "crowds ... gathered to flaunt their sexuality, play guitars, smoke marijuana, and hurl Frisbees."[21] As she puts it, "We just tripped.

And there were some people that were out of school that used to trip all the time. We used to just sit on blankets and just take LSD and just – I remember just kind of running through the fountain."[22]

Richard Goldstein likewise felt that Central Park was a fantastic place to visit under the influence. He remembers taking acid at the Metropolitan Museum of Art by the park, but there was something wrong about the setting. "It just seemed stony to me," he recalls. "The art had no meaning. The floors of the museum are marble or something. I wanted to get out. It was like a tomb." Outside, the park's "trees were vibrating, I saw Blakean clouds ... I realized that 'Wow! I need to be around organic things. Stone is not organic.'" He allegedly found a new connection with nature as a result of this experience, but unlike Edwards he always stayed away from the fountain because he found it too artificial.[23]

The gradual shift toward Central Park coincides with the rise of the Brotherhood of Eternal Love, a dealing network with strong connections to Leary, the Grateful Dead, and talented underground chemists. These idealistic acid heads believed that psychedelics, marijuana, and hashish were sacred drugs and that extensive use would lead to global peace, so when Nick Sand teamed up with Tim Scully to create the highly potent Orange Sunshine, the brotherhood was only too happy to facilitate the distribution. Sand had since divorced to dedicate his life to psychedelic chemistry, and Leary had dubbed him the league's official supplier. By the spring of 1967, Sand's Bell Perfume Labs' front in Brooklyn had relocated to California, where he and Scully began making Sunshine in 1968.[24] Half a year later, Sand and Scully had made more than 3.5 million tablets, which reached consumers across the entire country.[25]

The brotherhood's first known involvement in the New York drug scene was a delivery of half a ton of marijuana from California to Manhattan Island in late 1967,[26] but they remained discreet locally. A couple of years later, the *East Village Other* interviewed two dealers who believed that Sunshine was a godsend. "Sunshine LSD is pure sacramental LSD," claimed one of them. "The people who make it don't have money as their prime objective." While some former LSD users had moved on thanks to Indian gurus, they still listened to Leary's preaching. "Unlike Maharishi [Mahesh Yogi] who says 'if you want to see god follow me,' as said Meher Baba and others, Timothy Leary says 'Get into yourself and you will see God.' That's where Sunshine is at. It enables you to see the God within you."[27] Both dealers made no mention of the brotherhood and had no actual connection with Leary, and this likely illustrates the effectiveness of their underground distribution ring.

Sometime after the Woodstock festival, some brotherhood members, who looked "like secret agent guys," approached Chad Stickney, a fourteen-year-old acid head hanging out by the fountain. They were immediately taken by him, and they asked him if he would like to distribute large quantities of LSD. Before he knew it, Stickney was making far more money than he could spend,[28] and this was probably down to his role in the middle of the distribution hierarchy, involving moderately large transactions. In 1970, the EVO was running a column indicating the going rates for drugs in the city. A dose of Sunshine cost as little as 85¢ and should not be sold for more than $2,[29] which would seem to back the claims the two dealers had made in the paper the previous year.

Around that time, Stickney took on another hobby: graffiti. He was particularly enamoured by the art of Peter Max, and as he joined the brotherhood he began to write his name on walls around Central Park.[30] In 1971, he quit dealing and changed his name to "LSD-OM" and signed off on the South Bronx walls. Soon he was a hero in the local graffiti subculture.[31] By 1975, he had become the leader of a graffiti crew and was painting on subway cars all over the city. According to a rival (but friendly) leader, psychedelics were a major source of influence for the local scene. "They did acid or, a lot of the poor kids would do the poor man's psychedelic, unfortunately, PCP. Even though it's terrible stuff, it took them to other realms. They were amazing."[32]

In 1973, authorities caught up with the brotherhood and indicted the major players. Among them was Billy Hitchcock, who was charged with tax evasion and who cut a deal by testifying against his former associates. Although Sand was sentenced to fifteen years in 1974, he fled to Canada two years later, where he continued to make LSD until he was finally caught in 1996. In a 2009 interview, he estimated that he had produced approximately 140 million doses of LSD over the course of his career,[33] and if that was the case, then there is a good chance that some of that acid made it across the border to New York City.

Regardless, LSD continued to appear in Central Park. Steve Bloom, a sixteen-year-old high school student from the Bronx who went on to become a marijuana activist, was another young lad to take acid there. In August 1974, he attended a free concert by the New Riders of the Purple Sage with a friend and his older brother. They sat on the grass and smoked pot while waiting for the band to play, and then someone passed around an "orange-looking drink" in a glass jug. Whatever the drink was, they took several gulps. After a while, they were too stoned to catch the gig and could only watch the clouds zoom by.[34]

Before 1975, most of the acid available in the park was of superior quality. One acid dealer, a seventeen-year-old graffiti artist, remembers all the different brands of the time that had their own specific illustrations on the acid tabs: "Some of it was produced by guys right in the city, out of liquid stashes in their freezers, using micro-screens. Some of the better ones we had were the rainbow blotters, little booklets of 5,000, perforated sheets with little rainbows. As that whole thing picked up, they started to produce them in orange and black. I remember pink Windowpane came around. And the little barrels that were, at that point, still the real thing. I vividly remember seeing the Empire State Building blast off."[35]

The barrels came from the interstate network of the Grateful Dead. Born in 1965, the California band had become a popular feature in New York's psychedelic rock scene in the second half of the Sixties, with shows at the Café Au Go Go, in Tompkins Square Park, at the Village Theater, and for the 1968 Columbia strikes,[36] followed by several gigs in Central Park. Their concerts provided the platform for a close circle of dealer friends, so the fans had access to a virtually unlimited supply of quality acid whenever they set foot in a city. Tellingly, the Dead took a year off the road to write an album in 1975, and doses suddenly became less powerful. But the more knowledgeable "Parkies" knew they could get their hands on magic mushrooms upstate[37] or peyote from the Native American Church branch in the East Village.[38]

As these stories illustrate, acid was still popular among a new generation of teenagers who liked to hang out in Central Park. But as the Seventies carried on, New Yorkers of all ages remained interested in LSD, and for those who did not follow the Grateful Dead or who were unacquainted with the brotherhood, there were always other channels – and other drugs.

New Scenes, New Drugs

As acid heads rallied in Central Park, New York's downtown was still dominated by heroin, which found a new audience in the punk scene. The subculture was the most visible one in the Lower East Side, "with its portent of collapse, its hint of anarchy, its obvious misery in one of the nation's wealthiest cities, and its collection of burned-out buildings and open-air drug markets." In East Village clubs and Lower Manhattan, cocaine, alcohol, heroin, and quaaludes (methaqualone) became the punks' choice drugs, and junk even displaced booze on the Bowery.[39] On that street, many gravitated around the "Bunker," the loft where William Burroughs was still shooting up.[40] That did not stop Isaac Abrams from making incursions into that area and engaging with the decaying metropolis, however. In 1973, he created *Death Comes to the City*, a dark painting that resulted from his LSD use on the streets, and around the same time, he also painted *Rat World*, a bleak depiction of life on the Bowery.[41]

While Abrams carried on most of his work in Woodstock, Alex Grey began a painting career of his own. When he was twenty-one, Grey was invited to a party by his future wife Allyson, and they both took a strong dose of LSD. Grey had long been interested in anatomy and the human body, and his use of LSD triggered visions that deeply influenced his art. "I started having visions of glowing bodies with the acupuncture meridians and points, chakras and auras all inter-relating," he remembers. In 1979, Grey began the *Sacred Mirrors* series, which consisted of several paintings meant to explore human anatomy from a physical and metaphysical perspective (mind, body, and spirit). Each "Mirror" depicts a human-sized figure that allows the viewer so see a mirror image.[42]

Although psychedelic art was rather discreet in the early Seventies, there were other ways for New York's surviving psychedelic culture to influence the dying metropolis in a positive fashion. At a time when the city's psychedelic discotheques were all closing, New York City's nightlife was about to change dramatically under the influence of disco music, and the transition from psychedelia to disco would not have been the same without David Mancuso's acid parties in downtown Manhattan.

Born in 1944, Mancuso grew up in a children's home in Utica, New York, and by the age of sixteen he had dropped out of high school and was working various jobs in Manhattan. After favourably experimenting with acid, he began hosting parties in his loft at 647 Broadway in 1965. At first, these were carefully prepared LSD sessions with a limited number of participants. Mancuso built a "yoga shrine" for the purpose and placed a Buddha statue between the loudspeakers of his stereo, which played his homemade mix-tapes. Gradually, more and more New Yorkers were taken by the atmosphere, and in the second part of the Sixties his parties began to incorporate mixed-media and featured a much larger dance floor.[43]

By the early 1970s, Mancuso's invitation-only parties were drawing hundreds of New Yorkers. "You had to climb all these stairs and then you'd get a tab of acid ... at the door," remembers Judy Weinstein, who became Mancuso's manager in the mid-Seventies: "there was salad and fruit and the punchbowl, which was spiked with acid."[44] Mancuso liked to structure his parties as a three-stage psychedelic experience whereby invitees would enter the night in a smooth and calm way, go through a much longer and far more intense dancing phase, and finally re-enter the outside world in a more tranquil fashion.[45] This contrasted with Sybil Burton's Arthur in the previous decade, where the DJ would work toward a build-up with a few upbeat tunes, only to have everything come crashing down with Elvis Presley's "Love Me Tender."[46]

The LSD may well have played a part in dissolving the racial and sexual boundaries of the time. Indeed, these weekly get-togethers were probably the first to host Blacks and Hispanics, as well as some of the homosexual New Yorkers who wanted their own open nightlife following the 1969 Stonewall Riots, though Mancuso claimed that this was not the result of a conscious effort; he just happened to know many people.[47] In any event, Goldstein loved the absence of exclusivity, which was not always the case in the city's gay clubs. "Many gay discos of that era had door policies that appalled me," he remembers. "One place, Paradise Garage, rejected a prominent feminist whom I had taken there, because there were 'too many women' in the house. When I objected, they gave some excuse about attracting straight men, but, really, it was a homocentric excuse."[48]

Outside Mancuso's loft, dancing and socializing were enhanced by drugs that quickly became the symbols of the hedonism of the time. The first was cocaine, which had been much more discreet than heroin and the amphetamines in the postwar era. But from the mid-Sixties onward, the market expanded, and throughout the Seventies many rock stars like Eric Clapton carried on its popularization through praising lyrics. The drug soon reached high society, and by the end of the decade a staggering 20 per cent of Americans between eighteen and twenty-five years of age had taken coke at least once in the previous year.[49]

Isaac Abrams remembers how ubiquitous it had become in the upper spheres of the city. "The whole coke scene was happening everywhere. In bathrooms. But then they even invented a restaurant, cooking style, to serve the coke trade. Nouvelle Cuisine. Which was really tiny amounts of food on really big plates, mainly decorated with bits of sauce. A sprinkle of parsley. Little baby corn, maybe. And these were restaurants where people kept going to the bathroom to snort coke."[50]

The other two key drugs of the disco era were amyl nitrite, better-known as "poppers," and quaaludes. When inhaled, poppers cause a quick drop in blood pressure, resulting in a short-acting but powerful high, and for Goldstein, "they are the key to disco the way acid is the key to the acid rock scene … All the swoops of the music are a signal and you wore the drug in an amulet around your neck. You unscrewed it and did a popper when you knew that the swoop was coming. Because the popper lasts as long as the swoop." But gay men also found that poppers could massively enhance sexual experiences and that they naturally led to "orgiastic behaviours … It's also a male orgasm drug. So if you do it just before orgasm it's much more intense … So the club would reek of poppers. It smelt like a swimming pool."[51]

Quaalude, on the other hand, is a synthetic barbiturate that was first used to treat insomnia and anxiety, but in the early Seventies medical doctors were freely prescribing it to their patients, and Congress made it a Schedule II drug in 1973 and Schedule I in 1983, after which it basically disappeared from the psychoactive landscape.[52] On the dance floor, methaqualone turned people's arms and legs into jelly, and both quaalude and poppers could be counterbalanced by cocaine.[53] Meanwhile, some disco-goers continued to party on acid.[54]

The climate of hedonism also permeated the offices of the *Village Voice* headquarters over on Sheridan Square. Although "someone pretty high up at the paper" was a regular smack user and ended up getting fired for stealing typewriters, the *Voice* was mostly filled with the heady scent of marijuana, thanks to an intern who became the paper's go-to dealer. "So we often put out the paper stoned," remembers Goldstein. "We'd go to the roof and get stoned and put out the paper." At that time, the staff was also enjoying a great deal of casual sex. "Everyone sleeping with everyone. I mean, I once got hepatitis and had to warn half a dozen people to get gamma globule shots. Of both sexes." It was also around that time that Goldstein encountered the energizing and mood-elevating MDA. "We called it Miracle Drug of America. That was our name for it. I remember giving a party where everyone was on MDA. I had to worry that they wouldn't jump off my terrace, actually."[55]

Acid and quaaludes might have originated from a most unlikely local source. In 1979, the chairman of NYU's Department of Anthropology, John Buettner-Janusch, was arrested on charges that he was manufacturing LSD, methaqualone, and other drugs in his university lab with the assistance of both knowing and unknowing students and with university funds to purchase the raw materials. Buettner-Janusch created an organization called Simian Expansions Inc. to raise funds in order to support the study of lemurs. In reality, this move was designed to channel the profits of the illicit drug trade. During the trial, one witness told the court that back in 1977 Buettner-Janusch wanted to make LSD because the drug was fashionable again and there was money to be made.[56]

In the 1980s, the production of cocaine increased substantially in the Andes, and soon it began to appear in the form of crack, causing heroin use to decrease noticeably.[57] Throughout the decade and in the early 1990s, New York's Black working class was particularly beset by crack, a combination of coke and baking soda cooked into a pellet and smoked in a pipe. In an era of deregulated economics, the crack trade became a dark mirror image of American neoliberalism but one that nevertheless spurred many Blacks to deal to both earn a living and spend their money on flashy consumer goods. In keeping with the city's long tradition of overlapping drug and music subcultures, hip-hop artists praised crack dealers "as underground heroes in a racist society that left too many black men with too little dignity and too few opportunities for exuberant economic success."

At the heart of Nancy Reagan's "Just Say No" to drugs campaign, the crack problem led to the 1986 Anti–Drug Abuse Act that mandated an automatic five-year prison sentence for the distribution of five grams or more. Critics of the new law charged that it had blatantly racist implications because poor urban Blacks were the chief users. They only needed to look at the cocaine penalties to prove their point: cocaine traffickers were mostly white or Hispanic, and they catered to the upwardly mobile white consumers. For a similar prison sentence, they had to be caught peddling five *hundred* grams of powdered cocaine.[58] Once more, New York's working-class Blacks were massively affected by this new drug problem at a time when they were suffering from gross economic inequalities and racism.

As a meagre consolation, people living in the South Bronx found the unexpected support of a group of psychedelic idealists from rural Tennessee. From 1978 to 1984, they set up a relief program in an area that was notorious for its slow ambulance response time. To the South Bronx residents urgently needing medical assistance, they offered a free emergency care and transportation service and trained more than 200 "emergency medical technicians" to take over from them as they left. This social awareness emanated from the "psychedelically inspired mystical teachings of Stephen Gaskin" – the leader of the commune whence they originated. He and his followers "interpreted the oneness of mystical consciousness as a catalyst for local and global engaged activism."[59] Such an involvement with the community found itself at the crossroads of relief and spirituality "through real-world projects of social justice"[60] rather than utopian fancies of psychedelic revolution.

But perhaps the greatest hope of alleviating widespread addiction in the city came from ibogaine and Howard Lotsof. Ibogaine had joined LSD as a Schedule I drug, but Lotsof had since drawn a broad coalition ranging from former addicts to the radical left, and in December 1981 he received his first donation ($4,000) from a woman whose boyfriend was addicted. With these funds, he reviewed a century of work on ibogaine and found promising leads hinting at a relationship between the biochemical actions of ibogaine and opiates.

Public backing, by contrast, was non-existent. In 1983, he approached the National Institute for Drug Abuse (NIDA), but after he told them about his first ibogaine experience and subsequent heroin release, they did not take him seriously, probably because memories of Leary touting LSD as a cure-for-all were still fresh. In 1983, Lotsof and his wife Norma set up the Dora Weiner Foundation, a charity named after his grandmother designed to provide ibogaine as an alternative treatment for opiate addiction. But as they reached out to drug education organizations, they were stunned by the lack of empathy for addicts.[61]

Toward the end of the decade, Bob Sisko, a friend of Lotsof's who had relinquished his cocaine and tobacco habits thanks to ibogaine, began treating heroin users in New York. When he gave the drug to a long-time addict in April 1989, the improvement was so dramatic that marijuana activist Dana Beal decided to give ibogaine the same priority as legalizing cannabis. Around the same time, a cocaine user who had been interested in ibogaine since the late 1970s used his connections in the club scene to secure the endorsement of Madonna and Billy Idol.[62]

Meanwhile, there were signs that acid and like drugs were resiliently sailing through the narcotics storm. In 1983, the DEA reported seizures of LSD and other psychedelics in most US cities, including New York. The doses were significantly milder than in the Sixties and were often mixed with other chemicals, and the acid was mostly used in nightclubs.[63]

But Brad, who had been occasionally experimenting since 1970, had more ambitious plans. In the winter of 1980, he wanted to impress an acquaintance he was courting, "one of the most decadent people" he had ever met. Brad wanted to show him a good time on a visit to New York, so they both took psilocybin for a performance featuring the acclaimed dancers Rudolph Nureyev and Mikhail Baryshnikov. "I had to behave the way my friend wanted to behave," he admits. "And I had to come across as almost as decadent as he was … I also thought that I would have absolutely no chance of a relationship unless I extended myself, if that's a proper term." His strategy of seduction worked, though the relationship soon went out of control because that man took many other drugs indiscriminately.

A few years later, Brad attended Wagner's "extremely long, mytho-logical, and spiritual" *Parsifal* at the Metropolitan Opera House of the Lincoln Center. He took psilocybin again, and under the influence he was deeply moved and experienced something close to transcendence. "It starts at 6:00," he recalls. "The climax of the opera is about 11:30 at night. So the audience is usually asleep by then. Because it's very slow. I was slightly speeding at the most beautiful music imaginable."[64]

Outside the Opera House, LSD was back in multimedia theatre. In 1984, the controversial SoHo-based Wooster Group performed an experimental play: *L.S.D. (… Just the High Points …)*. *L.S.D.* featured audio excerpts from psychedelic luminaries, and it was partly intended to dramatize the Sixties without giving in to nostalgia. But the play was more than a work of art documenting history, and, for the third part, the crew had taken acid for a rehearsal and videotaped themselves under the influence. They then watched the tape and attempted to recreate

THE SIXTIES HAPPENED IN THE SEVENTIES | 193

their actions and moods on stage, where they depicted the initial rush of the drug, followed by the inevitable coming down.[65]

Back in Greenwich Village, there was an even stronger nod to the psychedelic culture of the Sixties. In 1988, Jacaeber Kastor, an acquaintance of Isaac Abrams, organized an art exhibition at the Psychedelic Solution Gallery. But rather than involving classic canvas, this was "blotter art," a collection of sheets of small squares with drawings on them. Here, the acid was chemically neutralized, and the art works were not for sale. The sheets were decorated with various symbols like "zodiac signs, whirling planets, silver bolts of lightning and purple half-moons."[66]

The gallery was a successful venture and a popular place for acid heads. Its customers included celebrities like Whoopi Goldberg, Iggy Pop, and John McEnroe. However, a lot of the art available had come a long way from the classic psychedelic paintings of the Sixties and had acquired a somewhat unsettling touch. "Spiders and severed limbs are motifs of choice for many ... artists" and could be found on a wide range of supports such as "rod-riding, surfing, tattooing, carny art, and, of course, commix." Charles Manson's favourite artist, Joe Coleman, had a painting that displayed "an intricately executed study in rotting, carbuncular flesh" that sold for a staggering $7,000. For Kastor, this aesthetic shift resulted from the demise of psychedelic idealism, and perhaps it was an attempt to convey the feeling of decay that prevailed in the metropolis.[67]

With the relative scarcity of quality psychedelics, a new generation of drugs with no legal status entered New York's psychoactive bazaar. These drugs could be used for recreational purposes, but others, probably familiar with the history of drug-based religions, used them in structured rituals. In 1980, Alan Birnbaum founded the Temple of the True Inner Light and took participants through psychedelic sessions. This occurred after Birnbaum had a revelatory experience with DET, which convinced him that "the psychedelic is a pure light being and primeval ... also being God the Creator." Subsequently, he guided sessions using DPT (N,N-Dipropyltryptamine) in the temple's Lower East Side storefront. Its catechism was a kind of Christian revisionism that held DPT "as an actual manifestation or physical form of God." By 1987, however, DPT had been outlawed.[68]

Ed Rosenfeld remembered that people were trying compounds like 2-CB (2,5-dimethoxy-4-bromophenethylamine) and the energizing, euphoria-inducing, and mildly psychedelic MDMA. The drug, also known as ecstasy, was synthesized some time before 1912 by Merck, but it was only in the 1950s that it became reconsidered for the purpose of chemical brainwashing. MDMA did not enjoy the same fate as LSD, however. In the 1960s, it was eclipsed by the similar MDA, but MDMA enjoyed a major comeback in the 1980s after it crossed the Atlantic courtesy of British DJs and landed in New York's gay club scene. Soon after, the rave phenomenon was underway in the UK and likewise reached New York in 1989. In the meantime, MDMA had become a Schedule I drug.[69]

On one occasion, Rosenfeld took it in the East Village, which was finally undergoing urban renewal and cashing in on its subcultural edge.[70] "I took it at my apartment with a friend," he remembered, "and I lived where you can see this development, which has red brick. And I've never seen a brick face [laughs], like I did on ADAM ... I had a friend who did light-shows here in the City. And there was a huge scene. An ecstasy scene. I was never part of that. I knew what was going on. I wasn't taking ecstasy and dancing."[71]

In the following decade, New Yorkers were using MDMA along with LSD and marijuana to enhance the pleasure of dancing in waist-high foam at the Limelight in Chelsea. A few years later, however, the nightclub routinely found its doors padlocked by the police because of rampant MDMA use,[72] while another Manhattan club needed to hire private ambulances to take overdosed users to hospital.[73] During the mid-1990s rave scene, an LSD-MDMA cocktail appeared, but dealers soon discarded acid because MDMA was far more profitable.[74] It was cheap to manufacture, and a dose sold for around $20 in New York City clubs. Later, the police dismantled an Israeli drug ring that had reportedly sold 100,000 tablets weekly.[75]

Meanwhile, Lotsof's movement gathered even more support after Black Panther and practising Muslim Dhoruba al-Mujahid bin Wahad was released from prison on 23 March 1990 after the State Supreme Court overturned his twenty-five-year-to-life prison sentence for attempted murder of two NYPD officers. Wahad had been actively involved in curbing heroin use among Black New Yorkers, and he met Dana Beal, who gave him a summary of information on ibogaine.[76] Entangled with legal issues over pot trafficking, Beal nonetheless organized a protest to "Storm NIDA for Ibogaine" on 10 July.[77]

THE SIXTIES HAPPENED IN THE SEVENTIES | 195

After the first hints of favourable media coverage, Wahad openly endorsed the ibogaine movement in 1992 when he claimed that ibogaine did not violate Muslim teachings and that it could be used to cure addiction.[78] In August 1992, Beal prepared an ibogaine workbook for a Harlem Hospital workshop[79] and made plans to lobby for a community-based ibogaine trial in Harlem a year later. Wahad was also keen to show the Black community the existing data on ibogaine, which suggested that the drug had little potential for abuse.[80]

Of course, Lotsof could not hold back the tide of addiction, but his movement nonetheless allowed ibogaine to re-enter the conversation about the medical potential of psychedelics. For NYU professor of psychiatry and neurology Kenneth Alper, "[Lotsof's] greatest achievement was in inducing the National Institute on Drug Abuse to undertake a research project on ibogaine that produced scores of peer-reviewed publications and paved the way for FDA approval of a clinical trial," even though the trial was never completed because of a lack of funding and ibogaine remains a federally banned substance.[81] For all its potential, then, ibogaine could not find a place in New York's drug scene.

Around the same time, several drug experts suggested that LSD was enjoying a mild comeback among young people, like a teenager who claimed that the drug was easy to acquire in those days.[82] A twenty-one-year-old musician who experimented with LSD declared that it was "something akin to Eastern meditation" and that it had put him "in harmony with the earth." But not all of them enjoyed the experience. In Manhattan, one twenty-year-old tried the drug and underwent a spell of mild paranoia, with visions of a white spider crawling up a friend's back.[83]

In 1992, NIDA investigated the supposed resurgence of LSD at the time but concluded that a nationwide epidemic was highly unlikely.[84] However, the drug was still available in New York. In 1997, the police arrested a drug suspect in Queens after discovering an LSD factory in the Far Rockaway area. It was the biggest bust in more than a decade. There, agents found 700,000 doses with an estimated retail value of between $2 and $3 million, and they subsequently discovered another house where psilocybin mushrooms were grown.[85] In 2011, thirteen were caught selling acid to Columbia students. The undercover agent responsible for the arrests reported that one suspect had made plans to kidnap a rival dealer from Queens and torture him with LSD.[86]

The continued availability of acid was accompanied by the rise of "designer drugs." After psychedelics were prohibited in the United States and controlled by the United Nations' Convention on Psychotropic Substances in the early 1970s, chemists developed derivatives that circumvented the legislation and allowed dealers to stay one step ahead of the law. The Internet has since played a critical role in the worldwide distribution of these substances, and authorities have struggled to effectively curb access to them on "Dark" websites, in spite of the 1986 Federal Analog Act and the 2012 Synthetic Drug Abuse Prevention Act.[87] This legal loophole allowed Rosenfeld to discover 4-ACO-DET (3-[2-(Dimethylamino)ethyl]-1H-indol-4-yl acetate). Following Albert Hofmann's injunction to take 25μgrs of LSD daily, he took 5mlgrs of 4-ACO daily for a while (the recommended does is closer to 20mlgrs) and had "a grand old time."[88]

In the 2010s, these grey market substances became popular alternatives to the "classic" psychedelics because they allowed prospective users to choose from one or more according to their effects and according to the setting at the time of consumption. In a context of urban density, some might want to enjoy a short-acting trip with minimum visions or without introspective moments. For instance, New Yorkers could turn on with an "N-bomb" that was close to LSD in its effects but much shorter (and a dose cost a measly dollar). "In New York," one user claimed, "you can't give acid away – it's an entire day: 'I have to do laundry,' 'I need to see this person,' it sucks. The N-bomb is less intellectual and about giant God questions than LSD, and a little bit more in your body – great for dates or art museums."[89]

In fact, museums and galleries continued to offer an important platform for psychedelia. In 2007, the Whitney hosted the *Summer of Love* exhibition (initially organized by the Tate Liverpool), which featured the works of several psychedelic artists. Abrams's *All Things Are One Thing* was hung up on banners on Park Avenue, "almost like an icon." Abrams immensely enjoyed the show, not least for its absence of anything by Warhol.[90] Gerd Stern was equally enthusiastic, praising the exhibition's "very complete catalogue of experiences by artists and other persona."[91]

In spite of psychedelia's apparent unravelling at the turn of the 1960s, it did not leave the metropolis. Isaac Abrams, the historian rather than the painter, believes that an extensive focus on the Sixties significantly diminishes what happened in the following decade. "From 67 and so on, into the 70s, was really where a lot of things were happening," he comments. "I think people were probably taking more acid in the 70s, than they were in 65, definitely. So the 60s happened in the 70s, really."[92]

Still, there is an element of truth in Brad's observation that the Seventies were "a terrible time"[93] because the drug scenes were then dominated by heroin and cocaine. The following decade only added to this impression. The crack epidemic among Black working-class communities was another gruesome illustration of survival and escapism through narcotics. The tragedy of addiction and the social problems that came along naturally drew most of the attention of the time, and it is no surprise that very few histories of psychedelia are set after the Sixties. For even as scores of New Yorkers shot up, snorted, and smoked, others continued to explore the old and new psychedelic drugs and to find meaning in them.

In fairness, the idea that psychedelics were inherently part of the 1960s and that they disappeared with that decade is nothing new. That heroin, crack, and coke dominated the Manhattan drug scene so strongly in the 1970s and 1980s undoubtedly cemented this impression, and this is probably what spurred the art world to examine psychedelia as a thing of the past. The exhibitions at the Psychedelic Solution Gallery as well as the Wooster Group's take on the psychedelic Sixties approached LSD retrospectively as a cultural phenomenon firmly rooted in a particular era. Besides, the negative responses Lotsof drew from NIDA in relation to ibogaine also suggest that Leary's dream of a chemical revolution had survived the Sixties and was preventing sober reappraisals of psychedelic substances.

After New Yorkers discovered these vision-inducing plants and chemicals during the Cold War, they never left the city's unique, broad, and perpetually evolving psychoactive marketplace. As these drugs move inexorably out of illegality and promise improved mental health and spiritual life, the story of psychedelic New York illustrates the fascination and enthusiasm they exerted for more than half a century and points to a viable psychedelic future.

A Wave That Never Rolled Back

There is an oft-quoted moment in Hunter Thompson's *Fear and Loathing in Las Vegas* when his fictitious alter ego Raoul Duke reflects on the San Francisco acid scene of the mid-Sixties. "There was madness in any direction, at any hour ... You could strike sparks anywhere. There was a fantastic universal sense that whatever we were doing was *right*, that we were winning." Those who were fortunate enough to have lived through the era were filled with a sense of momentum that would lead to their inevitable triumph over the forces of evil. They were riding a powerful wave that seemed unstoppable at the time. But the wave did not quite reach the capital of gambling.

"So now, less than five years later, you can go up on a steep hill in Las Vegas and look West, and with the right kind of eyes you can almost *see* the high water mark – that place where the wave finally broke and rolled back."[1]

Although Thompson was more intent on literary licence than historical accuracy, this is the kind of reflection that has strengthened San Francisco's position as the psychedelic Mecca of the Sixties. His metaphor has another obvious implication: the acid wave that came from the West Coast was powerful enough to reach the outer rim of Nevada but not what he saw as the dark underbelly of the American

Dream. Nixon's silent majority had won. The psychedelic revolution had failed.

Had Thompson looked east instead, admittedly with a pair of even sharper eyes, he might have seen a different kind of wave: one that began in the early 1950s with experimental investigations into psychedelic compounds; gathered momentum as Bohemian New Yorkers encountered psychoactive plants and chemicals; swelled in the early Sixties as they discovered LSD; and seemed to pull back after the crest of the final years of the decade, revealing burnt-out acid heads on the shoreline.

But it never actually retreated, and in the following decades New York was still riding the initial wave of the Sixties, albeit without Thompson's psychedelic exceptionalism. The idea that psychedelia was a powerful revolutionary force that was ultimately crushed by a conservative backlash and the war on drugs ignores a much deeper history of LSD and psychedelics that reveals that these drugs permeated just about every facet of American society from the postwar period onward.

And it is a story that involves a number of people who would have taken Thompson by surprise. Where psychedelia has often been associated with colourful rock bands and wide-eyed baby boomers, New York's psychedelic culture features a broad cast of characters like Diane di Prima, Isaac and Rachel Abrams, Jean Houston, Henry Luce, Jackie Cassen and Rudi Stern, Lauretta Bender, Richard Goldstein, Bernard Friedman, Mabel Dodge Luhan, Paul Hoch, Peggy Hitchcock, Howard Lotsof, Ed Rosenfeld, and Nina Graboi.

It is a story that involves an equally wide array of locations like the Natural Church, the *East Village Other*, Cerebrum, the Department of Experimental Psychiatry, Madison Avenue, the Center for the League of Spiritual Discovery, as well as all the apartments, head shops, bars, nightclubs, lofts, and penthouses in which New Yorkers were navigating the confines of their consciousness. All these places allowed this rich psychedelic culture to nurture supportive space for drug use, explore syncretic forms of spirituality, create alternative media outlets, treat mental illness, dance to the latest hits, and earn a living.

Such diversity is a fitting reflection of this prominent landing spot for Jews, Britons, and Indians, who significantly shaped the local psychedelic culture. Thanks to the under- and above-ground media, New Yorkers from very diverse backgrounds became interested in the psychedelic experience. Well-off New Yorkers who wished to sample LSD only needed to speak to their analyst or mingle with high society, while Bohemians could simply wander around Greenwich Village or Central Park to make contact. Drug dealers easily moved acid in and out of the city, and in some instances they received the help of the upper class. But in a city that has harboured gross socio-economic inequalities over the centuries, psychedelia did little to reach out to working-class and ethnic New Yorkers.

New York's distinctive influence on psychedelia only explains this level of sophistication in part, however. Just as important was the power of the psychedelic drug experience to obliterate ontological certainties and cultural frames of references, and many New Yorkers gave new directions to their lives after experimenting with LSD and like drugs. It allowed Nina Graboi to see through the veil of the American Dream and become a bridge between young experimenters and their troubled parents. It allowed Isaac Abrams to develop a highly original type of art, even though he had never painted anything beforehand. It allowed Bernard Friedman to leave a highly successful position in real estate to become a full-time writer. These drugs certainly magnified the psyches of their users and the environment in which they took these drugs, but there was nevertheless something fundamentally unpredictable at the heart of the experience.

Even then, these fascinating stories point to an unnerving question: what of the countless number of New Yorkers who have experimented with LSD and psychedelics over the decades? On the one hand, they are further proof that a limited focus on radical psychedelia overlooks this incredibly broad range of users, their ways of taking drugs, and their incentives for taking drugs. On the other hand, they suggest that psychedelic drug use was so commonplace that there was nothing particularly controversial or subterranean about it, in spite of the legislative attacks that made these drugs illegal. In this way, the notion of a psychedelic "drug culture" reads like a tautology.[2]

As cannabis moves toward legalization in the United States and as some local jurisdictions begin to decriminalize psychedelics, the idea that LSD, MDMA, DMT, and psilocybin will soon be legally available for consumption no longer seems like a pipe dream. Present-day New York features psychedelic research centres, ayahuasca ceremonies, conferences, and grass-roots activism, which echo the enthusiasm that swept similar circles during the postwar period. Although disputes surrounding the ultimate purpose of the psychedelic experience remain, contemporary psychedelia is unfolding in a far more serene way and points to a gradual integration of psychedelic knowledge into society. But that should not come as a surprise, given that the Sixties happened sixty years ago.

When psychedelics entered New York's psychoactive marketplace, by contrast, very little was known about the effects they might have on society. Given the cultural context of the time, however, they appealed to curious New Yorkers who were looking for meaningful experiences. As a woman who began taking drugs at the heart of the Cold War, Diane di Prima felt incredibly lucky to have been able to engage in boundless psychoactive experimentation. "It is hard," she wrote decades later, "in our present era of self-righteousness, to even begin to imagine what drugs and the taking of drugs meant to us in the late 1950s. How special and, indeed, precious it was – what promise it held."[3]

Nina Graboi would have agreed. On a personal level, she immensely benefitted from exploring her inner space and became a much happier person as a result. But she also believed that LSD had allowed so many Americans to reach previously unattainable heights of consciousness. "More people than ever before have entered states of awareness that were formerly reserved to mystics, saints, and the rare inspired artist … a bridge to the divine has been built."[4] Isaac Abrams, for one, enjoyed several psychedelic experiences that were profoundly unifying: "Such as the unity of the planet, the unity of the biosphere, and the actual consciousness of the biosphere – the sense that the biosphere has consciousness."[5]

As an artist who has been painting psychedelic art for more than five decades, Abrams has hugely profited from his life-changing psychoactive experimentation, and so has Susun Weed, who happens to live five minutes away from his home in upstate New York. After the 1960s, she became fascinated by herbal medicine, and she has since authored six books, the Wise Woman Herbal Series. LSD showed Susun the deeply interconnected web of life and helped her to craft a new – but ancient – mindset around healing and health. The Wise Woman tradition, as she articulates in *Healing Wise*,[6] encourages the use of simple, local healing agents, especially weeds, to nourish health. "Herbal medicine is people's medicine," says Weed. "That's what LSD taught me and I've been teaching others to recognize and use green blessings ever since."[7]

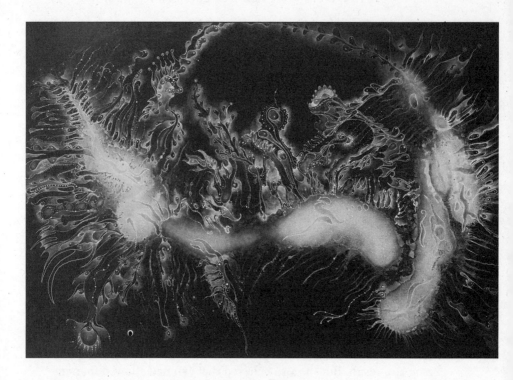

Figure 9.1 White Light Fungal Delight, 2022

Others have more nuanced views on the benefits of the psychedelic experience, but all acknowledge its unique power. Ed Rosenfeld was thrilled when he discovered psychedelics, but in hindsight he may have been a bit careless. "I was naïve and over-enthusiastic and oversimplified the result that I had expected," he admitted. "So in that sense I have changed. I still think psychedelics are wonderful. I don't think they are for everybody. At the time, I was much more indiscriminative and I thought probably everybody could take them. Now I see that that may not be the case and be more judicious."[8] Stanley Krippner is even more cautious and believes in a more restricted use for these drugs. "My position is very conservative," he openly concedes. "It only should be used for research, especially creativity and psychotherapy. And that was my position then, it's my position now. There are other ways of having fun, which are less dangerous, legal, and more productive."[9]

Amelie Edwards certainly had a lot of fun with LSD. In retrospect, she regrets some aspects of her life as a runaway, but in spite of her misfortunes in the East Village, she also sees long-lasting positive changes. "It just made me less afraid of taking chances overall," she believes. "Just the fact that I could handle it led me to believe that I could handle almost anything. I've been to war, to front-lines in wars in my life, and everything. I've been to Sarajevo, to the front-lines there. And I was able to handle that." But on the other hand she still gets upset about little things.[10]

Rachel Abrams did not face the horror of war zones, but she did manage to deal with her fear of snakes, thanks to mescaline. Perhaps more important, she believes that her life-changing psychedelic experiences awakened her spirituality. "In a certain way [pauses], you can never get back there," she claims. "Even with a spiritual path, doing whatever the spiritual work I do, which is not very much anymore – a little meditation here and there. Mainly it's following something here inside." Although her ex-husband made the most of the psychedelic visions by becoming an artist, the otherworldly colours and lights have never left her: "When I make my jewellery, I love to work with these iridescent jewels – I don't even like to wear jewellery, but iridescence. Color. Sparkling color."[11] Almost seventy year after Huxley's writings, then, gemstones and diamonds continue to offer a transcendental bridge into the visionary world.

This points to an even longer tradition of transcendentalism, according to Richard Goldstein. Ideas of non-violence, pantheism, and anti-Puritanism are "embedded in American consciousness," and they were rekindled at the height of psychedelia. And the instant Nirvana of the psychedelic experience also has a much longer tradition of shortcuts that he traces right back to Alexis de Tocqueville's observations on American culture. "He writes about the grandiosity of American culture. Acid culture is grandiose. Look at Tocqueville you can see acid culture in its proto state. Certainly in the Transcendentalists."[12]

Regardless of its origins, Ed Rosenfeld had envisioned a bright future for psychedelia, and he was delighted to learn that historians were taking the topic seriously: "Well, I'm pleased to see that people are still doing research in the field and trying to select and make clear some of the things that went on, because there is a rich history … So I'm excited. These are good times. Things are looking up."

LSD and psychedelics indeed have a rich legacy, and the story of psychedelic New York does reveal an incredibly broad impact on postwar society. But these drugs were also significant in other, less obvious ways, according to writer Paul Krassner. "LSD was influencing music, painting, spirituality – and the stock market. Tim Leary once let me listen in on a call from a Wall Street broker thanking him for turning him on to acid because it gave him the courage to sell short."[13] And that, I hope, is a fitting quote to end this book.

Acknowledgments

This book results from research I began in the early 2010s at the University of Saskatchewan. I had the immense pleasure of working with Professor Erika Dyck, who saw potential in my project early on, fully supported it with her Canada Research Chair funds, and expertly guided me through the process. Over the years, we continued to work together, but more important, she continued to offer her help, kindness, generosity, and enthusiasm.

At Usask, my academic training was greatly enhanced by the classes I took with Erika Dyck, Martha Smith-Norris, and Keith Carlson, who introduced me to historical research. I also benefitted from the intellectual support of Lindsey Banco, Frank Klaassen, Mark Meyers, and Martha Smith-Norris. Many thanks, as well, to the friendly staff and colleagues of the History Department at Usask.

At the University of Queensland, another influential scholar I would like to acknowledge is Sylvie Shaw, who introduced me to the scientific study of altered states of consciousness through rigorously empirical scholarship. My thanks also go to Chris Dixon (then also at UQ) for his class on the 1960s, which gave me an early taste of the complexity of that decade.

This book greatly benefitted from the feedback of David Farber, who offered constructive suggestions to improve it by underscoring how New York's unique cultural landscape influenced its psychedelic culture.

206 | ACKNOWLEDGMENTS

My gratitude goes to the helpful staff at the archives that I consulted for this project – UC Santa Cruz, UC Berkeley, Stanford, CUNY, NYU, NYPL, Columbia, Kent State, and Purdue. I would also like to thank all the people who were interviewed for this book. Some interviewees, however, did a little more than just share their recollections, and Gerd Stern, Isaac Abrams, Stanley Krippner, and Amelie Edwards helped me to identify new leads. Ed Rosenfeld was another fascinating source of knowledge, but he did not live to see this book finished. I hope that his family and friends have enjoyed reading about his involvement in psychedelic New York. I would also like to thank all the people who have uploaded their transcripts of interviews and digitalized other sources on the Internet.

This manuscript has immensely benefitted from the blind reviewers of McGill-Queen's University Press, who saw promise in the first draft but rightly advised a complete rewriting. Many thanks to Kyla Madden for her continued editorial support and her thoughtful suggestions for improvements and to the helpful staff at MQUP.

Over the course of my research, I had the opportunity to meet people who helped in various ways and with whom I had productive conversations: Jeremy Varon, Nicolas Langlitz, Matt Oram, Peter Collopy, Lucas Richert, Tehseen Noorani, Thomas Lannon, Dan Graboi, Ivo Gurschler, Nicholas Meriwether, Ido Hartogsohn, Torsten Passie, Rex Weiner, John McMillan, Ralph Abraham, Jesse Jarnow, Larry Vigus, Stephen Snelders, Susun Weed, Kali Carrigan, Graham Mushnik, Rodolphe Catoire, and Amy Fletcher. Apologies to those I might have forgotten.

Many thanks as well to my family for their support over the years. I am particularly grateful to my parents, Steve and Annick, who were farsighted enough to bring me up speaking both French and English. A particular mention also goes to my English grandmother Barbara. Her enthusiasm over the years was a major source of inspiration.

For the index of this book, I received the invaluable help of my friend Audrey Meunier, who was only too happy to oblige.

Finally, a very special acknowledgment goes to my old friend Pierre Morel, who introduced me to the topic back in 2006. Sans ton étincelle, ce livre n'aurait pas vu le jour.

Notes

IF YOU'RE GOING TO NEW YORK CITY

1 William O'Neill, *Coming Apart: An Informal History of America in the 1960's* (New York: Times Books, 1971); Edward J. Bacciocco, *The New Left in America: Reform to Revolution: 1956–70* (Stanford: Hoover Institution Press, 1974); Todd Gitlin, *The Sixties: Years of Hope, Days of Rage* (New York: Bantam Books, 1987); Maurice Isserman and Michael Kazin, *America Divided: The Civil War of the 1960s* (New York: Oxford University Press, 2003).

2 As an exception based on some outstanding oral histories, see Jesse Jarnow, *Heads: A Biography of Psychedelic America* (Philadelphia: Da Capo Press, 2016).

3 Albert Hofmann, LSD, *My Problem Child: Reflections on Sacred Drugs, Mysticism and Science* (New York: McGraw-Hill, 1980).

4 Steven J. Novak, "LSD before Leary: Sidney Cohen's Critique of 1950s Psychedelic Drug Research," *Isis* 88, no. 1 (1997): 87–110; Erika Dyck, *Psychedelic Psychiatry: LSD: From Clinic to Campus* (Baltimore: Johns Hopkins University Press, 2008); Matthew Oram, *The Trials of Psychedelic Therapy: LSD Psychotherapy in America* (Baltimore: Johns Hopkins University Press, 2018); Ido Hartogsohn, *American Trip: Set, Setting, and the Psychedelic Experience in the Twentieth Century* (Cambridge, MA: MIT Press, 2020); Jesse Donaldson and Erika Dyck, *The Acid Room: The Psychedelic Trials and Tribulations of the Hollywood Hospital* (Vancouver: Anvil Press, 2022).

208 | NOTES TO PAGE 7

5 John Marks, "Intelligence or 'Witches' Potion,'" in *The Search for the "Manchurian Candidate": The CIA and Mind Control: The Secret Story of Behavioural Sciences* (New York: W.W. Norton, 1988), 54–130.

6 John Higgs, *I Have America Surrounded: The Life and Times of Timothy Leary* (Fort Lee, NJ: Barricade Books, 2006); Robert Greenfield, *Timothy Leary: A Biography* (Orlando: Harcourt, 2006); Don Lattin, *The Harvard Psychedelic Club: How Timothy Leary, Ram Dass, Huston Smith, and Andrew Weil Killed the Fifties and Ushered in a New Age for America* (New York: HarperOne, 2011); Chris Elcock, "The Fifth Freedom: The Politics of Psychedelic Patriotism," *Journal for the Study of Radicalism* 9, no. 2 (2015): 17–40.

7 David Farber, "The Intoxicated/Illegal Nation: Drugs in the Sixties Counterculture," in *Imagine Nation: The American Counterculture of the 1960s and '70s*, ed. Peter Braunstein and Michael William Doyle (New York: Routledge, 2002), 17–40.

8 Robert C. Fuller, "Psychedelics and the Metaphysical Illumination," in *Stairways to Heaven: Drugs in American Religious History* (Boulder, CO: Westview, 2000), 51–89; Devin R. Lander, "Start Your Own Religion: New York State's Acid Churches," *Nova Religio: The Journal of Alternative and Emergent Religions* 14, no. 3 (2011): 64–80; Morgan Shipley, *Psychedelic Mysticism: Transforming Consciousness, Religious Experiences, and Voluntary Peasants in Postwar America* (Lanham, MD: Lexington Books, 2015).

9 Aldous Huxley, *The Doors of Perception and Heaven and Hell* (New York: Harper, 2004).

10 Robert E.L. Masters and Jean Houston, eds, *Psychedelic Art* (New York: Grove Press/Balance House, 1968); Christoph Grunenberg and Jonathan Harris, eds, *Summer of Love: Psychedelic Art, Social Crisis and Counterculture in the 1960s* (Liverpool: Liverpool University Press, 2005); Scott B. Montgomery, "Radical Trips: Exploring the Political Dimension and Context of the 1960s Psychedelic Poster," *Journal for the Study of Radicalism* 13, no. 1 (2019): 121–54.

11 The peyote cactus that contains the mescaline alkaloid could still be used by Native American Indians only. Alexander S. Dawson, *The Peyote Effect: From the Inquisition to the War on Drugs* (Oakland: University of California Press, 2018); Mike Jay, *Mescaline: A Global History of the First Psychedelic* (New Haven, CT: Yale University Press, 2019).

12 John R. Neill, "'More Than Medical Significance': LSD and American Psychiatry – 1953 to 1966," *Journal of Psychoactive Drugs* 19, no. 1 (1987): 41; Leigh A. Henderson and William J. Glass, eds, LSD: *Still with Us after All These Years* (New York: Lexington Books, 1994). A sizeable majority of Jesse Jarnow's *Heads* focuses on the psychedelic culture after the 1960s.

13 Oram, *The Trials of Psychedelic Therapy*.

14 Myron Stolaroff, ed., *The Secret Chief: Conversations with a Pioneer of the Underground Psychedelic Therapy Movement* (Charlotte: MAPS, 1997).

NOTES TO PAGES 7–9 | 209

15 Nicolas Langlitz, *Neuropsychedelia: The Revival of Hallucinogen Research Since the Decade of the Brain* (Berkeley: University of California Press, 2013).

16 Robert Forte, ed., *Entheogens and the Future of Religion* (San Francisco: CSP, 1997); William A. Richards, *Sacred Knowledge: Psychedelics and Religious Experiences* (New York: Columbia University Press, 2015).

17 To date, journalists have been the chief investigators of the social history of LSD. See in particular Martin A. Lee and Bruce Shlain, *Acid Dreams: The Complete Social History of LSD: The CIA, the Sixties, and Beyond* (New York: Grove Weidenfeld, 1985); Jay Stevens, *Storming Heaven: LSD and the American Dream* (New York: Perennial Library, 1988); Jarnow, *Heads.*

18 George J. Lankevich, *American Metropolis: A History of New York City* (New York: New York University Press, 1998), ix.

19 Kim Phillips-Fein, *Fear City: New York's Fiscal Crisis and the Rise of Austerity Politics* (New York: Metropolitan Books, 2017).

20 Eric C. Schneider, *Smack: Heroin and the American City* (Philadelphia: University of Pennsylvania Press, 2008); Nicolas Rasmussen, *On Speed: The Many Lives of Amphetamine* (New York: New York University Press, 2009).

21 An exception is Carlo McCormick's short history of New York's psychedelic culture, though his celebratory tone is uncalled for, as is his dismissal of the San Francisco scene, which he sees as "backward" because the work of one New York multimedia art group was dismissed by art critics there. See "The Urban Trip: New York's Psychedelic Moment," in *Summer of Love*, 228.

22 Charles Perry, *The Haight-Ashbury: A History* (New York: Random House, 1984); Jay Stevens, *Storming Heaven: LSD and the American Dream* (New York: Perennial Library, 1988).

23 Christine Stansell, *American Moderns: Bohemian New York and the Creation of a New Century* (New York: Metropolitan Books/Henry Holt & Company, 2000); Ross Wetzsteon, *Republic of Dreams: Greenwich Village, the American Bohemia, 1910–1960* (New York: Simon and Schuster, 2002).

24 Masters and Houston, *Psychedelic Art.*

25 Tom Wolfe, *The Electric Kool-Aid Acid Test* (New York: Picador, 2008).

26 Rick Dodgson, *It's All a Kind of Magic: The Young Ken Kesey* (Madison: University of Wisconsin Press, 2013), 7.

27 Quoted in ibid., 23.

28 Ibid., 140. The fact that Kesey's discovery of LSD was made possible by covert drug testing has added a layer to his legend.

29 Howard D. Fabing, "Fenquel, a Blocking Agent against Experimental LSD-25 and Mescaline Psychosis: Preliminary Note on its Clinical Applications," *Neurology* 5, no. 319 (1955): 328; James L. Goddard, "Injunction Action," *FDA Papers* 2, no. 1 (1968): 44.

30 Anthony K. Busch and Warren C. Johnson, "L.S.D. 25 an Aid in Psychotherapy," *Diseases of the Nervous System* 11, no. 8 (1950): 243; Gordon R. Forrer and Richard D. Goldner, "Experimental Physiological Studies with Lysergic Acid Diethylamide (LSD-25)," *Archives of Neurology* 65, no. 5 (1951): 581; Charles Savage, "Lysergic Acid Diethylamide (LSD-25). A Clinical-Psychological Study," *American Journal of Psychiatry* 108, no. 12 (1952): 900.

31 Peter Stafford, *Psychedelics Encyclopedia* (Berkeley: Ronin, 1992), 42.

32 For biographies of Ginsberg, see Barry Miles, *Ginsberg: A Biography* (New York: Simon & Schuster, 1989); Michael Schumacher, *Dharma Lion: A Biography of Allen Ginsberg* (Minneapolis: University of Minnesota Press, 2016).

33 Tim Scully, "Nick Sand: May 10, 1941–April 24, 2017," Erowid.org, 4 May 2017, https://www.erowid.org/culture/characters/sand_nick/sand_nick_biography2.shtml.

34 As an outstanding exception that focuses on a group of Tennessee acid users and their involvement in New York, see Morgan Shipley, "'This Season's People': Stephen Gaskin, Psychedelic Religion, and a Community of Social Justice," *Journal for the Study of Radicalism* 9, no. 2 (2015): 41–92; as well as Jarnow's *Heads*.

35 This was the case for cannabis smokers, who needed the guidance of peers to learn how to experience the drug. See Howard S. Becker, "Becoming a Marihuana User," in *Outsiders: Studies in the Sociology of Deviance* (New York: Free Press, 1973), 41–58.

36 "New York Medical Unit Says LSD More Dangerous than Heroin," *Jamestown (NY) Post-Journal*, 31 March 1966.

37 Schneider, Smack, 149–50.

38 David T. Courtwright, "The Rise and Fall and Rise of Cocaine in the United States," in *Consuming Habits: Drugs in History and Anthropology*, ed. Jordan Goodman, Paul E. Lovejoy, and Andrew Sheratt (London: Routledge, 2007), 224–5.

39 In the broader history of the Sixties, what are commonly believed to be the trademark movements of the decade, whether progressive or radical, likewise drew most of the attention back then, to a point where conservative activism went barely noticed. As an excellent illustration, see Lisa McGirr, *Suburban Warriors: The Origins of the New American Right* (Princeton, NJ: Princeton University Press, 2001).

40 In this way, this book joins the "long Sixties" scholarship. See, for example, John D'Emilio, *Sexual Politics, Sexual Communities: The Making of a Homosexual Minority in the United States, 1940–1970* (Chicago: University of Chicago Press, 1983); Arthur Marwick, *The Sixties: Cultural Revolution in Britain, France, Italy, and the United States, c.1958–c.1974* (Oxford: Oxford University Press, 1998); Tom Hayden, *The Long Sixties: From 1960 to Barack Obama* (Boulder, CO: Paradigm, 2009).

NOTES TO PAGES 11–13 | 211

41 Oram, *The Trials of Psychedelic Therapy.*

42 Rick Strassman, DMT: *The Spirit Molecule* (Rochester, VT: Park Street Press, 2001).

43 For a focused study on the importance of these variables, see Hartogsohn, *American Trip.*

44 The word has been used freely in a number of books. See, for example, Lee and Shlain, *Acid Dreams*; Timothy Miller, *The Hippies and American Values* (Knoxville: University of Tennessee Press, 1991); Gerald DeGroot, *The 60s Unplugged A Kaleidoscopic History of a Disordered Decade*, 301–6. In his excellent history of Toronto's hip Yorkville quarter, Stuart Henderson points out that "hippie" is a cultural construct and an identity category that fails "to convey much agency on the part of the actor thus labelled." See *Making the Scene: Yorkville and Hip Toronto in the 1960s* (Toronto: University of Toronto Press, 2011), note 2 on page 279.

45 Brad (real name obscured at interviewee's request), interview by the author, interviewee's home, New York City, 16 March 2013.

46 Chuck Gould interviewed by Jay Babcock, Diggers Docs, 2010, Gould's home in Petrolia, CA, https://diggersdocs.home.blog/tag/peggy-hitchcock.

47 For a discussion on the problem of media distortion in the 1960s, which occasionally examines the coverage of "hippies" in the media, see Edward P. Morgan, *What Really Happened to the 1960s: How Mass Media Culture Failed American Democracy* (Lawrence: University Press of Kansas, 2010). See in particular pages 150–2.

48 As quoted in Karen M. Staller, *Runaways: How the Sixties Counterculture Shaped Today's Practices and Policies* (New York: Columbia University Press, 2006). On pages 36–41, Staller offers an informative overview of the media coverage of the word.

49 Art Kleps, "Freemen!" in Kleps, *Millbrook: A Narrative of the Early Years of American Psychedelianism, Recension of 2005* (San Francisco: Original Kleptonian Neo-American Church, 2005), page unavailable, accessed 10 November 2014, http://okneoac.org/millbrook. David Courtwright and colleagues have also pointed out that none of the former heroin addicts they interviewed ever considered themselves to be "junkies." David Courtwright, Herman Joseph, and Don Des Jarlais, eds, *Addicts Who Survived: An Oral History of Narcotic Use in America before 1965* (Knoxville: University of Tennessee Press, 2012), 31–2.

50 Ernie Barry to editor, *Village Voice*, 3 July 1969.

51 Ann Ward, letter to the *East Village Other* 2, no. 12, 15 May–1 June 1967.

52 As a prime example, see Lewis S. Feuer, *The Conflict of Generations: The Character and Significance of Student Movements* (New York: Basic Books, 1969). Many of the protest movements have been remembered as inherently youthful, and age was a convenient explanation for their failure. For more on the young and politics in the Sixties, see Holly V.

Scott, *Younger Than That Now: The Politics of Age in the 1960s* (Amherst: University of Massachusetts Press, 2016).

53 Stansell, *American Moderns*, 93.

54 Dick Schaap, "The Cure for All Their 'Hang-ups,'" *World Journal Tribune*, 13 October 1966, folder "College Drug Scandals," box 3, Peter Stafford papers, Rare Book & Manuscript Library, Columbia University in the City of New York [hereafter "Stafford papers"].

55 Dick Schaap, "College Drug Scene: Almost Anything Goes," *World Journal Tribune*, 14 October 1966, folder "College Drug Scandals," box 3, Stafford papers.

56 See for instance Reginald G. Smart and Dianne Fejer, "Illicit LSD Users: Their Social Backgrounds, Drug Use and Psychopathology," *Journal of Health and Social Behavior* 10, no. 4 (1969): 297–308.

57 The Leary papers reveal that Americans of all ages and backgrounds were interested in his work. Timothy Leary papers, Manuscripts and Archives Division, New York Public Library [hereafter "Leary papers"].

58 Stephen Siff, *Acid Hype: American News Media and the Psychedelic Experience* (Urbana: University of Illinois Press, 2015), 1–2. For a biography of Henry Luce, see Alan Brinkley, *The Publisher: Henry Luce and His American Century* (New York: Alfred A. Knopf, 2010).

59 Erika Dyck, "'Just Say Know': Criminalizing LSD and the Politics of Psychedelic Expertise, 1961–8," in *The Real Dope: Social, Legal, and Historical Perspectives on the Regulation of Drugs in Canada*, ed. Edgar-André Montigny (Toronto: University of Toronto Press, 2011), 169–206; Marcel Martel, "Setting Boundaries: LSD Use and Glue Sniffing in Ontario in the 1960s," in *The Real Dope*, 197–218.

60 See endnote 1.

61 M.J. Heale, "The Sixties as History: A Review of the Political Historiography," *Reviews in American History* 33, no. 1 (2005): 136–7.

62 For similar approaches that pay attention to the complexity and pluralism of the New Left in the 1960s, see Doug Rossinow, *The Politics of Authenticity: Liberalism, Christianity, and the New Left in America* (New York: Columbia University Press, 1998); Joshua Clark Davis, *From Headshops to Whole Foods: The Rise and Fall of Activist Entrepreneurs* (New York: Columbia University Press, 2017).

63 Hartogsohn, *American Trip*.

64 See Nicholas Bromell, *Tomorrow Never Knows: Rock and Psychedelics in the 1960s* (Chicago: University of Chicago Press, 2000); Michael J. Kramer, *The Republic of Rock: Music and Citizenship in the Sixties Counterculture* (New York: Oxford University Press, 2017).

CHAPTER ONE

1 For more on the pharmaceutical industry's role in the spread of drug abuse, see David Herzberg, *White Market Drugs: Big Pharma and the*

Hidden History of Addiction in America (Chicago: University of Chicago Press, 2020).

2 Ted Gioia, *The History of Jazz* (New York: Oxford University Press, 1998), 204. See also Scott DeVeaux, *The Birth of Bebop: A Social and Musical History* (Berkeley: University of California Press, 1997); Eddie S. Meadows, *Bebop to Cool: Context, Ideology, and Musical Identity* (Westport, CT: Greenwood, 2003).

3 Schneider, *Smack*, 24.

4 Leslie Fishbein, "The Culture of Contradiction: The Greenwich Village Rebellion," in *Greenwich Village: Culture and Counterculture*, ed. Rick Beard and Leslie Berlowitz (New Brunswick, NJ: Rutgers University Press, 1993), 220.

5 Mel van Elteren, "The Subculture of the Beats: A Sociological Revisit," *Journal of American Culture* 22, no. 3 (1999): 82.

6 David T. Courtwright, *Dark Paradise: Opiate Addiction in America before 1940* (Cambridge, MA: Harvard University Press, 1982), 64.

7 H.H. Kane, "American Opium-Smokers," *Harper's Weekly*, 24 September 1881.

8 Harry Hubbell Kane, "A Hashish House in New York," *Harper's Monthly*, November 1883.

9 Courtwright, *Dark Paradise*, 84. The opium smoking subculture has a less obvious linguistic heritage: the word "hip" actually refers to the opium pipe that lies on the hip of the smoker. In the postwar era, the word evolved to signify being privy to drug use. See Ned Polsky, *Hustlers, Beats, and Others* (New York: Lyons Press, 1998), 145–6.

10 Courtwright, *Dark Paradise*, 36.

11 Joseph F. Spillane, *Cocaine: From Medical Marvel to Modern Menace in the United States, 1884–1920.* (Baltimore: Johns Hopkins University Press, 2002).

12 Ibid., 91.

13 Courtwright, *Dark Paradise*, 98.

14 David F. Musto, "The Harrison Act," in *The American Disease: Origins of Narcotic Control* (New York: Oxford University Press, 1999), 54–68.

15 Harrington had studied with Franz Boas at Columbia University at a time when New York City was a major hub for anthropology. Beginning in 1842, the metropolis was the home of the American Ethnological Society, which was formally incorporated in 1916 as it was becoming closely associated with Columbia and developing new ties at home and abroad. A brief overview is offered here: https://americanethnologist. org/about/history (accessed 17 June 2022).

16 Wetzsteon, *Republic of Dreams*, 62.

17 Ferenc Erős, "Psychoanalysis and the Emigration of Central and Eastern European Intellectuals," *American Journal of Psychoanalysis* 76, no. 4 (2016): 399–413.

214 | NOTES TO PAGES 21–5

18 Wetzsteon, *Republic of Dreams*, 22.

19 Ibid., 34.

20 Mabel Dodge Luhan, excerpt from *Movers and Shakers*, in *Shaman Woman, Mainline Lady: Women's Writings on the Drug Experience*, ed. Cynthia Palmer and Michael Horowitz (New York: William Morrow, 1982), 113–18.

21 Dawson, *The Peyote Effect*, 38–9.

22 Alwyn Knauer and William J.M.A. Maloney, "A Preliminary Note on the Psychic Action of Mescalin, with Special Reference to the Mechanism of Visual Hallucinations," read before the New York Neurological Society, 6 March 1913. Published in the *Journal of Nervous and Mental Disease* 40 (1913): 425–36.

23 Carleton Simon, "Survey of the Narcotic Problem," *Journal of the American Medical Association* 82, no. 9 (1924): 675–9.

24 Schneider, *Smack*, 5. By contrast, most nineteenth-century morphine addicts were women. See Courtwright, *Dark Paradise*, 36–41.

25 Courtwright et al, *Addicts Who Survived*, 289–90.

26 Schneider, *Smack*, 6.

27 Lankevich, *American Metropolis*, 146.

28 Stansell, *American Moderns*, 82.

29 George Chauncey, "Long-Haired Men and Short-Haired Women," in *Greenwich Village*, 155–6.

30 Stephen R. Duncan, *The Rebel Café: Sex, Race, and Politics in Cold War America's Nightclub Underground* (Baltimore: Johns Hopkins University Press, 2018), 59.

31 Schneider, *Smack*, 9.

32 David T. Courtwright, "A Century of American Narcotic Policy," in *Treating Drug Problems*, vol. 2: *Commissioned Papers on Historical, Institutional, and Economic Contexts of Drug Treatment*, ed. Dean R. Gerstein and Henrick J. Harwood (Washington, DC: National Academies Press, 1992), 4.

33 Siff, *Acid Hype*, 22–6.

34 O.W., excerpt from *No Bed of Roses: The Diary of a Lost Soul*, in *Shaman Woman*, 130. Though urban working-class men supplanted middle-class women as the most visible category beset by narcotics in the early twentieth century, medical authorities continued to ascribe an inherently feminine quality to addiction as late as the 1930s. See Mara L. Keire, "Dope Fiends and Degenerates: The Gendering of Addiction in the Early Twentieth Century," *Journal of Social History* 31, no. 4 (1998): 809–22.

35 Lankevich, *American Metropolis*, 163.

36 Michael Hotz, ed., *Holding the Lotus to the Rock: The Autobiography of Sokei-an, America's First Zen Master* (New York: Four Walls Eight Windows, 2002), 11–14. Quotation on p. 13.

NOTES TO PAGES 25–8 | 215

37 For more on this, see Nellie L. Thompson, "The Transformation of Psychoanalysis in America: Emigré Analysts and the New York Psychoanalytic Society and Institute, 1935–1961," *Journal of the American Psychoanalytic Association* 60, no. 1 (2012): 9–44.
38 Sue A. Shapiro, "The History of the William Alanson White Institute Sixty Years after Thompson," *Contemporary Psychoanalysis* 53, no. 1 (2017): 48.
39 Kenneth Eisold, "The Splitting of the New York Psychoanalytic Society and the Construction of Psychoanalytic Authority," *The International Journal of Psycho-Analysis* 79, no. 5 (1998): 871–85.
40 Ronald Sukenick, *Down and In: Life in the Underground* (New York: Collier Books, 1988), 32.
41 Duncan, *The Rebel Café*, 37–8.
42 Ibid., 43.
43 William D. Armstrong and John Parascandola, "American Concern over MARIHUANA in the 1930's," *Pharmacy in History* 14, no. 1 (1972): 25–35. For a biography of Harry Anslinger, see Alexandra Chasin, *Assassin of Youth: A Kaleidoscopic History of Harry J. Anslinger's War on Drugs* (Chicago: University of Chicago Press, 2016).
44 DeVeaux, *The Birth of Bebop*, 188.
45 Schneider, *Smack*, 18–21.
46 Mayor LaGuardia's Committee on Marihuana, "The Marihuana Problem in the City of New York," The New York Academy of Medicine, City of New York, 1944, available at http://www.druglibrary.org/schaffer/library/studies/lag/lagmenu.htm.
47 Rasmussen, *On Speed*, 87.
48 Ibid., 91–3.
49 Florrie Fisher, excerpt from *The Lonely Trip back*, in *Shaman Woman*, 153.
50 Rasmussen, *On Speed*, 94–5.
51 Barry Miles, "The Beat Generation in the Village," in *Greenwich Village*, 169.
52 Jerome Poynton, "Biographical Sketch," in *The Herbert Huncke Reader*, ed. Benjamin G. Schaffer (New York: Morrow, 1997), xx–xxiii.
53 Rasmussen, *On Speed*, 96.
54 Carolyn Cassady, *Off the Road: Twenty Years with Neal Cassady, Jack Kerouac, and Allen Ginsberg* (New York: Overlook Press, 2008), 23.
55 Gerd Stern, interview by the author, Greenwich Village apartment, New York City, 5 March 2013. For more on this, see Janet Hadda, "Ginsberg in Hospital," *American Imago* 65, no. 2 (2008): 229–59.
56 Gerd Stern, "From Beat Scene Poet to Psychedelic Multimedia Artist in San Francisco and Beyond, 1948–1978," interview by Victoria Morris Byerly, 2001, 7, The Bancroft Library, University of California, Berkeley, Regional Oral History Office.

216 | NOTES TO PAGES 29–32

57 Miles, "The Beat Generation in the Village," 170.

58 Duncan, *The Rebel Café*, 70.

59 Mason Currey, "Auden, Sartre, Graham Greene, Ayn Rand: They Loved Amphetamines," *Slate*, 22 April 2013, https://slate.com/culture/2013/04/auden-sartre-graham-greene-ayn-rand-they-loved-amphetamines.html.

60 Sukenick, *Down and In*, 35–6.

61 Gioia, *The History of Jazz*, 295.

62 Hotz, *Holding the Lotus to the Rock*, 17–18.

63 Stephen A. Kent, *From Slogans to Mantras: Social Protest and Religious Conversion in the Late Vietnam War Era* (Syracuse, NY: Syracuse University Press, 2001), 9. For a more substantial discussion on the Beats and Buddhism, see Carl T. Jackson, "The Counterculture Looks East: Beat Writers and Asian Religion," *American Studies* 29, no. 1 (1988): 51–70.

64 Alan Watts, *The Way of Zen* (New York: Vintage Books, 1989).

65 Millicent Brower, "The Rigid Road to Unbeat Zen," *Village Voice* 6, no. 11, 5 January 1961.

66 Carlos S. Alvarado et al., "Fifty Years of Supporting Parapsychology: The Parapsychology Foundation (1951–2001)," *International Journal of Parapsychology* 12, no. 2 (2001): 1–5.

67 Eileen J. Garrett, *Many Voices: The Autobiography of a Medium* (New York: Putnam, 1968), 169.

68 Chester Anderson, "Two Page Racial Rap," printed by the Communication Company, 9 February 1967, folder 2 Jan. 1967, box 1, Chester Anderson papers, circa 1963–1980, BANC MSS 92/839 c, Bancroft Library, University of California, Berkeley.

69 Wini Breines, "The 'Other' Fifties: Beats and Bad Girls," in *Not June Cleaver: Women and Gender in Postwar America, 1945–1960*, ed. Joanne Meyerowitz (Philadelphia: Temple University Press, 1996), 382–408.

70 Diane di Prima, *Memoirs of a Beatnik* (San Francisco: Last Gasp of San Francisco, 1988), 10–13. For more on the history of gays in New York, see George Chauncey, *Gay New York: Gender, Urban Culture, and the Makings of the Gay Male World, 1890–1940* (New York: Basic Books, 1994).

71 Christopher Mele, *Selling the Lower East Side: Culture, Real Estate, and Resistance in New York City* (Minneapolis: University of Minnesota Press, 2000), 122, 135.

72 Di Prima, *Memoirs of a Beatnik*, 53–4.

73 Janet L. Abu-Lughod, *From Urban Village to East Village: The Battle for New York's Lower East Side* (Oxford, UK; Cambridge, MA: Blackwell, 1994), 123.

74 Di Prima, *Memoirs of a Beatnik*, 63–5.

75 Ibid., 67–8.

76 Ibid., 83.

77 Daniel Wolf, "Delinquency in the Village," *Village Voice* 3, no. 5, 27

November 1957.

78 Di Prima, *Memoirs of a Beatnik*, 126–7.

79 Charles Winick, "The Use of Drugs by Jazz Musicians," *Social Problems* 7, no. 3 (1959): 242.

80 Siff, *Acid Hype*, 41.

81 Aldous Huxley, *The Perennial Philosophy* (New York: Harper Perennial Modern Classics, 2009).

82 Di Prima, *Memoirs of a Beatnik*, 126–7.

83 Diane Di Prima, *Recollections of My Life as a Woman* (New York: Viking, 2001), 159.

84 Ibid., 130–3.

85 LeRoi Jones, *The Autobiography of LeRoi Jones* (New York: Freundlich Books, 1984), 133.

86 Ibid., 134.

87 Ibid., 150.

88 Ibid., 153.

89 van Elteren, "The Subculture of the Beats," 73.

90 As quoted in Breines, "The 'Other Fifties,'" 392.

91 The word "beatnik" should also be used cautiously. Neil Cassady, for one, took issue with it: "While some have called me beatnik … I prefer to identify as wandering poet, amateur philosopher, autopilot outlaw." Quoted in Timothy Leary, *Flashbacks: A Personal and Cultural History of an Era* (Los Angeles: Jeremy P. Tarcher, 1990), 51.

92 Miles, "The Beat Generation in the Village," 175.

93 Interview with Allen Ginsberg, "Contra Speedamos Ex Cathedra and Other Subjects," from *Electric Newspaper*, Liberation News Service, date unavailable, folder "Drugs Crackdown (2)," box 5, Stafford papers.

94 Jones, "The Autobiography of LeRoi Jones," 166–7.

95 Sukenick, *Down and In*, 128.

96 Ellen Sander, *Trips: Rock Life in the Sixties* (New York: Charles Scribner's Sons, 1973) 16–17.

97 Di Prima, *Recollections*, 204–5.

98 Ed Rosenfeld, interview by the author, Cooper Square apartment, New York City, 4 April 2013.

99 George Andrews to Timothy Leary, 26 June 1961, folder 11, box 46, Leary papers.

100 Polsky, *Hustlers, Beats, and Others*, 163.

101 Ibid., 166–70.

102 Peter Stafford, *Psychedelics Encyclopedia* (Berkeley: Ronin Publishing, 1992), 16.

103 Polsky, *Hustlers, Beats, and Others*, 165.

104 "Habit-Forming Drug Sold by N.Y. Beatnik Coffee Shops," *Washington Post*, 19 June 1960. Peyote, though, is neither habit-forming nor a stimulant, as the article claims.

218 | NOTES TO PAGES 36–9

105 Edward C. Burks, "Peyote Peddler at Odds with U.S.," *New York Times*, 23 June 1960.

106 Quoted in Jarnow, *Heads*, 4.

107 Ed Rosenfeld, interview by the author, Cooper Square apartment, New York City, 4 April 2013.

108 Di Prima, *Recollections*, 210–12.

109 Allan Hunt Badiner and Alex Grey, eds, *Zig Zag Zen: Buddhism on Psychedelics* (San Francisco: Chronicle Books, 2002); Lucas Richert and Matthew DeCloedt, "Supple Bodies, Healthy Minds: Yoga, Psychedelics and American Mental Health," *Medical Humanities* 44, no. 3 (2018): 193–200.

110 Herbet Scheidt to International Foundation for Internal Freedom, 28 February 1964, folder 6, box 56, Leary papers.

111 Harold Naiderman to Timothy Leary, 4 January 1963, folder 5, box 47, Leary papers.

112 James L. Goddard, "Injunction Action," *FDA Papers* 2, no. 1 (February 1968): 44.

113 Art Kleps, "King Arthur's Court," in Kleps, *Millbrook*.

114 "Court Orders Drug Firm to Set up Records, Permit Inspection, Hire Trained Personnel," *1962 Report on Enforcement and Compliance* (Washington, DC: US Government Printing Office, 1962), 10.

115 Annette Hollander to Timothy Leary, 20 November 1966, folder 1, box 47, Leary papers.

116 Audrey Beck to Richard Alpert, 18 June 1963, folder 12, box 51, Leary papers.

117 David Solomon, "Editor's Preface," in *LSD: The Consciousness-Expanding Drug*, ed. David Solomon (New York: G.P. Putnam's Sons, 1966), viii.

118 Jed Birmingham, "William Burroughs and David Solomon," *RealityStudio*, accessed 7 May 2021, https://realitystudio.org/bibliographic-bunker/william-burroughs-and-david-solomon.

119 Loren Glass, *Counterculture Colophon: Grove Press, the Evergreen Review, and the Incorporation of the Avant-Garde* (Stanford: Stanford University Press, 2013), 168.

120 Puckett Johnson (Robert Bashlow) to Timothy Leary, 20 May 1963, folder 11, box 47, Leary papers. A more detailed account is provided in a letter likely addressed to John Beresford in the same folder. See Robert to J., 19 May 1963, in the same box and folder.

121 Robert Bashlow to Timothy Leary, 7 September 1963, folder 9, box 48, Leary papers.

122 James J. Peterson to Timothy Leary, 18 December 1963, folder 1, box 49, Leary papers.

123 Arthur Roberts, "Consciousness Expanding Drugs," *Clyde*, January 1965, 79, folder "Morning Glory," box 10, Stafford papers.

124 Saskatchewan-based psychiatrist Humphry Osmond unsuccessfully

NOTES TO PAGES 40–5 | 219

tried to place an order in the 1950s. See "Research on Schizophrenia," *Neuropharmacology: Transactions of the 2nd Conference, May 25–27, 1955. Princeton, N.J.*, ed. H.A. Abramson (New York: Josiah Macy Jr Foundation, 1956), 197.

125 Paul De Rienzo and Dana Beal, "Howard Lotsof," in *The Ibogaine Story: Report on the Staten Island Project*, page unavailable, accessed 22 May 2021, http://ibogaine.mindvox.com/articles/ibogaine-story-staten-island-project.

126 Howard Lotsof, interview by Geert Lovink, Amsterdam, date unavailable, page unavailable, accessed 17 November 2014, https://archive.org/details/InterviewMetHowardLotsofAboutIbogaine.

127 De Rienzo and Beal, "Howard Lotsof."

128 Solomon, "Editor's Preface," viii; Robert Bashlow to J., 19 May 1963, folder 11, box 47, Leary papers.

129 Rosenfeld, interview. For a complete discussion on the role of psychedelic guidebooks, see Shipley, *Psychedelic Mysticism*.

CHAPTER TWO

1 Siff, *Acid Hype*, 73–4.

2 Rosenfeld, interview.

3 Keith Angier to International Foundation for Internal Freedom. 29 October 1963, folder 9, box 51, Leary papers.

4 Jane Ross to editors, *Life* 3, no. 22, 3 June 1957, 16.

5 As quoted in *Shaman Woman*, 215.

6 For an assessment of Leary the psychologist, see David C. Devonis, "Timothy Leary's Mid-Career Shift: Clean Break or Inflection Point?" *Journal of the History of the Behavioral Sciences* 48, no. 1 (2012): 16–39.

7 Stern, "From Beat Scene Poet," 90.

8 Higgs, *I Have America Surrounded*, 20–1.

9 For the prison psychologist who later observed Leary behind bars in the early 1970s, Leary was a classic megalomaniac who was ready to sacrifice others in his interest. See ibid., 219.

10 Ibid., 18–19.

11 Ibid., 24–7.

12 Timothy Leary to Arthur Koestler, January 1961 (exact day unavailable), box 45, folder 14, Leary papers.

13 Leary, *Flashbacks*, 44.

14 Allen Ginsberg to Timothy Leary, 10 November 1960, reproduced in Jennifer Ulrich, *The Timothy Leary Project* (New York: Abrams Press, 2018), 47.

15 See William S. Burroughs and Allen Ginsberg, *The Yage Letters Redux* (London: Penguin, 2008).

16 Timothy Leary, "In the Beginning, Leary Turned on Ginsberg and Saw That It Was Good ...," *Esquire*, July 1968, 84, Stafford papers.

17 Leary, *Flashbacks*, 49–50.
18 B.H. Friedman, *Tripping: A Memoir* (Provincetown, MA: Provincetown Arts Press, 2006), 48. Another less-known source of supplies was a biochemical company named Argyll based in Toronto, which was also carrying out modest clinical investigations into psilocybin. Argyll was appreciative of Leary's work at Harvard and promised to send him drug samples for his research. Peter D. Bayne to Timothy Leary, 4 February 1961, folder 15, box 45, Leary papers. In March 1961, he received a shipment containing psilocybin, ibogaine, and bufotenine, though what he did with the latter two is not known. See Argyll Laboratories Company to Timothy Leary, 20 March 1962, folder 9, box 45, Leary papers.
19 Leary, *Flashbacks*, 53–5.
20 Hartogsohn, *American Trip*, 96.
21 The history of psychedelics reveals that many "bad trips" could have positive meaning ascribed to them nonetheless. See Erika Dyck and Chris Elcock, "Reframing Bummer Trips: Scientific and Cultural Explanations to Adverse Reactions to Psychedelic Drug Use," *The Social History of Alcohol and Drugs* 34, no. 2 (2020): 271–96.
22 Leary, *Flashbacks*, 65–6.
23 "Allen Ginsberg," box 35, folder 11, Leary papers.
24 Leary, *Flashbacks*, 66–7.
25 Greenfield, *Timothy Leary*, 136–7.
26 Leary, *Flashbacks*, 67–8.
27 As quoted in Glass, *Counterculture Colophon*, 23.
28 Leary, *Flashbacks*, 68.
29 Ibid., 68–9.
30 As quoted in Greenfield, *Timothy Leary*, 139.
31 Masters and Houston, *Psychedelic Art*.
32 Leary, *Flashbacks*, 70.
33 As quoted in Greenfield, *Timothy Leary*, 140–1.
34 The exact dates vary according to different primary sources and journalistic accounts, which point to initiations of Kerouac, Lowell, Rosset, and Black jazz musicians occurring during the winter of 1960–61.
35 As quoted in Lee and Shlain, *Acid Dreams*, 79.
36 Greenfield, *Timothy Leary*, 142.
37 In *Flashbacks*, Leary indicates going to the Fergusons' house for the first time in spring 1962, but this is highly unlikely because multiple sources point to his presence there in 1961.
38 Greenfield, *Timothy Leary*, 142.
39 Leary, *Flashbacks*, 110–14.
40 Friedman, *Tripping*, 30.
41 Ibid., 51.
42 Ibid., 3.

NOTES TO PAGES 52–8 | 221

43 B.H. Friedman to Timothy Leary, 9 April 1961, folder 10, box 46, Leary papers.
44 A critical assessment of their study was published almost forty years later. See Rick Doblin, "Dr. Leary's Concord Prison Experiment: A 34-Year Follow-up Study," *Journal of Psychoactive Drugs* 30, no. 4 (1998): 419–26.
45 Friedman, *Tripping*, 11.
46 "Newsletter #1," February 1962, 14, folder 19, box 33, Leary papers.
47 B.H. Friedman to Timothy Leary, 28 June 1961, folder 19, box 45, Leary papers.
48 John Wilcock to Timothy Leary, 30 May 1961, box 46, folder 11, Leary papers.
49 Sukenick, *Down and In*, 109.
50 John McMillian, *Smoking Typewriters: The Sixties Underground Press and the Rise of Alternative Media in America* (New York: Oxford University Press, 2011), 33–4. Quotation on p. 33.
51 Saundra Sorenson, "Mr. Underground," *VC Reporter*, 17 October 2006, https://web.archive.org/web/20061017065058/http://www.vcreporter.com/article.php?id=3762&IssueNum=88.
52 John Wilcock, *Manhattan Memories: An Autobiography* (self-published memoir, 2009), 26.
53 John Wilcock to Timothy Leary, 11 July 1961, folder 20, box 45, Leary papers.
54 John Wilcock, "The Village Square," *Village Voice*, 27 July 1961.
55 John Wilcock, "The Village Square," *Village Voice*, 8 August 1961.
56 Friedman, *Tripping*, 60.
57 B.H. Friedman psilocybin report, 6 September 1961, 38, folder 11, box 34, Leary papers.
58 Friedman, *Tripping*, 43–6.
59 Ibid., 48–53.
60 Aldous Huxley to Humphry Osmond, 1 June 1957, in *Psychedelic Prophets: The Letters of Aldous Huxley and Humphry Osmond*, ed. Cynthia Carson Bisbee, Paul Bisbee, Erika Dyck, Patrick Farrell, James Sexton, and James W. Spisak (Montreal and Kingston: McGill-Queen's University Press, 2018), 337.
61 Leary, *Flashbacks*, 93.
62 Robert Forte, "A Conversation with R. Gordon Wasson," in Forte, *Entheogens*, 81–4.
63 Greenfield, *Timothy Leary*, 156–7.
64 Ibid., 161–2.
65 Stanley Krippner, interview by the author, Hyatt Regency, Albuquerque, 15 February 2013.
66 Stanley Krippner, *Song of the Siren: A Parapsychological Odyssey* (New York: Harper Colophon Books, 1977), 21.

222 | NOTES TO PAGES 58–64

67 Stanley Krippner, "The Psychedelic Adventures of Alan Watts," personal website, accessed 29 July 2021, https://stanleykrippner.weebly.com/the-psychedelic-adventures-of-alan-watts.html.

68 Krippner, interview.

69 B.H. Friedman psilocybin report, 15 September 1961, 15, folder 11, box 34, Leary papers.

70 John Beresford, "To Tim from John," in *Timothy Leary: Outside Looking In*, ed. Robert Forte (Rochester, VT: Park Street Press, 1999), 31–2.

71 Jolie Braun, "A History of Diane di Prima's Poets Press," *Journal of Beat Studies* 6 (2018): 3.

72 Jones, *The Autobiography of LeRoi Jones*, 170.

73 Ibid., 178.

74 Robert Rowe to Timothy Leary, 7 September 1961, folder 6, box 45, Leary papers.

75 Friedman, *Tripping*, 73.

76 B.H. Friedman to Timothy Leary, 4 October 1961, folder 23, box 45, Leary papers.

77 Friedman, *Tripping*, 74.

78 Ibid., 83–98.

79 Ibid., 112–15.

80 Ibid., 132.

CHAPTER THREE

1 Knauer and Maloney, "A Preliminary Note."

2 Hartogsohn, *American Trip*, 31–2.

3 Max Rinkel, "Discussion at Annual Meeting of the American Psychiatric Association in Detroit," *Journal of Clinical and Experimental Psychopathology* 12 (May 1950): 42. As referenced in Hartogsohn, *American Trip*, 390; Paul H. Hoch, "Experimentally Produced Psychoses," *American Journal of Psychiatry* 107, no. 8 (1951): 607–11. Hoch's paper states that it was read at the annual conference in May 1950.

4 Oram, *The Trials of Psychedelic Therapy*, 22.

5 Hans Pols, "Anomie in the Metropolis: The City in American Sociology and Psychiatry," *Osiris* 18 (2003): 206; Dennis Doyle, "Slums, Race and Mental Health in New York (1938–1965)," *Palgrave Communications* 4, no. 1 (2018): 1–11. At the same time, academics increasingly believed that urban mental illness was acutely linked to poverty, and the view of the city as inherently pathogenic basically disappeared after the 1960s.

6 R.E. Mogar and R.W. Aldrich, "The Use of Psychedelic Agents with Autistic Schizophrenic Children," *Behavioral Neuropsychiatry* 1, no. 8 (1969): 44–50; Jeff Sigafoos et al., "Flashback to the 1960s: LSD in the Treatment of Autism," *Developmental Neurorehabilitation* 10, no. 1 (2007): 75–81.

NOTES TO PAGES 64–7 | 223

7 A notable exception was Betty Eisner, whose work is documented in Hartogsohn's *American Trip.*

8 Oram, *The Trials of Psychedelic Therapy*, 109.

9 See, for example, Roland R. Griffiths et al., "Psilocybin Produces Substantial and Sustained Decreases in Depression and Anxiety in Patients with Life-Threatening Cancer: A Randomized Double-Blind Trial," *Journal of Psychopharmacology* 30, no. 12 (2016): 1181–97.

10 Oram, *The Trials of Psychedelic Therapy*, 18–19. Quotation on p. 19.

11 "Paul Hoch Dies," *New York Times*, 16 December 1964.

12 Paul H. Hoch, James P. Cattel, and Harry H. Pennes, "Effects of Mescaline and Lysergic Acid (d-LSD-25)," *American Journal of Psychiatry* 108, no. 8 (1952): 579–84.

13 Hoch, "Experimentally Produced Psychoses," 609.

14 James P. Cattel, "The Influence of Mescaline on Psychodynamic Material," *Journal of Nervous & Mental Disease* 119, no. 3 (1954): 233–44.

15 "$700,000 Awarded to Estate of Army Drug Test Victim," *Los Angeles Times*, 6 May 1987.

16 "Harold Blauer MDA Death," accessed 10 October 2021, https://www.youtube.com/watch?v=4rLOoydB9ec. In *Acid Dreams*, Lee and Shlain have a slightly different but basically similar quote on page 38. This story is also discussed by Torsten Passie and Udo Benzenhöfer in "MDA, MDMA, and Other 'Mescaline-like' Substances in the US Military's Search for a Truth Drug (1940s to 1960s)," *Drug Testing and Analysis* 10, no. 1 (2018): 72–80.

17 John M. Doyle, "U.S. Held Responsible for Death in Street Army Drug Testing," *AP News*, 6 May 1987. Later in 1953, Frank Olson, a CIA scientist, was also unwittingly dosed in rural Maryland and committed suicide in Manhattan. See "Family in LSD Case Gets Ford Apology," *New York Times*, 22 July 1975; and Marks, "Intelligence or 'Witches' Potion.'"

18 Siff, *Acid Hype*, 51.

19 Dyck, *Psychedelic Psychiatry*, 53–78.

20 Humphry Osmond to Aldous Huxley, 14 April 1955, in *Psychedelic Prophets*, 178.

21 Don Lattin, *Distilled Spirits: Getting High, Then Sober, with a Famous Writer, a Forgotten Philosopher, and a Hopeless Drunk* (Berkeley: University of California Press, 2012), 4.

22 Stacy Horn, *Unbelievable: Investigations into Ghosts, Poltergeists, Telepathy, and Other Unseen Phenomena, from the Duke Parapsychology Laboratory* (New York: Ecco, 2010), 185.

23 Alvarado et al., "Fifty Years of Supporting Parapsychology," 9.

24 Humphry Osmond to Aldous Huxley, 11 June 1959, in Bisbee et al., *Psychedelic Prophets*, 419–20; Robert Sommer, Humphry Osmond, and Lucille Pancyr, "Selection of Twins for ESP experimentation," *International Journal of Parapsychology* (Autumn 1961): 55–73. A year

later, Osmond took part in two mediumistic sessions, including one hosted by Wilson and his group. See Bisbee et al., *Psychedelic Prophets*, 445–6.

25 Timothy Leary and Walter Houston Clark, "Religious Implications of Consciousness Expanding Drugs," *Religious Education* 58, no. 3 (1963): 251. That study was also funded by the Uris Brothers, which confirms Bernard Friedman's story in the previous chapter.

26 Frank Fremont-Smith, "Introductory Remarks," in *The Use of LSD in Psychotherapy*, ed. Harold A. Abramson (New York: Josiah Macy Jr Foundation, 1960), 8.

27 L.H. Geronimus, H.A. Abramson, L.J. Ingraham, and B. Sklarofsy, "Effects of LSD-25," in *Annual Report of the Biological Laboratory, Cold Spring Harbor, NY*, 1954, 36–9. This was followed by several studies involving snails and fighting fish.

28 H.A. Abramson, M.E. Jarvik, M.R. Kaufman, C. Kornetsky, A. Levine, and M. Wagner, "Lysergic Acid Diethylamide (LSD-25): I. Physiological and Perceptual Responses," *Journal of Psychology* 39, no. 1 (1955): 3–60. In several papers published in this journal, Abramson reported on the administration of several tests and psychometric scales to healthy individuals under the influence.

29 Harold A. Abramson, "Lysergic Acid Diethylamide (LSD-25): III. As an Adjunct to Psychotherapy with Elimination of Fear of Homosexuality," *The Journal of Psychology* 39, no. 1 (1955): 127–55; quotation on p. 153.

30 David K. Johnson, *The Lavender Scare: The Cold War Persecution of Gays and Lesbians in the Federal Government* (Chicago: University of Chicago Press, 2006). As well, this study occurred just as similar investigations were underway in Canada and a few years before another was initiated in France. See, respectively, Andrea Ens, "'Wish I Would Be Normal': LSD and Homosexuality at Hollywood Hospital, 1955–1973," MA thesis, University of Saskatchewan, 2019; Zoë Dubus, "Utiliser les psychédéliques pour « guérir » des adolescents homosexuels ? Essai de thérapie de conversion, France, 1960," *Annales Médico-psychologiques, revue psychiatrique* 178, no. 6 (2020): 650–6.

31 "Artificial psychoses," *Time*, 19 December 1955.

32 Oram, *The Trials of Psychedelic Therapy*, 31–3.

33 Harold A. Abramson, "Discussion," in *The Use of LSD in Psychotherapy and Alcoholism*, ed. Harold A. Abramson (New York: The Bobbs-Merrill Company, 1967), 42.

34 Archie A. Silver, "Lauretta Bender's Contribution to Understanding Language Disorders," *Annals of Dyslexia* 39 (1989): 24–33.

35 Rasmussen, *On Speed*, 50.

36 "Lauretta Bender, 1897–1987," The Autism History Project, accessed 12 April 2021, https://blogs.uoregon.edu/autismhistoryproject/people/lauretta-bender-1897-1987.

NOTES TO PAGES 69–74 | 225

37 Bender, "Children's Reactions to Psychotomimetic Drugs," 272.
38 Alfred M. Freedman, Eva V. Ebin, and Ethel A. Wilson, "Autistic Schizophrenic Children. An Experiment in the Use of d-Lysergic Acid Diethylamide (LSD-25)," *Archives of General Psychiatry* 6, no. 3 (1962): 205.
39 Heinrich Waelsch, "Paul H. Hoch, M.D. (1902–1965)," *American Journal of Psychiatry* 121, no. 9 (1965): 935–6.
40 Muriel K. Gibbon to Lauretta Bender, 15 November 1963, folder 12, box 17, Bender papers.
41 As quoted in Lee and Shlain, *Acid Dreams*, 69.
42 Bender, "Children's Reactions to Psychotomimetic Drugs," 268–70.
43 Sydney Malitz et al., "Some Observations on Psilocybin, a New Hallucinogen, in Volunteer Subjects," *Comprehensive Psychiatry* 1 (1960): 15.
44 Harold Esecover, Sidney Malitz, and Bernard Wilkens, "Clinical Profiles of Paid Normal Subjects Volunteering for Hallucinogen Drug Studies," *American Journal of Psychiatry* 117, no. 10 (1961): 912.
45 Humphry Osmond to Aldous Huxley, 2 June 1955, in Bisbee et al., *Psychedelic Prophets*, 185.
46 Harriet Linton Barr et al., *LSD: Personality and Experience* (New York: Wiley-Interscience, 1972), xi.
47 Robert R. Holt, "History of the Research Center for Mental Health," paper presented at the annual meeting of the Rapaport-Klein Study Group on 10 June 2006 at New York University. Full transcript available at http://www.psychomedia.it/rapaport-klein/holt06.htm.
48 Harriet B. Linton and Robert J. Langs, "Placebo Reactions in a Study of Lysergic Acid Diethylamide (LSD-25)," *Archives of General Psychiatry* 6, no. 5 (1962): 382.
49 Joseph Berger, "Performing Seances? No, Just 'Pushing the Membrane of the Possible,'" *New York Times*, 25 June 1996.
50 Jean Houston, *A Mythic Life: Learning to Live our Greater Story* (San Francisco: HarperOne, 1996), 172–3.
51 Ibid., 179.
52 Ibid., 181.
53 Jean Houston, "A Different Kind of Mysticism," *Jubilee* 14, no. 6 (1967): 17.
54 Oram, *The Trials of Psychedelic Therapy*, 8.
55 Houston, *A Mythic Life*, 183–4. For a comprehensive history of the Esalen Institute, see Jeffrey J. Kripal, *Esalen: America and the Religion of No Religion* (Chicago: University of Chicago Press, 2007).
56 Houston, *A Mythic Life*, 185.
57 Ibid., 186. This story contrasts with the standard narrative, whereby the *Island* manuscript was the only one Huxley and his second wife Laura were able to retrieve from the blaze. A few months later, Houston received the visit of another English intellectual and close friend of Huxley's, Gerald Heard.

226 | NOTES TO PAGES 74–7

58 Multiple sources conflict over the exact date: 1961, 1962, or 1963.

59 Chris Elcock, "Psychedelic Philanthropy: The Nonprofit Sector and Timothy Leary's 1960s Psychedelic Movement," *Journal of the History of the Behavioral Sciences* 57, no. 1 (2021): 4.

60 Robert E.L. Masters and Jean Houston, *The Varieties of Psychedelic Experience: The Classic Guide to the Effects of LSD on the Human Psyche* (Rochester, VT: Park Street Press, 2000), 134–5.

61 Andy Roberts, *Divine Rascal: On the Trail of LSD's Cosmic Courier Michael Hollingshead* (London: Strange Attractor Press, 2019), 34. Beresford claimed that "Bobby Kennedy was known to be taking LSD or psilocybin and providing psychedelic entertainment for foreign dignitaries in a fashionable New York apartment" in 1963. While this is certainly a sensational claim, it may explain why Kennedy subsequently defended psychedelic science when it came under attack. Peter Stafford and Bruce Eisner, "Who Turned on Whom?," *High Times*, October 1977.

62 Corinne Gilb, "In Memoriam: Roger Williams Wescott, 1925–2000," *Comparative Civilizations Review* 44, no. 44 (2001): 115–18.

63 Roger Wescott to Timothy Leary, 14 February 1964, folder 5, box 61, Leary papers.

64 Sigrid Radulovic, "John Spencer Beresford: March 28, 1924 – September 2, 2007," 19, accessed 10 October 2021, https://erowid.org/culture/characters/beresford_john/beresford_john_obituary1.pdf.

65 John Beresford to Timothy Leary, 3 April 1963, folder 10, box 47, Leary papers.

66 Quoted in Masters and Houston, *The Varieties of Psychedelic Experience*, 93–4.

67 Charles Clay Dahlberg, "The 100 Minute Hour," *Contemporary Psychoanalysis* 4, no. 1 (1967): 2. (Presidential address to the William Alanson White Psychoanalytic Society, 17 May 1967).

68 Charles C. Dahlberg, "Pharmacologic Facilitation of Psychoanalytic Therapy," *Current Psychiatric Therapies* 3 (1963): 91–9; quotation on p. 91.

69 Charles Clay Dahlberg, "LSD as an Aid to Psychoanalytic Treatment," in *Science and Psychoanalysis*, vol. 6: *Violence and War*, ed. J.H. Masserman (St Louis, MO: Grune Stratton, 1963), 256.

70 See, for example, D.B. Blewett and N. Chwelos, *Handbook for the Therapeutic Use of Lysergic Acid Diethylamide-25: Individual and Group Procedures* (Santa Cruz, CA: MAPS, 1959), http://www.erowid.org/psychoactives/guides/handbook_lsd25.pdf.

71 Carl Aldo Marzani, "LSD Experience Typescript," date unavailable, 1–10; quotation on p. 5, box 33, folder "LSD," Carl Aldo Marzani Papers, Tamiment Library/Robert F. Wagner Labor Archives, New York University. Unfortunately, there are no hints as to who that psychiatrist was.

72 Ibid., 17.

NOTES TO PAGES 77–81 | 227

73 Ibid., 74.

74 Ibid., 62.

75 Bob Gaines, "LSD: Hollywood's Status-Symbol Drug," *Cosmopolitan*, November 1963, 80, folder "Hollywood," box 7, Stafford papers. The doctor remained anonymous during his interviews, reasoning that his trade was too controversial.

76 Robert Cullen to IF-IF, 28 March 1963, folder 41, box 52, Leary papers.

77 Robert Cullen to Timothy Leary, 3 May 1963, folder 41, box 52, Leary papers.

78 Quoted in Ram Dass, Ralph Metzner, and Gary Bravo, *Birth of a Psychedelic Culture: Conversations about Leary, the Harvard Experiments, Millbrook and the Sixties* (Santa Fe, NM: Synergetic Press, 2010), 42.

79 Levin, "LSD in New York," *New York Post*, 7 June 1966, folder "LSD – New York Post," box 8, Stafford papers. In the 1970s, some American commune-dwellers understood child-labouring along the lines of a psychedelic experience. See Wendy Kline, "Psychedelic Birth: Bodies, Boundaries and the Perception of Pain in the 1970s," *Gender & History* 32, no. 1 (2020): 70–85.

80 Harold Naiderman to Timothy Leary, 13 October 1963, folder 4, box 47, Leary papers.

81 Eve Babitz, "Statement of Walter H. Bowart, Publisher, The East Village Other; Paula Sherwood, New York, N.Y.; and Eve Babitz, New York, N.Y.," The Narcotic Rehabilitation Act of 1966, Hearings before a Special Subcommittee of the Committee on the Judiciary, United States Senate, 89th Congress, 2nd Session, January 25–7, May 12, 13, 19, 23 and 25, June 14 and 15, July 19, 1966 (Washington, DC: US Government Printing Office, 1966), 550.

82 Oram, *The Trials of Psychedelic Therapy*, 10.

83 John Beresford to Timothy Leary, 3 April 1963, folder 10, box 47, Leary papers. The next day, the FDA made what was probably the first arrest for illegal LSD distribution in California after two individuals attempted to sell a gram and a half to two undercover agents. Geo. P. Larrick to L.H. Fountain, 17 September 1963, in *Hearings before a Subcommittee of the Committee on Government Operations. House of Representatives Eighty-ninth Congress, Second Session, March 9, 10; May 25, 26; June 7, 8, and 9, 1966* (Washington, DC: US Government Printing Office, 1966), 260. This is also mentioned by Oram in *The Trials of Psychedelic Therapy*, 70.

84 Ibid., 51–3. By then, Abramson was working full-time on Long Island.

85 Ibid., 69–70.

86 Paul Lowinger to Editor, *Science* 153, no. 3,732 (8 July 1966): 121.

87 Carlo Henze to Editor, *Science* 153, no. 3,737 (12 August 1966): 688.

88 Masters and Houston, *The Varieties of Psychedelic Experience*, vi.

89 Houston, *A Mythic Life*, 192.

228 | NOTES TO PAGES 81–3

90 Houston, "A Different Kind of Mysticism," 17.

91 Masters and Houston, *The Varieties of Psychedelic Experience*, 66. Oram has similar figures: approximately twenty grams of Sandoz LSD and twelve research groups working with that brand of acid. Oram, *The Trials of Psychedelic Therapy*, 76.

92 Oram, *The Trials of Psychedelic Therapy*, 47.

93 "New and Notes," *Contemporary Psychoanalysis* 2, no. 1 (1965): 85–6.

94 Dahlberg, "The 100 Minute Hour," 14.

95 Charles Clay Dahlberg to Editor, *Science* 153, no. 3,744 (30 September 1966): 1595. Dahlberg and colleagues actually investigated the impact of media publicity on psychedelic research. See Charles C. Dahlberg, Ruth Mechaneck, and Stanley Feldstein, "LSD Research: The Impact of Lay Publicity," *American Journal of Psychiatry* 125, no. 5 (1968): 685–9.

96 Charles Clay Dahlberg, "LSD Facilitation of Psychoanalytic Treatment: A Case Study in Depth," in Abramson, *The Use of LSD in Psychotherapy*, 237–58.

97 Dahlberg, "The 100 Minute Hour," 10–11.

98 H.B. Linton and R.J. Langs, "Empirical Dimensions of LSD-25 Reaction," *Archives of General Psychiatry* 10 (1964): 469–85.

99 Leo Goldberger, "Cognitive Test Performance under LSD-25, Placebo and Isolation," *The Journal of Nervous and Mental Disease* 142, no. 1 (1966): 4–9.

100 Barr et al., *LSD*, ix.

101 Sydney Malitz, "The Role of Mescaline and D-Lysergic Acid in Psychiatric Treatment," *Diseases of the Nervous System* 27, no. 1 (1966): 39.

102 Herman C.B. Denber and Sidney Merlis, "A Note on Some Therapeutic Implications of the Mescaline-Induced State," *The Psychiatric Quarterly* 28, no. 1 (1954): 637. It was Denber who had cautioned *Village Voice* journalist John Wilcock about unsupervised mescaline experimentation in the early Sixties.

103 Herman C.B. Denber, "Mescaline and Lysergic Acid Diethylamide: Therapeutic Implications of the Drug-Induced State," *Diseases of the Nervous System* 30, no. 2 (1969): 26.

104 Harold A. Abramson, "The Use of LSD (d-Lysergic Acid Diethylamide) in the Therapy of Children (a Brief Review)," *The Journal of Asthma Research* 5, no. 2 (December 1967): 139–43.

105 Harold A. Abramson, "Lysergic Acid Diethylamide (LSD 25): XXXXI The Use of LSD as an Adjunct to Psychotherapy: Fact and Fiction," *Journal of Asthma Research* 10, no. 4 (January 1973): 227–35. Abramson continued to publish his data on LSD into the late 1970s.

106 Harold A. Abramson, "LSD Spelled Out," *Mademoiselle* 64, no. 3 (January 1967): 53.

107 Robert E.L. Masters and Jean Houston, "Psychedelic Art and Society," in Masters and Houston, *Psychedelic Art*, 19.

NOTES TO PAGES 83–5 | 229

108 Robert E.L. Masters to the Foundation for Mind Research, 11 October 1967, folder "LSD – research," box 8, Stafford papers.

109 R.E.L. Masters, "Sex, Ecstasy and the Psychedelic Drugs," *Playboy* 14 (11), November 1967, folder "Personalities," box 11, Stafford papers. Masters had taken issue with Leary's infamous *Playboy* interview in which the former Harvard professor had claimed that a woman could have over a hundred orgasms under the influence of LSD, and he had also touted the drug as the ultimate cure for what was then commonly called frigidity. See "Timothy Leary: A Candid Conversation with the Controversial Ex-Harvard Professor, Prime Partisan and Prophet of LSD," *Playboy*, September 1966, pages unavailable, http://www.archive.org/details/playboylearyinteooplayrich.

110 Bender, "Children's Reactions to Psychotomimetic Drugs," 268–70. Dahlberg also took part in a major study that reached similar conclusions in the 1970s. See L.F. Jarvik et al., "Chromosome Examinations after Medically Administered Lysergic Acid Diethylamide and Dextroamphetamine," *Diseases of the Nervous System* 35, no. 9 (1974): 399–407.

111 Krippner, interview. Tellingly, she had read Huxley's "Doors of Perception" and was using the word psychedelic by 1966. Lauretta Bender, "D-Lysergic Acid in the Treatment of the Biological Features of Childhood Schizophrenia," *Diseases of the Nervous System*, Monograph Supplement 27, no. 7, 1, 1968. Reprint found in box 13, folder 4, Bender papers.

112 Box 9, folder 4, Bender papers.

113 Oram, 183–5. Quotation on p. 183.

114 J. Jaffe et al., "Speech Rhythms in Patient Monologues: The Influence of LSD-25 and Dextroamphetamine," *Biological Psychiatry* 4, no. 3 (1972): 243–6; J. Jaffe et al., "Effects of LSD-25 and Dextroamphetamine on Speech Rhythms in Psychotherapy Dialogues," *Biological Psychiatry* 6, no. 1 (1973): 93–6.

115 Charles C. Dahlberg, "Effects of LSD-25 on Psychotherapeutic Communication," *Psychopharmacology Bulletin* 10, no. 2 (1974): 64–5.

116 M. Natale et al., "Effect of Psychotomimetics (LSD and Dextroamphetamine) on the Use of Figurative Language during Psychoanalysis," *Journal of Consulting and Clinical Psychology* 46, no. 6 (1978): 1579–80.

117 Michael Natale, Charles Clay Dahlberg, and Joseph Jaffe, "The Effects of LSD-25 and Dextroamphetamine on the Use of Defensive Language," *Journal of Clinical Psychology* 35 (1979): 250–4.

118 Levin, "LSD in New York," *New York Post*, 7 June 1966.

119 Dahlberg, "The 100 Minute Hour," 12.

230 | NOTES TO PAGES 86–9

CHAPTER FOUR

1 David Herzberg, *Happy Pills in America: From Miltown to Prozac* (Baltimore: Johns Hopkins University Press, 2009); David Healy, *The Creation of Psychopharmacology* (Cambridge, MA: Harvard University Press, 2002).

2 Aldous Huxley to Humphry Osmond, 20 October 1956, in Bisbee et al., *Psychedelic Prophets*, 300.

3 Michael Augustine Itkin to IF-IF, 23 May 1963, folder 2, box 54, Leary papers.

4 Imrich J. Feldman to Richard Alpert, 27 November 1964, folder 9, box 64, Leary papers.

5 Siff, *Acid Hype*, 2.

6 Audrey Jewett to Timothy Leary, 25 February 1963, folder 6, box 47, Leary papers.

7 Roberts, *Divine Rascal*, 34.

8 Peter Stafford, "Re-Creational Uses of LSD," *Journal of Psychoactive Drugs* 17, no. 4 (1985): 222. The initial batch of LSD Beresford ordered was used in the trust's own drug sessions.

9 Quoted in ibid., 224.

10 Rosenfeld, interview.

11 Jeff Perkins, interview by the author, Upper West Side apartment, New York City, 12 April 2013.

12 Melinda Parks to Timothy Leary, 26 December 1963, folder 1, box 49, Leary papers.

13 Rosenfeld, interview.

14 Michael Francis Itkin, "Psychedelic Artist Survey," No. 15, folder 4, box 5, Stanley Krippner papers (MS-0063), University of West Georgia Special Collections [hereafter "Krippner papers"]. Perusal of the papers was undertaken before they were transferred from Kent State University in March 2016.

15 Michael Augustine Itkin to IF-IF, 23 May 1963, folder 2, box 54, Leary papers. Note: Itkin's full name was Michael Francis Augustine Itkin.

16 Mark Oppenheimer, *Knocking on Heaven's Door: American Religion in the Age of Counterculture* (New Haven, CT: Yale University Press, 2003), 30.

17 "Bishop Michael Francis Augustine Itkin," LGBTQ Religious Archives Network, accessed 29 June 2021, available at https://lgbtqreligiousarchives.org/profiles/michael-francis-augustine-itkin. In *Knocking on Heaven's Door*, Oppenheimer argues that the protest and countercultural movements of the 1960s changed the ways Americans worshipped God. For more on independent Catholics, see Julie Byrne, *The Other Catholics: Remaking America's Largest Religion* (New York: Columbia University Press, 2016).

18 Jon Butler, "Religion in New York City: Faith That Could Not Be," *U.S. Catholic Historian* 22, no. 2 (2004): 52.

19 Ibid., 58.

20 Michael Augustine Itkin to IF-IF, 23 May 1963, folder 2, box 54, Leary papers.

21 Clifton Hood, *In Pursuit of Privilege: A History of New York City's Upper Class & the Making of a Metropolis* (New York: Columbia University Press, 2017), x–xi.

22 Dass, Metzner, and Bravo, *Birth of a Psychedelic Culture*, 42–3.

23 Elcock, "Psychedelic Philanthropy."

24 Ronald F.S. Forbes to Timothy Leary, 26 April 1963, folder 8, box 53, Leary papers.

25 Ron Hewson to George Litwin, 22 March 1963, folder 29, box 53, Leary papers.

26 Alan Harington, "The Pros and Cons, History and Future Possibilities of Vision-Inducing Psychochemicals," *Playboy*, November 1963, 168, folder "Playboy," box 28, Stafford papers.

27 Quoted in Peter G. Stafford, chapter 4 "Everyday Problems (part 1)," in *LSD, the Problem-Solving Psychedelic* (New York: Award Books, 1967), page unavailable, http://www.druglibrary.org/schaffer/lsd/staf4.htm.

28 Alan Harrington, "A Visit to Inner Space," in Solomon, *LSD: The Consciousness-Expanding Drug*, 73–4.

29 Linda Sontag, "The Eyes of the Child-Corpse Were Open Wide," in *The Ecstatic Adventure: Reports of Chemical Explorations of the Inner World*, ed. Ralph Metzner (New York: McMillan, 1968), http://www.psychedelic-library.org/books/ecstatic15.htm.

30 Perkins, interview.

31 Siff, *Acid Hype*, 128.

32 Interview by Nina Graboi in Nina Graboi, *One Foot in the Future: A Woman's Spiritual Journey* (Santa Cruz, CA: Aerial Press, 1991), 250.

33 Lander, "Start Your Own Religion."

34 Timothy Leary, Ralph Metzner, and Richard Alpert, *The Psychedelic Experience: A Manual Based on the Tibetan Book of the Dead* (New York: Citadel Press, 1995).

35 Rosenfeld, interview.

36 Tim Lawrence, *Love Saves the Day: A History of American Dance Music Culture, 1970–1979* (Durham, NC: Duke University Press, 2003), 9–10.

37 Tom Schneider to Timothy Leary, 1966 (full date unavailable), folder 7, box 76, Leary papers.

38 Levin, "LSD in New York," *New York Post*, 6 June 1966. The author altered their real names.

39 Callum G. Brown, "What Was the Religious Crisis of the 1960s?" *Journal of Religious History* 34, no. 4 (2010): 468–79.

232 | NOTES TO PAGES 93–9

40 Robert S. Ellwood, *The Sixties Spiritual Awakening: American Religion Moving from Modern to Postmodern* (New Brunswick, NJ: Rutgers University Press, 1994).

41 Fuller, "Psychedelics and the Metaphysical Illumination," 77–8.

42 As quoted in Sukenick, *Down and In*, 127.

43 Di Prima, *Memoirs of a Beatnik*, 81.

44 For more on the Village folk revival, see Stephen Petrus and Ronald D. Cohen, *Folk City: New York and the American Folk Music Revival* (New York: Oxford University Press, 2015).

45 Duncan, *The Rebel Café*, 220.

46 Robert Nichols, "Geometry No Answer to Washington Sq.," *Village Voice*, 21 May 1964.

47 Emily Kies Folpe, *It Happened on Washington Square* (Baltimore: Johns Hopkins University Press, 2002), 312.

48 Stephanie Gervis Harrington, "City Puts Bomb under Off-Beat Culture Scene," *Village Voice*, 26 March 1964. A week later, the charges against Le Metro were dismissed, however.

49 Joseph P. Viteritti, "Times a-Changin': A Mayor for the Great Society," in *Summer in the City: John Lindsay, New York, and the American Dream*, ed. Joseph P. Viteritti (Baltimore: Johns Hopkins University Press, 2014), 8–13.

50 Suze Rotolo, *A Freewheelin' Time: A Memoir of Greenwich Village in the Sixties* (New York: Broadway Books, 2008), 18.

51 Osha Neumann, *Up against the Wall Motherf**ker: A Memoir of the '6os, with Notes for Next Time* (New York: Seven Stories Press, 2008), 35–6.

52 Mele, *Selling the Lower East Side*," 153–5.

53 Sukenick, *Down and In*, 58.

54 Di Prima, *Recollections*, 373–5.

55 Lander, "Start Your Own Religion," 65.

56 "nccc," 2 June 1965, folder 5, box 64, Leary papers.

57 Sukenick, *Down and In*, 108.

58 Ed Rosenfeld, email to the author, 26 March 2015.

59 Perkins, interview.

60 McMillian, *Smoking Typewriters*, 6.

61 Ed Sanders, "Ed Sanders on EVO and 'the New Vision,'" *East Village Other*, accessed 21 July 2021, http://eastvillageother.org/recollections/sanders.

62 Dan Rattiner, "Founding of the East Village Other," *East Village Other*, accessed 21 July 2021, http://eastvillageother.org/recollections/rattiner.

63 John Wilcock, "EVO Columnist John Wilcock Interviews John Wilcock," *East Village Other*, accessed 21 July 2021, http://eastvillageother.org/recollections/wilcock.

64 As quoted in McMillian, *Smoking Typewriters*, 73.

NOTES TO PAGES 99–103 | 233

65 "Psychedelic Art," *Life*, 9 September 1966, 68.
66 Clarence Newman, "Call It Psychedelic and It Will Sell Fast, Some Merchants Say," *Wall Street Journal*, 9 February 1967.
67 Al Van Starrex, "Hippie Businessmen," *Mr. Magazine* 12, no. 7, May 1968, 39, folder "Drugs Crackdown," box 4, Stafford papers.
68 Joshua Clark Davis, "The Business of Getting High: Head Shops, Countercultural Capitalism, and the Marijuana Legalization Movement," *The Sixties* 8, no.1 (2015): 28. Davis also argues that head shops made important contributions to movements seeking to reform drug laws.
69 Krippner, interview.
70 Schwartz, "Context, Value and Direction," 150.
71 Krippner, interview.
72 D.A. Latimer, "Chanel One," *East Village Other* 2, no. 16, 15 June–1 July 1967.
73 For an overview of the debates opposing subculture and post-subculture theories, see Andy Bennett, "The Post-subcultural Turn: Some Reflections 10 Years on," *Journal of Youth Studies* 14, no. 5 (2011): 493–506.
74 Schaap, "College Drug Scene."
75 Sarah Thornton, *Club Cultures: Music, Media, and Subcultural Capital*, 1st US edn, Music/Culture (Middletown, CT: Wesleyan University Press, 1996).
76 "Being," *East Village Other* 2, no. 9, 1 April–15 April 1967, folder "Be-ins," box 2, Stafford papers.
77 Edward Edelson, "For $5, Teen-Agers Buy Drugs in Greenwich Village," *New York World-Telegram*, 29 November 1965, folder "College Drug Scandals," box 3, Stafford papers.
78 Levin, "LSD in New York," *New York Post*, 8 June 1966.
79 David Walley, "Heads and Dopers: A Continuing Saga," *East Village Other* 5, no. 24, 12 May 1970.
80 Levin, "LSD in New York," *New York Post*, 9 June 1966.
81 Richard Goldstein, *Another Little Piece of My Heart: My Life of Rock and Revolution in the '60s* (New York: Bloomsbury USA, 2015), 142.
82 Levin, "LSD in New York," *New York Post*, 7 June 1966.
83 Rosetta Reitz to Timothy Leary, 5 January 1961, folder 14, box 45, Leary papers.
84 John Cashman, *The LSD Story* (Greenwich, CT: Fawcett, 1966), 83.
85 Levin, "LSD in New' York," *New York Post*, 7 June 1966.
86 Amelie Edwards (real name obscured at interviewee's request), interview by the author, midtown apartment, 22 March 2013.
87 Susan Szekely, "Teen Talk," *World of Women*, 15 September 1966, 8, folder "Masters + Houston," box 9, Stafford papers.

234 | NOTES TO PAGES 103–8

88 Levin, "LSD in New York," *New York Post*, 8 June 1966.
89 Quoted in Lewis Yablonsky, *The Hippie Trip* (New York: Pegasus, 1968), 121.
90 Levin, "LSD in New York," *New York Post*, 7 June 1966.
91 Peter Stafford, "Re-creational Uses of LSD," *Journal of Psychoactive Drugs* 17, no. 4 (1985): 224.
92 Brackman, "Four Ways to Go."
93 Edelson, "For $5."
94 Sherwood, "Statement of Walter H. Bowart," 549.
95 Schneider, *Smack*, xiii.
96 Quoted in Cashman, *The LSD Story*, 119.
97 Levin, "LSD in New York," *New York Post*, 10 June 1966.
98 Sherwood, "Statement of Walter H. Bowart," 559.
99 Levin, "LSD in New York," *New York Post*, 9 June 1966.
100 Levin, "LSD in New York," *New York Post*, 10 June 1966.
101 Levin, "LSD in New York," 9 June 1966.
102 Edelson, "For $5."
103 H.S.K., letter to the *East Village Other* 2, no. 15, 1 July–15 July 1967, folder "Drugs Crackdown," box 4, Stafford papers.
104 Sander, *Trips*, 29.
105 Lenni Brenner, "Sitting in with Mingus," *Couinterpunch*, 17 July 2003, https://www.counterpunch.org/2003/07/17/sitting-in-with-mingus.

CHAPTER FIVE

1 Braunstein and Doyle, *Imagine Nation*; Gretchen Lemke-Santangelo, *Daughters of Aquarius: Women of the Sixties Counterculture* (Lawrence: University Press of Kansas, 2009); David Kaiser and Patrick McCray, eds, *Groovy Science: Knowledge, Innovation, and American Counterculture* (Chicago: University of Chicago Press, 2016); Davis, *From Headshops to Whole Foods*; Damon R. Bach, *The American Counter-culture: A History of Hippies and Cultural Dissidents* (Lawrence: University Press of Kansas, 2020).
2 For more on this tension, see Elcock, "The Fifth Freedom."
3 Gerald Rothberg, "LSD," *Clyde*, December 1965, 19, folder "LSD Experiences," box 8, Stafford papers.
4 David Farber, "The Counterculture and the Antiwar Movement," in *Give Peace a Chance: Exploring the Vietnam Antiwar Movement*, ed. Melvin Small, William D. Hoover, and Charles DeBenedetti (Syracuse, NY: Syracuse University Press, 1992), 8–9.
5 David McReynolds, "An Open Letter to: Richard Alpert," *Win*, July 1967, 10, folder "Drugs Crackdown," box 4, Stafford papers.
6 Huxley, *The Doors of Perception and Heaven and Hell*, 17.
7 Peter Braunstein, "Forever Young: Insurgent Youth and the Sixties Culture of Rejuvenation," in Braunstein and Doyle, *Imagine Nation*, 253.

NOTES TO PAGES 108–12 | 235

8 "Drug Addict," *Look*, May 1967, 58, folder "Look", box 24, Stafford papers.

9 Lemke-Santangelo, *Daughters of Aquarius*, 2009), 116–23. These two memoirs would fall into that category: Jane Dunlap (Adelle Davis), *Exploring Inner Space: Personal Experiences under LSD-25* (New York: Harcourt, Brace & World, 1961); and Constance Newland, *Myself and I* (New York: Coward-McCann, 1962).

10 Debra Michals, "From 'Consciousness Expansion' to 'Consciousness Raising': Feminism and the Countercultural Politics of Self," in Braunstein and Doyle, *Imagine Nation*, 41–68; Lemke-Santangelo, *Daughters of Aquarius*, 2–3; Kim Hewitt, "Psychedelic Feminism: A Radical Interpretation of Psychedelic Consciousness?" *Journal for the Study of Radicalism* 13, no. 1 (2019): 75–120.

11 David Farber, "Building the Counterculture, Creating Right Livelihoods: The Counterculture at Work," *The Sixties* 6, no. 1 (2013): 3.

12 See, for example, Pedro Galán Lozano, "The Counterculture on Stage: Radical Theater and the Reclamation of the Public Space in 1960s San Francisco," *Journal for the Study of Radicalism* 12, no. 2 (2018): 35–53.

13 Elaine Tyler May, *Homeward Bound: American Families in the Cold War Era* (New York: Basic Books, 1988).

14 Graboi, *One Foot in the Future*, 109.

15 Rick Doblin, "Pahnke's 'Good Friday Experiment': A Long-Term Follow-up and Methodological Critique," *The Journal of Transpersonal Psychology* 23, no. 1 (1991): 1–28.

16 Graboi, *One Foot in the Future*, 130.

17 Chris Elcock, "A New Perspective on Harm Reduction: George Peters and the Chicago LSD Rescue Service," in *Pleasures and Panic: New Essays on the History of Alcohol and Drugs*, ed. Dan Malleck and Cheryl Krasnick (Vancouver: UBC Press, 2022), 191–216.

18 May, *Homeward Bound*.

19 Frank F. Furstenberg, "History and Current Status of Divorce in the United States," *The Future of Children* 4, no. 1 (1994): 34.

20 Nadine Weidman, "Between the Counterculture and the Corporation: Abraham Maslow and Humanistic Psychology in the 1960s," in Kaiser and McCray, *Groovy Science*, 109.

21 Nina Graboi to Paul Noble, 24 September 1965, box 7, Nina Graboi papers, 1960–99, McHenry Library Special Collections NRLF, University of California at Santa Cruz [hereafter "Graboi papers"].

22 Graboi, *One Foot in the Future*, 142–3.

23 For a historical analysis of the case, see Devin R. Lander, "'Legalize Spiritual Discovery': The Trials of Dr. Timothy Leary," in *Prohibition, Religious Freedom, and Human Rights: Regulating Traditional Drug Use*, ed. Beatriz Caiuby Labate and Clancy Cavnar (Heidelberg; New York; Dordrecht; London: Springer, 2014), 165–87.

24 Elcock, "Psychedelic Philanthropy."

25 Graboi, "Changing His Mind," 1.

26 Graboi, *One Foot in the Future*, 149.

27 Weidman, "Between the Counterculture and the Corporation," 110.

28 Graboi, *One Foot in the Future*, 161.

29 Ibid., 177.

30 Ibid., 188–90.

31 Dass, Metzner, and Bravo, *Birth of a Psychedelic Culture*, 206–9.

32 Graboi, *One Foot in the Future*, 188–90.

33 Ibid., 200.

34 Ibid., 201.

35 A copy of the Natural Church's statement of purpose is available in the Leary papers, but it is not clear when it was sent to him and whether Leary paid any attention. See "nccc," 2 June 1965, folder 5, box 64, Leary papers.

36 Robert E. Dallos, "Dr. Leary Starts New 'Religion' with 'Sacramental' Use of LSD," *New York Times*, 20 September 1966.

37 Peter Weinberg, "'On This Cube Will I Build My Church,'" *East Village Other* 1, no. 21, 1–15 October 1966.

38 Graboi, *One Foot in the Future*, 202.

39 Janah Loprest to Timothy Leary, 19 October 1966, folder 1, box 75, Leary papers.

40 Joel Levine to Timothy Leary, 16 December 1966, folder 2, box 75, Leary papers.

41 Graboi, *One Foot in the Future*, 214.

42 Ibid., 207.

43 Ibid., 208–9.

44 Nina Graboi, "Ecstatic Housecleaning," box 13, Graboi papers.

45 Graboi, *One Foot in the Future*, 219–20.

46 Ibid., 222.

47 Nina Graboi to Timothy Leary, 16 February 1967, folder 1, box 69, Leary papers.

48 Richard Goldstein, interview by the author, La Rotonde, Paris, 16 June 2017.

49 Don McNeill, "An Opening to the West: Ashram on Hudson Street," *Village Voice*, 23 February 1967, folder "League for Spiritual Discovery," box 9, Stafford papers.

50 Clyde Haberman, "That New-Time Religion: The Rites of LSD," *New York Post*, 14 March 1967, folder "League for Spiritual Discovery," box 9, Stafford papers.

51 Graboi, *One Foot in the Future*, 229.

52 Ibid., 227.

53 Ibid., 235.

54 Langlitz, *Neuropsychedelia*, 12–13.

55 Graboi, *One Foot in the Future*, 240.

56 Gerard DeGroot, "In Bed: Sex and Love," in *The 60s Unplugged: A Kaleidoscopic History of a Disorderly Decade* (London: Pan, 2009), 215–21.

57 Graboi, *One Foot in the Future*, 241.

58 Goldstein, interview.

59 Perkins, interview.

60 Graboi, *One Foot in the Future*, 225.

61 Ibid., 231.

62 Ibid., 226.

63 Ibid., 223. Timothy Miller has posited – tongue slightly in cheek – an "ethics of hair" to illustrate this in *The Hippies and American Values*, 116–8.

64 Graboi, *One Foot in the Future*, 229–30.

65 In Detroit, John Sinclair was arrested for giving two joints to undercover agents in 1969 and sentenced to ten years in prison, and head shops selling drug paraphernalia were likewise subjected to police harassment from the late 1960s on. See, respectively, Emily Dufton, *Grass Roots: The Rise and Fall and Rise of Marijuana in America* (New York: Basic Books, 2017), 18; and Davis, *From Headshops to Whole Foods*, 86.

66 Krippner, interview.

67 Graboi, *One Foot in the Future*, 245.

68 Ibid., 236.

69 Murray Levy, "The Psychedelic Showcase," undated, folder "Psychedelic Showcase," box 12, Stafford papers.

70 Graboi, *One Foot in the Future*, 237.

71 Ibid., 238.

72 Nina Graboi to Timothy Leary, 16 February 1967, folder 1, box 69, Leary papers.

73 Graboi, *One Foot in the Future*, 239–40.

74 "Scenes," *Village Voice*, 25 May 1967. For more on gangs, see Eric C. Schneider, *Vampires, Dragons, and Egyptian Kings: Youth Gangs in Postwar New York* (Princeton, NJ: Princeton University Press, 2001).

75 Greenfield, *Timothy Leary*, 313.

76 Graboi, *One Foot in the Future*, 247–9.

77 Don McNeill, *Moving through Here* (New York: Alfred A. Knopf, 1970), 21.

78 As quoted in Sukenick, *Down and In*, 158.

79 McNeill, *Moving through Here*, 27.

80 Timothy Miller, *The 60s Communes: Hippies and Beyond* (Syracuse, NY: Syracuse University Press, 1999), xiii–xiv.

81 Edwards, interview.

82 Mariana Mogilevich, "Arts as Public Policy: Cultural Spaces for Democracy and Growth," in Viteritti, *Summer in the City*, 195–201.

83 Brian Tochterman, *The Dying City: Postwar New York and the Ideology of Fear* (Chapel Hill: University of North Carolina Press, 2017), 145. As early as 1960, the future Lincoln Center for the Performing Arts was presented as "great fun." See Julia L. Foulkes, "Streets and Stages: Urban Renewal and the Arts after World War II," *Journal of Social History* 44, no. 2 (2010): 415.

84 Edwards, interview.

85 Peter Lefcourt, "Naked Lunch on Avenue A," *Village Voice*, 29 February 1968, folder "Drugs Crackdown," box 4, Stafford papers.

86 Lewis Yablonsky, *The Hippie Trip* (New York: Pegasus, 1968), 151.

87 On 6 October 1966, the day California moved to prohibit LSD, "a group of colourful kids came together in Tompkins Square park. 'Love,' the pink handbill read, 'A Psychedelic Celebration.'" McNeill, *Moving through Here*, 23.

88 Susun Weed, telephone interview with the author, 4 July 2022.

89 Trina Robbins, "Finding sanctuary at EVO," *East Village Other*, accessed 13 August 2021, http://eastvillageother.org/recollections/robbins.

90 Peter Leggieri, "Peter Leggieri's East Village Other," *East Village Other*, accessed 8 August 2021, http://eastvillageother.org/recollections/leggieri-2.

91 Don McNeill, "Central Park Rite Is Medieval Pageant," *Village Voice* 12, no. 24, 30 March 1967. Footage of the Be-in can be found at https://www.youtube.com/watch?v=37yTkaZM_u4.

92 Marvin Garson, "Electric Banana – Very Now Craze," *Village Voice*, 16 March 1967.

93 Yablonsky, *The Hippie Trip*, 138–9.

94 Garson, "Electric Banana."

95 McMillian, *Smoking Typewriters*, 91.

96 Ibid., 66–81.

97 "Oral History interview with Kim Deitch, 2007–2009," 26–7, box 5, folder 52, Series IV: Subject Files, Subseries A: Writers and Artists, Deitch, Kim, Ron Kolm Paper, The Fales Library & Special Collections, New York University. "Sunshine Girl" is not a reference to "Orange sunshine," a legendary brand of LSD that will be discussed in chapter 7.

98 Patrick Rosenkranz, "Where Underground Comix Lurched into Life," *East Village Other*, accessed 15 August 2021, http://eastvillageother.org/recollections/rosenkranz.

99 Richard Lacayo, "The Art of Being Critical: Robert Hughes (1938–2021)," *Time*, 7 August 2012, https://entertainment.time.com/2012/08/07/the-art-of-being-critical-robert-hughes-1938-2012.

100 Steven Heller, "Steven Heller's Dada," *East Village Other*, accessed 15 August 2021, http://eastvillageother.org/recollections/heller.

101 Goldstein, interview.

NOTES TO PAGES 130–3 | 239

102 John Garabedian, "New York's Hippies," *New York Post*, 15 September 1967, folder "Hippies, Yippies," box 7, Stafford papers.

103 Chuck Gould interviewed by Jay Babcock, "'The Do Was the Thing': A Lengthy Chat with Chuck Gould of the San Francisco Diggers," Diggers Docs, 2010, Gould's home in Petrolia, CA, https://diggersdocs.home. blog/tag/peggy-hitchcock.

104 See folder "Innerspace," box 21, Stafford papers.

CHAPTER SIX

1 The first part of this chapter, which focuses mostly on Isaac but also on Rachel Abrams, is based on two interviews carried out by the author, unless specified: Isaac Abrams, interview by the author, Montceaux, France, 22 May 2013; Rachel Abrams, interview by the author, Hotel La Louisiane, Paris, 18 May 2013. This chapter benefitted from Peter Collopy's comments, for which I am grateful.

2 Grunenberg and Harris, *Summer of Love*; Alastair Gordon, *Spaced Out: Radical Environments of the Psychedelic Sixties* (New York: Rizzoli, 2008); Robert J. Gluck, "Electric Circus, Electric Ear and the Intermedia Center in Late-1960s New York," *Leonardo* 45, no. 1 (2012): 50–7; Simon Rycroft, "Lightshows and the Cultural Politics of Light: Mid-Century Cosmologies," *The Sixties* 6, no. 1 (2013): 45–64.

3 See Donna M. Stein, *Thomas Wilfred: Lumia, a Retrospective Exhibition* (Washington, DC: Corcoran Gallery of Art, 1971).

4 Mogilevich, "Arts as Public Policy," 199–200; Kaprow quotation on p. 200.

5 Serge Guilbaut, *How New York Stole the Idea of Modern Art* (Chicago: University of Chicago Press, 1985); Rebeccah E. Welch, "Black Art and Activism in Postwar New York, 1950–1965," PhD thesis, New York University, 2002; Stephen J. Bottoms, *Playing Underground: A Critical History of the 1960s off-off-Broadway Movement* (Ann Arbor: University of Michigan Press, 2006); Foulkes, "Streets and Stages"; Allan Antliff, "Poetic Tension: The Aesthetic Politics of the Living Theatre," in *Radical Gotham: Anarchism in New York City from Schwab's Saloon to Occupy Wall Street*, ed. Tom Goyens (Urbana: University of Illinois Press, 2017), 142–60. The trend continued in the following decades. See Alan Moore, *Art Gangs: Protest and Counterculture in New York City* (Brooklyn, NY: Autonomedia, 2011).

6 Michael Oren, "USCO: 'Getting Out of Your Mind to Use Your Head,'" *Art Journal* 69, no. 4 (2010): 91.

7 New York City has a long tradition of theological art. See Meredith Massar Munson, "Babylon, New Jerusalem, and the Brooklyn Bridge: Modern Spirituality in American Art," PhD thesis, Graduate Theological Union, 2017.

240 | NOTES TO PAGES 134–41

8   "Isaac Abrams, peintures sous acides," *Tracks*, 2019, https://www.arte.tv/fr/videos/090747-006-A/isaac-abrams-peinture-sous-acides-tracks.

9   Rauschenberg discusses this role in the following interview: Dorothy Seckler, "Oral History Interview with Robert Rauschenberg," New York City, 21 December 1965, Smithsonian Archives of American Art, https://www.aaa.si.edu/collections/interviews/oral-history-interview-robert-rauschenberg-12870#overview. Rauschenberg's 1962 *Inside-Out*, for instance, used a combination of "oil, paper, fabric, wood, embossed tin, metal, wire, mirror, glass, bell, and wheel on structure mounted on four casters." Joshua Shannon, *The Disappearance of Objects: New York Art and the Rise of the Postmodern City* (New Haven, CT: Yale University Press, 2009), 95.

10 Bottoms, *Playing Underground*, 216–17. For more on experimental cinema, see Alison Lynn Wielgus, "You Had to Have Been There: Experimental Film and Video, Sound, and Liveness in the New York Underground," PhD thesis, University of Iowa, 2014; Wheeler Winston Dixon, *The Exploding Eye: A Re-visionary History of 1960s American Experimental Cinema* (Albany: State University of New York Press, 1997).

11 Scully, "Nick Sand."

12 Graham St John, *Mystery School in Hyperspace: A Cultural History of DMT* (Berkeley, CA: North Atlantic Books, 2015), 68.

13 Scully, "Nick Sand."

14 Masters and Houston, "Art and Psychedelic Experience," 119–20.

15 David Roman, "Psychedelic Art Survey," file 19, folder 4, 1967–1968," box 5, Krippner papers.

16 John A. Osmundsen, "Device Simulates Mind-Drug Effects," *New York Times*, 19 December 1964.

17 "Op Art: Pictures That Attack the Eye," *Time*, 23 October 1964.

18 David S. Rubin, "Stimuli for a New Millennium," in *Psychedelic: Optical and Visionary Art since the 1960s*, ed. David S. Rubin (San Antonio, TX : San Antonio Museum of Art; Cambridge, MA: MIT Press, 2010), 18.

19 Krippner, "The Psychedelic Artist," 171.

20 Masters and Houston, "Art and Psychedelic Experience," 122.

21 Ralph Metzner quoted in Dass, Metzner, and Bravo, *Birth of a Psychedelic Culture*, 127.

22 Howard Junker, "LSD: 'The Contact High,'" *The Nation*, 5 July 1965, page unavailable, http://www.thenation.com/article/156988/lsd-contact-high# (accessed 16 November 2013).

23 Michael Hollingshead to Alex Trochi, 22 May 1965, Trochi papers.

24 Greenfield, *Timothy Leary*, 217–18. Their marriage was short-lived. Von Schlebrugge remarried Bob Thurman, and they had a daughter, actor Uma Thurman.

25 Rosemary Woodruff Leary, *Psychedelic Refugee: The League for Spiritual*

Discovery, the 1960s Cultural Revolution, and 23 Years on the Run, ed. David F. Phillips (Rochester, VT: Park Street Press, 2021), 28.

26 Bonnie Marranca, "The Plays of Ronald Tavel: A Survey," *Performing Arts Journal* 3, no. 1 (1978): 55.

27 Isaac Abrams, telephone conversation with the author, 9 January 2021.

28 Bottoms, *Playing Underground*, 218.

29 Isaac Abrams, "Retour sur une carrière d'artiste psychédélique," talk given at the École des hautes études en sciences sociales, Paris, 14 February 2019, https://www.canal-u.tv/video/ehess/psychedelisme_punk_et_techno_experiences_croisees.48977.

30 Krippner, "The Psychedelic Artist," 177–8.

31 Abrams, "Retour sur une carrière d'artiste psychédélique."

32 For more on Erickson's legacy, see Aaron H. Devor and Nicholas Matte, "ONE Inc. and Reed Erickson: The Uneasy Collaboration of Gay and Trans Activism, 1964–2003," *GLQ: A Journal of Lesbian and Gay Studies* 10, no. 2 (2004): 179–209.

33 Levin, "LSD in New York," *New York Post*, 7 June 1966.

34 Krippner, "The Psychedelic Artist." To look at the files of the participants, see folder 4 "Psychedelic Artists Survey," 1966–1968," box 5, Krippner papers.

35 Graboi, *One Foot in the Future*, 223.

36 Ibid., 257–8.

37 For a critical appraisal of Leary's Psychedelic Celebrations, see James Penner, "Contesting the Stage of Reality: Timothy Leary's *The Psychedelic Celebrations* of 1966–1967, in *Playing Offstage: The Theater as a Presence or Factor in the Real World*, ed. Sidney Homan (Lanham, MD: Lexington Books, 2017), 101–19.

38 Michael Hollingshead to Alex Trocchi, 4 May 1965, item 55, folder 10–11: 1965, box 38, Sub-Series 1: Correspondence, Series 5: Sigma, box 38–45, Alexander Trocchi papers (MSS116), 1944–1984, Washington University Libraries, Department of Special Collections.

39 "Incense and Bass: LSD Show Is S.R.O.," *New York Times*, 11 April 1965.

40 Grace Glueck, "Multimedia: Massaging Senses for the Message," *New York Times*, 16 September 1967.

41 Quoted in Oren, "USCO: 'Getting out of Your Mind to Use Your Head,'" 78. But in the second half of the 1960s, they discarded this model because of the pain and disorientation that ultimately clashed with the meditation techniques the group was practising.

42 Naomi Feigelson, "Who R U?" *Cheetah*, May 1968, 35, folder "Drugs Crackdown," box 4, Stafford papers.

43 The word was coined by USCO and was based on a play on words – removing the "g" of "human being." Gerd Stern, email to the author, 3 March 2014.

44 "Psychedelic Art," *Life*, 9 September 1966, 65.

242 | NOTES TO PAGES 145–9

45 Quoted in Dass, Metzner, and Bravo, *Birth of a Psychedelic Culture*, 176.
46 Isaac Abrams, interview.
47 "Castalla Foundation and USCO Present: Psychedelic Explorations," folder "Castalla," box 3, Stafford papers.
48 Isaac Abrams, interview.
49 Stern, "From Beat Scene Poet," 91; Gerd Stern, interview.
50 Lisa Bieberman, "Bulletin," *Psychedelic Information Center*, 19, August 1968, 2, folder "Drugs Crackdown (2)," box 5, Stafford papers.
51 Stern, "From Beat Scene Poet," 92.
52 Friedman, *Tripping*, 54–5.
53 Isaac Abrams, interview.
54 Rudi Stern, interview by Davidson Gigliotti, December 1999, page unavailable, http://davidsonsfiles.org/rudisterninterview.html (accessed 7 November 2013).
55 Greenfield, *Timothy Leary*, 284.
56 Richard Goldstein, "Inside the Psychedelic Shell," *Village Voice*, 20 October 1966, folder "Leary, Timothy," box 9, Stafford papers.
57 Gerd Stern, interview.
58 Penner, "Contesting the Stage of Reality," 103.
59 Gerd Stern, interview.
60 Stephanie Harrington, "Dr. Leary's Formula: Turn on, Tune in, Drop Out," *Village Voice*, 29 September 1966, folder "League for Spiritual Discovery," box 9, Stafford papers.
61 Graboi, *One Foot in the Future*, 206.
62 "Psychedelic Art," *Life*, 9 September 1966, 68–9.
63 Krippner, interview.
64 Leary, *Flashbacks*, 255.
65 Ibid., 255–6. There was only one single performance, however, because, according to Metzner, the actor playing Jesus Christ confessed to being an undercover agent and promptly left. Ralph Metzner quoted in Dass, Metzner, and Bravo, *Birth of a Psychedelic Culture*, 204.
66 "Psychedelic Peace Fellowship Founded in New York," *Innerspace*, 1966, page unavailable, folder "Innerspace," box 21, Stafford papers.
67 Michael Francis Itkin, "An Open Letter to Timothy Leary," 27 November 1966, 2, folder "Itkin, Michael Francis," box 7, Stafford papers.
68 Walter Donald Kring, "Dr. Timothy Leary's 'Church,'" a sermon given at the Unitarian Church of All Souls, New York, 13 October 1966, folder "League for Spiritual Discovery," box 9, Stafford papers.
69 Mary Jo Warth, "The Acid Profiteers: Drop-out, Turn on, Cash In," *Village Voice*, 22 August 1974.
70 *Illumination* was followed by *The Trial of Giordano Bruno*, *The Mischief of Georges Gurdjieff*, *The Rebellion of Ralph Waldo Emerson*, and *The Assassination of Socrates*.
71 Ralph Metzner quoted in Dass, Metzner, and Bravo, *Birth of a Psychedelic Culture*, 205.

72 Dass, Metzner, and Bravo, *Birth of a Psychedelic Culture*, 206–9.

73 "Scenes," *Village Voice*, 13 April 1967. It is not entirely clear how this story ended, however. James Penner states that Hollywood producer Henry Saperstein took on the project but I could only find a short film called *Turn on, Tune in, Drop Out*, which was released in May 1967. See "Contesting the Stage of Reality," 115.

74 Leary, *Flashbacks*, 261–2.

75 Timothy Leary to Abigail Ferris Leary and Mary Ferris, 23 October 1968, folder 9, box 76, Leary papers.

76 Krippner, interview.

77 Peter Collopy, "The Revolution Will Be Videotaped: Making a Technology of Consciousness in the Long 1960s," PhD thesis, University of Pennsylvania, 2015, 100.

78 Ibid., 140–5.

79 Quoted in Gregory Zinman, "Dream Reeler: Jud Yalkut (1938–2013)," *The Brooklyn Rail*, 4 September 2013, http://www.brooklynrail.org/2013/09/film/dream-reeler-jud-yalkut-1938-2013.

80 Masters and Houston, "Art and Psychedelic Experience," 83.

81 Gerd Stern, email to the author, 8 November 2013. Yalkut also produced a film called *D.M.T.*

82 Rubin, "Stimuli for a New Millennium," 17.

83 See Jud Yalkut, "Kusama's Self-Obliteration," 1967, http://www.youtube.com/watch?v=n6wnhLqJqVE. This was scheduled at the Black Gate Theater in June 1967. See "Slumgoddess," *East Village Other* 2, no. 14, 15 June–1 July 1967.

84 Allan Katzman, "Jesus Runs Amok Crowd of Fags," *East Village Other* 3, no. 14, 8–14 March 1968.

85 Dan Sullivan, "Cerebrum: Club Seeking to Soothe the Mind," *New York Times*, 23 November 1968.

86 Larry Vigus, email to the author, 16 November 2013.

87 For a short video presentation of the Cerebrum, see "Cerebrum, Soho, 1968," accessed 8 November 2013, http://www.youtube.com/watch?v=VjozaLBbrUs.

88 Alastair Gordon, "What a Long, Strange Trip It's Been," *Interior Design*, 3 January 2007.

89 Gene Youngblood, "Part Six: Intermedia," in *Expanded Cinema* (New York: Dutton, 1970), 363.

90 Vigus, email to the author, 8 November 2013.

91 Dorothy Kalins, "Here's Looking at You: Voyeurism in New York," *New York*, 3 March 1969, 40.

92 Vigus, email to the author, 9 November 2013. Only one couple used LSD daily.

93 Vigus, email to the author, 16 November 2013.

94 Isaac Abrams, interview.

NOTES TO PAGES 155–7

CHAPTER SEVEN

1 William A. Frosch "Statement of Dr. William A. Frosch, Psychiatrist, Bellevue Hospital, New York, N.Y.," *The Narcotic Rehabilitation Act of 1966*, Hearings before a Special Subcommittee of the Committee on the Judiciary, United States Senate, 89th Congress, 2nd Session, January 25–7, May 12, 13, 19, 23, and 25, June 14 and 15, July 19, 1966 (Washington, DC: US Government Printing Office, 1966), 302–5.

2 Walter Bowart, "Leary's Politics and Ethics of Ecstasy," *East Village Other* 1, no. 10, 15 April–1 May 1966, 7. Some psychedelic drug users took issue with Leary's generalizations. One of Leary's "middle-agers" had begun his psychedelic experimentation in 1961 and had enjoyed forty-eight psychedelic experiences, mostly with LSD and mescaline, all under medical supervision. After reading Leary's *Politics of Ecstasy*, he told him that despite being forty-seven years of age, he believed "deeply in the truth and value of the psychedelic experience" and could "hardly be accused of the white middle-class revulsion [Leary spoke of]." See Andrew M. Underhill to Timothy Leary, 14 November 1968, folder 10, box 71, Leary papers.

3 For a history of runaways, see Staller, *Runaways*. As Staller shows, this occurred at a time when the media began to portray the act of running away as a social problem, whereas it had previously been characterized as a benign form of "Huck Finn" adventure-seeking.

4 Mele, *Selling the Lower East Side*, 174.

5 Ibid., 155.

6 Conor Hannan, "'We Have Our Own Struggle': Up Against the Wall Motherfucker and the Avant-Garde of Community Action, the Lower East Side, 1968," *The Sixties* 9, no. 1 (2016): 115–44.

7 Lankevich, *American Metropolis*, 206. In 1969, unemployment figures were lower than in any other city with the exception of Dallas.

8 Schneider, *Smack*, ix.

9 David Hoffman, telephone interview by the author, 8 March 2016.

10 Kent, *From Slogans to Mantras*, 7. On pages 107–13, Kent tells the story of a Berkeley student who embraced New Left activism but became increasingly disillusioned, particularly after experimenting with LSD in 1965. He ceased taking drugs when he joined the Church of Scientology in the East Village. See also Arthur Versluis, *American Gurus: From American Transcendentalism to New Age Religion* (Oxford, UK; New York: Oxford University Press, 2014).

11 Siff, *Acid Hype*, 170–3.

12 See, for example, "Electric Last Minute," *Eye*, April 1969, folder "Eye," 84–5, box 19, Stafford papers.

13 Peter Kerr, "Aaron E. Koota, 78, Is Dead; Former Judge and Prosecutor," *New York Times*, 23 July 1984.

NOTES TO PAGES 157–60 | 245

14 Murray Schumach, "New Laws Urged for LSD Pushers," *New York Times*, 16 April 1966. Koota, though, had no axe to grind with scientific study into LSD and psychedelics, which "may well serve a useful purpose in treating diseases of the mind."

15 "Koota Says Students Make LSD in Classes," *Daily News*, 20 April 1966, folder "College Drug Scandals," box 3, Stafford papers.

16 "The DA's LSD Cue Gives Schools Little to Go On," *New York Post*, 20 April 1966, folder "College Drug Scandals," box 3, Stafford papers.

17 "Principals Deplore Koota's LSD Charge," *New York Times*, 15 May 1966.

18 "Koota Urges LSD Crackdown," *Daily News*, 16 April 1966, folder "LSD – Legislation," box 8, Stafford papers.

19 Levin, "LSD in New York," *New York Post*, 9 June 1966.

20 Timothy Lee, "Students See No Rise in Use of Drugs," *New York Post*, 6 July 1966, folder "College Drug Scandals," box 3, Stafford papers.

21 Natalie Jaffe, "Stronger Curbs on LSD Proposed," *New York Times*, 30 April 1966.

22 Thomas J. Fleming, "Case of the Debatable Brooklyn D.A.," *New York Times Magazine*, 19 March 1967, page unavailable, folder "Koota, A.E.," box 7, Stafford Papers.

23 Richard L. Madden, "Legislature Gets Bills to Curb LSD," *New York Times*, 19 April 1966.

24 F. David Anderson, "Jury Acquits Kessler in LSD Murder," *New York Times*, 26 October 1967.

25 "Ban on LSD Voted by State Senate," *New York Times*, 29 April 1966.

26 "First LSD Casualty," *East Village Other* 2, no. 6, 15 February–1 March 1967.

27 De Rienzo and Beal, "Howard Lotsof."

28 Samuel Pearlman, "Drug Use and Experience in an Urban College Population," *American Journal of Orthopsychiatry* 38, no. 3 (1968): 503–14.

29 Jacob Brackman, "Four Ways to Go: The End of the Trip," *Esquire*, September 1966, folder "Esquire," box 18, Stafford papers.

30 Joseph Martin and john Quinn, "U.S.A. vs LSD: Hip (not Hippie) Unit Battling Drug Flood," *Daily News*, 29 January 1968, folder "Drugs Crackdown," box 4, Stafford papers.

31 Joseph Martin and john Quinn, "U.S.A. vs LSD: Special Agents Turn on the Heat in Drug War," *Daily News*, 30 January 1968, folder "Drugs Crackdown," box 4, Stafford papers.

32 (author unavailable), "LSD: Alarums and Excursions," *M.D.*, September 1968, 112, folder "LSD – Medical Accounts," box 8, Stafford papers.

33 David Brestid, "On LSDollars, Probers Told," *Daily News*, 28 June 1967, folder "LSD – Mafia," box 8, Stafford papers.

34 Richard (surname unreadable) to Timothy Leary, 24 May 1967, folder 1, box 74, Leary papers.

246 | NOTES TO PAGES 160–3

35 "Midipusher," interview by Jaakov Kohn, *East Village Other* 4, no. 8, 24 January 1969.

36 Fred Pincas to Timothy Leary, October 1969, folder 5, box 73, Leary papers.

37 David Walley, "Conversation with a Sixteen Year Old Junkie," *East Village Other* 5, no. 10, 11 February 1970.

38 Joseph Mulkern, "A Socialist Presidential Candidate – No, Not That One – Looks Back," *The Villager*, 27 August 2015.

39 "Interview: Rex Garvin," *Othersounds.com*, 31 January 2011, http://othersounds.com/interview-rex-garvin.

40 Courtwright, "The Rise and Fall and Rise of Cocaine in the United States."

41 Quoted in Edward Pouncey, "Laboratories of Light: Psychedelic Light Shows," in Grunenberg and Harris, *Summer of Love*, 176.

42 Ron Rosenbaum, "Leary's Final Dropout: 'This Time Around'?," *Village Voice*, 8 January 1970, folder "Village Voice," Stafford papers.

43 Szekely, "Teen Talk."

44 See Nicholas Schou, *Orange Sunshine: The Brotherhood of Eternal Love and Its Quest to Spread Peace, Love, and Acid to the World* (New York: Thomas Dunne Books, 2010).

45 "Sunshine Supermen," interview by Jaakov Kohn in the *East Village Other* 4, no. 28, 19 June 1969.

46 William Slattery, "Researcher Argues Pot Laws Hurt, Not Help, Society," *Staten Island Avenue*, 17 November 1969, folder "Krippner, Stanley," box 7, Stafford papers.

47 John Garabedian, "East Village: A Bad Trip," *New York Post*, 3 July 1968, folder "Drugs Crackdown," box 4, Stafford papers.

48 "Mafia Acid," New York Provo Statement, 20 July 1967, folder "LSD – Mafia," box 8, Stafford papers.

49 "Scenes," *Village Voice*, 23 March 1967. Nick Sand is credited for discovering this drug.

50 Don McNeill, "Is Acid Obsolete? The New Letters Are STP," *Village Voice*, 12 April 1967, folder "STP," box 13, Stafford papers. STP was created by Nick Sand.

51 Edwards, interview.

52 "Zonk," letter to the *East Village Other* 2, no. 22, 1–15 October 1967.

53 Eugene Schoenfeld, "Hip-pocrates," *East Village Other* 4, no. 22, 30 April 1969, folder, *East Village Other*, box 18, Stafford papers.

54 "Cyanara," *East Village Other* 2, no. 10, 15 April 15–1 May 1970, folder "Banana High, Pepper, etc.," box 2, Stafford papers. Ed Rosenfeld subsequently published a book offering 250 ways of altering consciousness without drugs. Edward Rosenfeld, *The Book of Highs: 250 Methods for Altering Your Consciousness without Drugs* (New York: Quadrangle, 1973).

NOTES TO PAGES 163–7 | 247

55 Mele, *Selling the Lower East Side*, 175.
56 Yuri Kapralov, *Once There Was a Village* (New York: St Martin's Press, 1974), 40.
57 Goldstein, interview.
58 John Kifner, "The East Village: A Changing Scene for the Hippies," *New York Times*, 11 October 1967. Marci Reaven and Jean Houck have dubbed the park "a sensitive barometer of the city's tensions." See "A History of Tompkins Square Park," in Janet L. Abu-Lughod, *From Urban Village to East Village*, 82. See also Herbert G. Gutman, "The Tompkins Square 'Riot' in New York City on January 13, 1874: A Re-examination of Its Causes and Its Aftermath," *Labor History* 6, no. 1 (1965): 44–70; Neil Smith, "'Class Struggle on Avenue B': The Lower East Side as Wild West," in *The New Urban Frontier: Gentrification and the Revanchist City* (London; New York: Routledge, 1996), 3–27.
59 Schneider, *Vampires, Dragons, and Egyptian Kings*, 218.
60 David Hardy and Judson Hand, "A Night in the East Village," *Daily News*, 11 October 1967, folder "Drugs Danger," box 5, Stafford Papers.
61 As quoted in Sukenick, *Down and In*, 183.
62 Sanders, *Fug You*, 241–2.
63 Edwards, interview.
64 Weed, interview.
65 "Hippie Delicatessen Is Raided by Police for Way-out Food," *New York Times*, 23 June 1968.
66 Weed, interview.
67 Quoted in Yablonsky, *The Hippie Trip*, 115.
68 Quoted in ibid., 145.
69 Kapralov, *Once There Was a Village*, 13. Contact followed in the footsteps of the better-known Covenant House. See Staller, *Runaways*, xvi–xxv.
70 Kapralov, *Once There Was a Village*, 43. Around 1968, a heroin addict mugged Goldstein and his then-wife in a Village hallway and took their money. Goldstein, interview by the author.
71 Kapralov, *Once There Was a Village*, 89.
72 Martin Gansberg, "Electric Circus Turns off Lights for the Last Time," *New York Times*, 8 August 1971.
73 Kapralov, *Once There Was a Village*, 111–18.
74 Peter Leggieri, "Peter Leggieri's East Village Other," *East Village Other*, accessed 8 August 2021, http://eastvillageother.org/recollections/leggieri-2.
75 Allen Ginsberg, "Renaissance or Die," *Los Angeles Free Press*, 23 December 1966, folder "Ginsberg, Allen," box 6, Stafford papers.
76 In San Francisco, a study reported that an overwhelming number of members had used LSD and marijuana prior to joining the church. See J. Stillson Judah, *Hare Krishna and the Counterculture* (New York: Wiley, 1974), as referenced in E. Burke Rochford, "Aligning Hare

Krishna: Political Activists, Hippies, and Hindus," *Nova Religio* 22, no. 1 (2018): 34–58.

77 Quoted in ibid., 43.

78 James R. Sikes, "Swami's Flock Chants in Park to Find Ecstasy," *New York Times*, 10 October 1966.

79 Margalit Fox, "Swami Bhaktipada Dies at Age 74," *New York Times*, 25 October 2011.

80 Kent, *From Slogans to Mantras*, 55.

81 McNeill, *Moving through Here*, 91–3.

82 Al Van Starrex, "Hippie Businessmen," *Mr. Magazine* 12, no. 7, May 1968, 39, folder "Drugs Crackdown," box 4, Stafford papers.

83 Jill Johnson, "Alpert's Third Life & the Chemistry of Divinity," *Village Voice*, 26 December 1968, folder "Village Voice," box 33, Stafford papers. Ram Dass also published a best-selling memoir: *Be Here Now* (Albuquerque, NM: Lama Foundation, 1971).

84 Graboi, *One Foot in the Future*, 271.

85 Linda Crawford, "Yoga," *East Village Other* 6, no. 26, 25 May 1971.

86 Don McNeill, "The Swami Makes the People Glow," *Village Voice* 12, no. 42, 3 August 1967.

87 Jeremy Varon, *Bringing the War Home: The Weather Underground, the Red Army Faction, and Revolutionary Violence in the Sixties and Seventies* (Berkeley: University of California Press, 2004), 159.

88 Sam Green and Bill Siegel, "The Weather Underground" (DVD, The Free History Project, 2002).

89 Duncan, *The Rebel Café*, 89–90.

90 Ibid., 111.

91 Ibid., 206.

92 Ibid., 231–2.

93 Graboi, *One Foot in the Future*, 294–5.

94 As quoted in Greenfield, *Timothy Leary*, 381.

95 Woodruff Leary, *Psychedelic Refugee*, 274.

96 Greenfield, *Timothy Leary*, 381.

97 Katzman, "Poor Paranoid's Almanac."

98 Graboi, *One Foot in the Future*, 295–7.

99 Woodruff Leary, *Psychedelic Refugee*, 275.

100 Art Kleps, "Sir Launcelot and Knights to the Rescue," in Kleps, *Millbrook*.

101 Art Kleps, "The Yankee and the King Sold as Slaves," in Kleps, *Millbrook*.

102 Abrams, interview.

103 Art Kleps, "The Battle of the Sand Belt," in Kleps, *Millbrook*.

104 Alfred Friendly Jr, "Police Fear Child Swallowed LSD," *New York Times*, 7 April 1966.

105 Siff, *Acid Hype*, 153. As in the Kessler case, the charges were dropped against the uncle because the poisoning was obviously an accident.

106 Warth, "The Acid Profiteers."

107 Art Kleps, "Sir Launcelot and Knights to the Rescue," in Kleps, *Millbrook*.

108 Warth, "The Acid Profiteers."

109 Hood, *In Pursuit of Privilege*.

110 Levin, "LSD in New York," *New York Post*, 7 June 1966.

111 Frank, *The Conquest of Cool*, 114.

112 Ibid., 35.

113 Ibid., 55.

114 Marlene Dobkin de Rios and Oscar Janiger, *LSD, Spirituality, and the Creative Process* (Rochester, VT: Park Street Press, 2003); Milana Aronov, "(Micro-) 'Psychedelic' Experiences: From the 1960s Creativity at the Workplace to the 21st Century Neuro-Newspeak," *Ethnologie française* 176, no. 4 (2019): 701–18.

115 Frank, *The Conquest of Cool*, 114.

116 "Insult Me, Comrade!" *Newsweek*, 14 April 1969, 112, folder "Art," box 2, Stafford papers.

117 "Peter Max: Mastering the Color Explosion," *Village Voice*, 31 August 1967, folder "LSD + Art," box 8, Stafford papers.

118 J. Anthony Lukas, "The Drug Scene," *New York Times Magazine*, 8–12 January 1968, 6, folder "Drugs," box 4, Stafford papers.

119 Leroy F. Adams, "LSD Is Taking a Trip Uptown," *New York Times*, 19 February 1967. LSD also inspired a fashion designer to make electronic dresses that allegedly recalled the psychedelic experience. Other leading garment manufacturers also realized the new trend and started to design "psychedelic fabrics."

120 Frank, *The Conquest of Cool*, 109.

121 Adams, "LSD Is Taking a Trip Uptown."

122 Glueck, "Multimedia." USCO collaborated with the Albert Einstein Medical Research Center in Philadelphia to work on an "overstimulator environment" to study endocrinological response.

123 Clive Barnes, "Dance: The Joffrey's Psychedelic Trip," *New York Times*, 21 September 1967. For an excerpt of the ballet, see "Film Excerpt: The making of Joffrey's 'Astarte,'" accessed 12 February 2014, http://www.pbs.org/wnet/americanmasters/episodes/joffrey/film-excerpt-the-making-of-joffrey%E2%80%99s-astarte/2395.

124 Glueck, "Multimedia."

125 Schwartz, "Context, Value and Direction," 149.

126 Levin, "LSD in New York," *New York Post*, 8 June 1966.

127 Levin, "LSD in New York," *New York Post*, 9 June 1966.

128 Peter Braunstein, "Disco," *American Heritage* 50, no. 7 (1999), pages unavailable, https://www.americanheritage.com/disco#2.

129 For example, Dynamite opened in Brooklyn in 1968 in an attempt to attract the same crowds. Alex Gross, "Dynamite Discotheque," *East Village Other* 4, no. 5, 3 January 1969.

130 "Clubs Offer Today's Youth 'Something to Do' at Night," *The Spokesman-Review*, 17 September 1967.

131 Barry N. Schwartz, "The Kinetic Scope of Cassen and Stern," in *Arts in Society: Tenth Anniversary Issue*, ed. Edward Kamarck (Madison: University of Wisconsin Press, 1969), 95–102, https://images.library.wisc.edu/Arts/EFacs/ArtsSoc/ArtsSocv06i1/reference/arts.artssocv06i1.bnschwartz.pdf.

132 John Gruen, "Cheetah – The Now Club," *New York/World Journal Tribune*, 29 January 1967, folder "Drugs Crackdown (2)," box 5, Stafford papers.

133 Newman, "Call It Psychedelic."

134 "Clubs Offer Today's Youth 'Something to Do' at Night."

135 "Hippies 'Integrate' with Puerto Ricans," *New York Times*, 16 August 1967.

136 "Scenes," *Village Voice*, 15 June 1967, folder "Be-ins," box 2, Stafford papers.

137 Vincent Canby, "A New Nightclub to Have 3 Stories," *New York Times*, 1 April 1966.

138 Mele, *Selling the Lower East Side*, 168.

139 Ibid., 157.

140 Ibid., 168.

CHAPTER EIGHT

1 Rasmussen, *On Speed*, 182–3.

2 Jessica Neptune, "Harshest in the Nation: The Rockefeller Drug Laws and the Widening Embrace of Punitive Politics," *Social History of Alcohol and Drugs* 26, no. 2 (2012): 170–91. For discussions on the opiate treatment models before these more punitive measures, see David T. Courtwright, "The Prepared Mind: Marie Nyswander, Methadone Maintenance, and the Metabolic Theory of Addiction," *Addiction* 92, no. 3 (1997): 257–65; Claire Clark, "'Chemistry Is the New Hope': Therapeutic Communities and Methadone Maintenance, 1965–71," *Social History of Alcohol and Drugs* 26, no. 2 (2012): 192–216.

3 Alice O'Connor, "The Privatized City: The Manhattan Institute, the Urban Crisis, and the Conservative Counterrevolution in New York," *Journal of Urban History* 34, no. 2 (2008): 333–53; Phillips-Fein, *Fear City*.

4 Nicholas Freudenberg, Marianne Fahs, Sandro Galea, and Andrew Greenberg, "The Impact of New York City's 1975 Fiscal Crisis on the Tuberculosis, HIV, and Homicide Syndemic," *American Journal of Public Health* 96, no. 3 (2006): 425–6.

5 In the Netherlands, psychiatrist Jan Baastians treated concentration camp survivors with LSD into the mid-1980s, which also suggests greater historical continuity than is currently assumed.

NOTES TO PAGES 182–5 | 251

6 Steven Conn, "Back to the Garden: Communes, the Environment, and Antiurban Pastoralism at the End of the Sixties," *Journal of Urban History* 36, no. 6 (2010): 831–48.

7 Adam Rome, "'Give Earth a Chance': The Environmental Movement and the Sixties," *Journal of American History* 90, no. 2 (2003): 541–2.

8 Rome concurs on page 543. This connection has since been underscored in several recent studies. See, for example, Matthias Forstmann and Christina Sagioglou, "Lifetime Experience with (Classic) Psychedelics Predicts Pro-Environmental Behavior through an Increase in Nature Relatedness," *Journal of Psychopharmacology* 31, no. 8 (2017): 975–88; Hannes Kettner et al., "From Egoism to Ecoism: Psychedelics Increase Nature Relatedness in a State-Mediated and Context-Dependent Manner," *International Journal of Environmental Research and Public Health* 16, no. 24 (2019): 5,147.

9 Babitz, "Statement," 561.

10 Quoted in Yablonsky, *The Hippie Trip*, 161–2.

11 Shelly Urso to Timothy Leary, 18 September 1967, folder 4, box 77; Leary papers.

12 Gray Henry quoted in Dass, Metzner, and Bravo, *Birth of a Psychedelic Culture*, 209.

13 Rachel Abrams, interview.

14 Graboi, *One Foot in the Future*, 294.

15 Nina Graboi, "I'm a Sixty Year Old Adolescent," date unavailable, 2, box 1, Graboi papers.

16 Carey, interview, 4.

17 "Midipusher," interview by Jaakov Kohn, *East Village Other* 4, no. 8, 24 January 1969.

18 Quoted in Graboi, *One Foot in the Future*, 226.

19 Roy Rosenzweig and Elizabeth Blackmar, *The Park and the People: A History of Central Park* (Ithaca, NY, and London: Cornell University Press, 1992), 489–97, quotation on p. 493.

20 Viteritti, "Times a-Changin'," 16–17.

21 Rosenzweig and Blackmar, *The Park and the People*, 494.

22 Edwards, interview.

23 Goldstein, interview.

24 Scully, "Nick Sand."

25 Schou, *Orange Sunshine*, 167.

26 Ibid., 72.

27 "Sunshine Supermen," interview by Jaakov Kohn in the *East Village Other* 4, no. 28, 19 June 1969.

28 Jarnow, *Heads*, 42.

29 "Intergalactic Union Doprogram," *East Village Other* 5, no. 16, 27 March 1970.

30 Jarnow, *Heads*, 42.

31 Ibid., 54.

32 Quoted in ibid., 104.

33 John Roger, "Brooklyn Native Nicholas Sand, Creator of Famous Orange Sunshine LSD, Dies," *Brooklyn Daily Eagle*, 17 May 2017.

34 Steve Bloom, "Flashback," in *Psychedelic Trips for the Mind*, ed. Paul Krassner (New York: Trans-High Corp., 2001), 142–3. Bloom refers to 1971 in this collection, but multiple sources indicate that the band played there in 1974.

35 As quoted in Jarnow, *Heads*, 118.

36 Hilton Obenzinger, "When the Grateful Dead Joined the Columbia Strike, Friday, May 3, 1968 – What Some Friends Heard, Saw, and Said," *The Sixties* 9, no. 2 (2016): 290–4. They only stopped touring in 1995 with the death of singer Jerry Garcia.

37 Jarnow, *Heads*, 118.

38 Ibid., 134.

39 Schneider, *Smack*, 188–9.

40 Goldstein, interview.

41 Abrams, "Retour sur une carrière d'artiste psychédélique."

42 Alex Grey, interview by David Jay Brown ("Reflections on a Sacred Mirror"), 1995, http://www.mavericksofthemind.com/grey-int.htm.

43 Lawrence, *Love Saves the Day*, 1–13.

44 Barry Walters, "David Mancuso's Message of Love," *Village Voice*, 22 November 2016.

45 "Love Saves the Day: An Interview with the Legendary NYC Club Pioneer and DJ David Mancuso," *Dangerous Minds*, 18 November 2016, https://dangerousminds.net/comments/love_saves_the_day_an_interview_with_the_legendary_nyc_club_pioneer_and_dj_.

46 Lawrence, *Love Saves the Day*, 19.

47 Ibid., 22.

48 Richard Goldstein, email to the author, 25 April 2022.

49 David Farber, *Crack: Rock Cocaine, Street Capitalism, and the Decade of Greed* (New York: Cambridge University Press, 2019), 30–3.

50 Isaac Abrams, interview.

51 Goldstein, interview.

52 David Herzberg, "Quaalude Nostalgia: A Retro Drug That Everyone Remembers Fondly," *The Atlantic*, 21 February 2021, https://www.theatlantic.com/health/archive/2012/02/quaalude-nostalgia-a-retro-drug-that-everyone-remembers-fondly/252285.

53 Braunstein, "Disco."

54 Lawrence, *Love Saves the Day*, 30.

55 Goldstein, interview.

56 Linda Wolfe, "The Strange Case of Dr. Buettner-Janusch," *New Yorker*, 15 September 1980, 18–22.

57 Schneider, *Smack*, 192–5.

58 Farber, *Crack*, 7–8. Quotation on p. 7.

59 Shipley, "This Season's People," 42.

60 Ibid., 44–5.

61 De Rienzo and Beal, "The Staten Island Project," in *The Ibogaine Story*.

62 De Rienzo and Beal, "Bob Sisko." Beal had been organizing "smoke-ins" in Tompkins Square Park in the late Sixties. See Dufton, *Grass Roots*, 21.

63 Thomas O'Toole, "LSD Found to Be Regaining Its Popularity," *Washington Post*, 21 July 1983.

64 Brad, interview.

65 Steve Grant, "Wooster Source," *Time Out*, 27 August–12 September 1986, 13, Wooster Group Ephemera, 1976–1999, Billy Rose Theater Division, New York Public Library for the Performing Arts. For a documentary on the play, see Alan Benson, "The Wooster Group," aired on "The South Bank Show" on 22 February 1987, available at http://ubu.com/film/wooster.html. For more on the Wooster Group and the play, see David Savran, *Breaking the Rules: The Wooster Group* (New York: Theatre Communications Group, 2005).

66 Patricia Leigh Brown, "Psychedelic-Art Show Is Reflection of Its Era," *New York Times*, 28 January 1988. CCN briefly reported on the gallery. See https://www.youtube.com/watch?v=ShdOjfEY5kc (accessed 14 February 2017).

67 Kramer, "Grooving out of Business."

68 Thomas Lyttle, "Drug Based Religions and Contemporary Drug Taking," *Journal of Drug Issues* 18, no. 2 (1988): 271–84.

69 Julie Holland, "The History of MDMA," in *Ecstasy: The Complete Guide*, ed. Julie Holland (Rochester, VT: Park Street Press, 2001), 11–17. See also Tim Pilcher, *E: The Incredibly Strange History of Ecstasy* (Philadelphia and London: Running Press, 2008).

70 Mele, *Selling the Lower East Side*, 220.

71 Rosenfeld, interview.

72 George James, "Limelight Goes Dark as Crackdown on Drugs Reaches Major Clubs," *New York Times*, 5 October 1995.

73 David Rohde, "Ecstasy Overdoses Continue despite Nightclub's Closing," *New York Times*, 4 September 2001.

74 Bill Werde, "Acid Test," *Village Voice*, 21 August 2001.

75 William K. Rashbaum, "Drug Experts Report a Boom in Ecstasy Use," *New York Times*, 26 February 2000.

76 De Rienzo and Beal, "Dhoruba Moore," in *The Ibogaine Story*.

77 De Rienzo and Beal, "Jon Parker," in *The Ibogaine Story*.

78 De Rienzo and Beal, "Carlo Contoreggi," in *The Ibogaine Story*.

79 De Rienzo and Beal, "Bwiti," in *The Ibogaine Story*.

80 De Rienzo and Beal, "Molliver's Travel," in *The Ibogaine Story*.

81 Dennis Hevesi, "Howard Lotsof Dies at 66; Saw Drug Cure in a Plant," *New York Times*, 17 February 2010.

82 Nancy S. Alexander, "Bouncing Back from Crack," *New Yorker*, 12 February 1990, 41.

83 Joseph B. Treaster, "A New Generation Discovers LSD, and Its Dangers," *New York Times*, 27 December 1991.

84 Henderson, "LSD Use and LSD Users: Questions and Answers about LSD," in *LSD: Still with Us after All These Years*, 97.

85 David M. Herszenhorn, "LSD Factory Is Discovered in Rockaway," *New York Times*, 6 April 1997.

86 Joseph Goldstein, "Under Cover in Drug Case at Columbia, Now Arrested," *New York Times*, 10 June 2011.

87 Mike Power, *Drugs Unlimited: The Web Revolution That's Changing How the World Gets High* (New York: Thomas Dunne Books, 2013).

88 Rosenfeld, interview.

89 Vanessa Grigoriadis, "Travels in the New Psychedelic Bazaar," *New York Magazine*, 7 April 2013, 3–4.

90 Isaac Abrams, interview.

91 Gerd Stern, interview.

92 Isaac Abrams, interview. Although some evidence supports these claims, one of the reasons that they are difficult to assess is that there is a significant dip in the quantity and quality of media coverage in the 1970s when it lost interest in LSD. Siff, *Acid Hype*, 3.

93 Brad, interview.

A WAVE THAT NEVER ROLLED BACK

1 Hunter S. Thompson, *Fear and Loathing in Las Vegas: A Savage Journey to the Heart of the American Dream* (London: Harper Perennial, 2005), 67–8.

2 Dave Boothroyd, *Culture on Drugs: Narco-Cultural Studies of High Modernity* (Manchester: Manchester University Press, 2007).

3 Di Prima, *Recollections*, 202.

4 Graboi, *One Foot in the Future*, 248.

5 Isaac Abrams, interview.

6 Susun S. Weed, *Healing Wise* (Woodstock, NY: Ash Tree Publishing, 1989).

7 Weed, interview.

8 Rosenfeld, interview.

9 Krippner, interview.

10 Edwards, interview.

11 Rachel Abrams, interview.

12 Goldstein, interview.

13 Paul Krassner, "My Acid Trip with Groucho Marx," in *Psychedelic Trips for the Mind*, 175.

Index

2-CB, 193
4-ACO-DET, 196
2001, 150

Abrams, Isaac, 17, 132, 143, 145, 154, 171, 182, 187, 189, 193, 196, 197, 199, 200, 201; becomes a painter, 138; early life, 134; first DMT experience, 136; first ibogaine experience, 137–8; first LSD experience, 137–8; first mescaline experience, 135; first psilocybin experience, 135; and jazz, 134, 135; meets Dalí, 142; meets Leary, 139; meets Lotsof, 137; psychedelic art exhibition, 139–42; religious freedom, 146
Abrams, Rachel, 17, 132, 143, 145, 154, 182, 199, 203; first DMT experience, 136; first LSD experience, 137–8; first mescaline experience, 135; first psilocybin experience, 135; psychedelic art exhibition, 139–42
Abramson, Harold, 64, 67–8, 80, 83, 85
abstract expressionism, 133, 134
Acid Test, 8, 9
addiction, 8, 10, 22, 28, 40, 78, 104, 105, 121, 156, 159, 160–1, 164, 165, 180, 181, 191–2, 195
Agora Scientific Trust, 74–5, 81, 84

Alcoholics Anonymous, 67
Aldcroft, Richard, 145
Alper, Kenneth, 195
Alpert, Richard (a.k.a. "Baba Ram Dass"), 7, 44, 87, 90, 91, 92, 107–8, 112, 117, 144, 167–8
Altamont Rock Festival, 6
altered states of consciousness, 58, 71, 72, 81, 111, 119
American Ethnological Society, 213n15
American Museum of Natural History, 42
American Psychiatric Association, 63
American Psychological Association, 57
American Society for Psychical Research, 110
American Weekly, 67
amphetamines, 8, 29, 40, 41, 105, 121, 135, 153, 159, 160, 161, 164, 166, 180, 188; and the Beats, 28, 34, 46; Benzedrine, 27, 28, 69; and jazz, 19, 26, 27; medical use of, 27, 69. *See also* methedrine
Anderson, Chester, 30
Andrews, George, 35–6, 52
Anslinger, Harry, 26
Anti-Drug Abuse Act, 190
anti-war movement, 6, 14, 39, 156, 169, 182

256 | INDEX

Argyll Laboratories Company, 220n18
Army Chemical Corps, 66
art galleries, 77, 125, 134, 139
Astarte, 175–6
astrology, 22
Atwell, Allen, 139
ayahuasca, 45, 200

Baastians, Jan, 250n5
Babitz, Eve, 79, 182
Balding, David, 187
banana hoax, 128–9
barbiturates, 29, 159, 160, 189
Bashlow, Robert, 39, 40
Bayer, 20
Beal, Dana, 192, 194, 195
Beatles, the, 161, 174, 175
beatnik, 217n91
Beats, 16, 27–9, 33, 34, 36, 46, 49, 57, 95, 98, 133, 145, 164, 217n91; and gender, 30–2, 33, 34, 42; publicity, 34, 35, 93; and race, 19, 33, 50
bebop, 18–9, 27, 41
Beckman, Bill, 129
Bellevue Hospital, 60, 61, 69, 155
Bender, Lauretta, 64, 68–70, 83, 199
Beresford, John, 74–5, 76, 80, 87, 88
Bernstein, Leonard, 147
Bethesda Fountain, 181, 183
Bick, Chuck, 88
Bieberman, Lisa, 131, 145
bin Wahad, Dhoruba al-Mujahid, 194–5
Bios Laboratories, 38
Birdland, 51, 52, 134
bisexuality, 29, 30, 92
Black Panthers, 181
Blacks, 19, 20, 33, 95, 97, 176, 180
Blauer, Harold, 66
Bleecker Street, 72, 96, 97, 169
Bloom, Steve, 185–6
Bogart, Larry, 112
Bohemians, 8, 9, 13, 18, 19, 21, 26–8,

31–6, 41, 44, 50, 58, 95, 97, 98
Bolton, Frances, 30
Book of Highs, The, 246n54
Book of Tao, The, 93
Bowart, Walter, 97–8, 127, 129, 166
Bowery, 182, 187
Brandeis University, 111, 112
Bridge Theater, 146
Brill, Abraham, 21, 25
Broadway, 95, 97, 123, 150, 152, 176, 188
Brooklyn, 9, 71, 92, 104, 135, 136, 137, 138, 143, 151, 155, 157, 158, 159, 172, 183, 184
Brotherhood of Eternal Love, 161, 184–6
Buddhist Society, 25, 29
Buettner-Janusch, John, 190
buffoteine, 88
bufotenine, 220n18
Bureau of Drug Abuse Control, 80, 158
Burroughs, William, 19, 27, 28, 35, 39, 187; at APA conference, 57

Café Au Go Go, 186
Canada, 104, 185, 224n30
cannabis, 5, 13, 16, 26, 27, 28, 32, 33, 39, 41, 52, 54, 112, 113, 122, 125, 135, 146, 149 152, 153, 159, 170, 171, 172, 180, 183, 184, 194; activism, 97, 120, 181, 185–6, 192, 200; and the Beats, 28, 31, 35, 36; in the East Village, 99, 129, 130, 163; in Greenwich Village, 35, 36, 130, 189; and jazz, 19, 26, 32; and Mexicans, 26; precursor of LSD, 88
Captain High, 129
Carey, Martin, 92, 130, 183
Cassady, Neal, 28; first psilocybin experience, 45–6
Cassen, Jackie, 133, 145, 175, 177, 199; collaborates with Leary, 146–8; rift with Leary, 149–50

INDEX | 257

Cattel, James, 65, 66
Center for the League for Spiritual
    Discovery, 17, 115–16, 131, 143, 168,
    169, 199; counselling, 116, 120;
    countercultural haven, 119–20;
    end of, 122; harm reduction,
    121; inauguration, 117–18;
    location, 116; and the police, 120;
    sexuality, 118–19; spirituality, 118
Central Intelligence Agency, 64, 67,
    69, 70, 87
Central Park, 25, 26, 73, 77, 101, 124,
    128, 133, 170, 178, 181; new home
    for psychedelia, 183–6
Central Park Easter Be-in, 128
Cerebrum, 134, 152–4, 199
Channel One, 100
Charles Theater, 135
Cheetah, 176–8
Chinatown, 20
Chinese immigrants, 20, 23, 55
City College of New York, 103
City Health Department, 36, 39
City Lights Books, 49
civil rights, 6, 61, 133, 156, 183
Clark, Walter Houston, 67
Clinton, Hillary, 72
cocaine, 10, 17, 20–1, 23, 27, 31, 32, 33,
    40, 41, 46
Coda galleries, 139–42
coffeehouses, 28, 36, 38, 97
Coltrane, John, 19
Columbia University, 19, 28, 29, 31,
    38, 63, 64, 68, 75, 88, 122, 149, 158,
    167, 182, 195
Columbia University strikes, 186
Committee to Legalize Marijuana, 97
conferences, 55, 57–9, 67, 69, 111, 113,
    115, 200
Contact, 165
Controlled Substance Act, 83
Cooper, Ruffin, 152
Cooper Square 96
Cooper Square Arts Theater 151

Coquelin, Olivier, 176–7
Cornell University, 139
Corner, Michael, 72
Corso, Gregory, 32, 35, 117
countercultural capital, 120, 124
counterculture, 7, 8, 11, 17,
    106; and academia, 118;
    embraced by Graboi, 114;
    and environmentalism, 182;
    and Indian gurus, 166; and
    the League for Spiritual
    Discovery, 115–19; and Maslow,
    112; migration to the East
    Village, 122–31; and progressive
    movements, 107–8, 157; and sex,
    119; and society, 109, 121; and
    women, 108
Covenant House, 247n69
crack, 17, 181, 190–1, 197
crash pads, 109, 118, 130, 156, 164
Creedmoor State Hospital, 69
Crumb, Robert, 129
Cuernavaca, Mexico, 44
Cullen, Robert, 78

Dahlberg, Charles, 65, 76, 81–2, 84, 85
Daoism, 96
dark net, 196
datura, 20
Davis, Miles, 19, 29
de Ropp, Robert, 40–1, 54
Death of the Mind, The, 147, 149
Deitch, Kim, 129
della-Cioppa, Mary, 43
Delta Chemical Works, 38
Denber, Herman, 82–3
Deneuve, Catherine, 178
depression, 29, 66, 69, 70, 77
DET, 113, 172, 193
Dexedrine, 34
Dharma Bums, 48
di Prima, Diane, 30–3, 34, 35, 58, 94,
    95, 96, 199, 201; tries marijuana,
    31; tries peyote, 37

258 | INDEX

disco, 11, 177, 187, 189
Displaced Persons Act, 31
Divine Comedy, 72
DMA, 66
DMT, 7, 9, 136, 142, 159, 200; effects of, 136; source, 9, 136; users, 136
Donovan, 128
Dora Weiner Foundation, 191
DPT, 193
Draper, Ray, 135
Drug Abuse Control Amendment, 80
drug dealers, 10, 23, 26, 36, 40, 54, 97, 101, 128, 129, 159, 160, 168, 183, 190, 194, 196, 200; and ethics, 101–2; and neighbourhoods, 23, 36, 176, 181, 186, 189, 195; and Orange Sunshine, 161, 184–5; profiles, 105
Drugs and the Mind, 40, 49
Dylan, Bob, 95, 125
Dynamite, 249n129

Eager, Allan, 78
East River, 55, 123
East Village, 8, 17, 125, 127, 135, 146–9, 157, 166–8, 170, 173, 178, 187, 194, 203; dealers, 105, 128; Electric Circus, 100; geography, 123; head shops, 99–100, 125–7; Native American Church, 186; new home for psychedelia, 96, 97–9, 106, 109, 131; real estate, 156, 194; runaways, 124–5, 156; tensions with the locals, 97; violence, 163–6
East Village Other, 106, 109, 123, 127, 129–30, 131, 147, 156, 160, 162, 185, 199; and banana hoax, 129; coverage of Eastern gurus, 166–7; and drugs, 129, 184; inception of, 97–9
Eastern spirituality, 12, 33, 37, 38, 46, 92, 96, 118, 139, 167, 168, 178, 195

Eastman, Max, 22
Ecstasy Review, 96
Edwards, Amelie, 102, 123–4, 162, 164, 183, 184, 202
Electric Circus, 100, 152, 165, 176
Electric Lotus, 99
environmentalism, 182, 251n8
Erickson, Reed, 142–3
Esalen Institute, 73
Escher, M.C., 146
ESP, 67, 110
Esquire, 38, 39
Evergreen Review, 49
experimental film, 135
Eye, 157

Fabrikant, Joel, 129
Far Rockaway, 195
Fear and Loathing in Las Vegas, 198
Federal Analog Act, 196
Federal Bureau of Narcotics, 26
Ferguson, Flora Lu and Maynard, 51–2, 54, 55, 58, 90, 92, 220n37
Fillmore East, 128, 165
first psychedelic art exhibition, 139–42
First Zen Institute of America, 29
Fisher, Florrie, 27
Fitzpatrick, Linda, 164
Five Spot, 50
Floating Bear, The, 58
Fonda, Peter, 178
Food and Drug Administration, 36, 39, 79, 80, 82, 128, 158, 159, 160, 195, 227n83
Foundation for Mind Research, 81
Frazer, Bonnie, 42
Freud, Sigmund, 21, 26, 71, 75
Friedman, Abby, 52, 59, 60, 62
Friedman, Bernard, 52–3, 54–6, 58–61, 62, 145, 199, 200
Frosch, William, 155
Fuchs, Ernst, 142
Fuck You magazine, 128

INDEX | 259

Galahad, 164
Garrett, Eileen, 30, 67
Garvin, Rex, 161
Gaskin, Stephen, 191
Gestalt, 64
Gilbert, Ronnie, 77
Gillespie, Dizzy, 39, 50
Ginsberg, Allen, 5, 9, 19, 27, 28, 29,
    30, 33, 34, 35, 41, 46–50, 57, 95, 117,
    169; and cannabis, 28; discovers
    Buddhism, 29; discovers
    psilocybin, 45; and jazz, 50–1;
    joins Hare Krishna, 167; meets
    Leary, 45
Girard, China, 54
Glenn, Virginia, 58, 110–13
Glick, Jeff, 99, 142
Goldstein, Richard, 102, 117, 130, 163,
    199, 203; and discos, 188–9; and
    nature, 184; and sex, 119, 190
Goldwater, Barry, 9
Gordon, Dexter, 28
Gordon, Waxy, 24
Gothic Blimp Works, 129
Gould, Chuck, 12
Gould, Stanley, 97
Graboi, Michel, 109–14, 116, 117
Graboi, Nina, 16, 108, 143, 147,
    168, 169–70, 183, 199, 200,
    201; becomes leader of the
    Center, 115–16; conference, 122;
    counsellor, 108–9, 116, 118–22;
    DET, 113–14; early life, 109–10;
    first cannabis experience, 113;
    first LSD experience, 114; and
    Leary, 111–12, 115–16, 116–17;
    and Maslow, 111; moves to
    Woodstock, 183; sexism, 108;
    spirituality, 110; transformed by
    psychedelics, 113, 114, 116, 117, 131
Graham, Bill, 128
Graham, Billy, 89, 93
Grateful Dead, the, 8, 178, 184, 186
Gray, Barry, 87

Greenwich Village, 16, 18, 53, 76, 93,
    95, 98, 102, 111, 112, 115, 122, 123,
    130, 131, 136, 147, 183, 193, 200;
    and alcohol, 24; and the Beats,
    27–9; as Bohemian capital, 8,
    30–4, 35; and Buddhism, 25, 29;
    and cannabis, 26, 35, 36; and
    heroin, 23; and ibogaine, 40; and
    jazz, 29, 50–1; Leary fundraiser,
    168–70; and LSD, 62, 87–8, 91,
    105, 106; and mescaline, 38–9;
    and peyote, 9, 21; psychoanalysis,
    25–6; and psilocybin, 42, 50–1
Grey, Alex, 17, 181, 187, 196
Group Image, 130–1, 178
Grove Press, 49

Haight-Ashbury, 5, 8
Haines, Bill, 171
Hair, 150
hallucinations, 25, 37, 66, 72, 151
Hamilton, George, 178
happenings, 8, 124, 128, 133, 145, 152
Harlem Hospital, 195
harm reduction, 110, 131
Harper's, 32
Harrington, Alan, 90–1
Harrington, Raymond, 21–2
Harrison Narcotics Tax Act, 21, 23
Harvard University, 42, 44–5, 51, 52,
    53, 54, 56, 57, 58, 59, 62, 91
hashish, 20, 33, 159, 168, 184
Hawaiian Baby Woodrose, 88
Head Shop, 99, 142
head shops, 99–100, 125, 164, 167,
    168, 199
Heard, Gerald, 225n57
Hearst, William Randolph, 24, 57, 67
Hell's Angels, 6
Henry, Gray, 113, 149, 182
heroin, 8, 10, 12, 17, 21, 23–4, 31–2, 32,
    33, 36, 40, 86, 104, 105, 121, 154,
    159, 160, 162–6, 187, 188, 190, 191–
    2, 194, 197; and the Beats, 27–8,

39, 46, 47–8, 97; and Blacks, 160–1, 180; distribution, 23–4, 97, 163; first released, 20; and jazz, 19, 27, 29, 78, 105–6, 135

hip, 213n9

hippie, 12, 75, 164

Hiskey, Clarence, 136

Hispanics, 180, 188. *See also* Puerto Ricans

Hitchcock, Aurora, 172

Hitchcock, Billy, 92, 112, 115, 122, 147, 172, 185

Hitchcock, Peggy, 78, 89–90, 127, 141, 170–2, 199

Hitchcock, Tommy, 92

Hitler, Adolf, 25, 114

Hoch, Paul, 199

Hoffman, Abbie, 64–6, 67, 68, 69–70, 76

Hoffmann-La Roche, 74

Hofmann, Albert, 6, 9, 126, 196

Holiday, Billie, 28

Hollingshead, Michael, 87, 89, 141, 144

Holt, Robert, 71

homosexuality, 29, 68, 89, 94, 119, 152, 183, 188, 189, 194

Hotel Albert, 111

Houston, Jean, 64, 71–6, 81, 82, 92, 103, 110; first LSD experience, 72; and Huxley, 73–4; training of guides, 74

Hoving, Thomas, 133

Howard Wise gallery, 151

"Howl", 30, 33, 34, 36, 49

Huautla de Jiménez, 42

Hudson River, 9, 33, 48, 62, 116

Hughes, Robert, 130

Huncke, Herbert, 28, 47, 97, 135

Hunter, Meredith, 6

Hutchinson, James (a.k.a. "Groovy"), 164

Huxley, Aldous, 52, 64, 73, 203; and Alcoholics Anonymous, 67; influence on the media, 16, 32, 49, 86–7; influence on psychedelia, 7, 14, 19, 38, 41, 42, 45, 54, 70, 74, 90, 110, 138; and "instant childhood", 108; *Island*, 73–4, 135; and Leary, 44–5, 51–2, 56, 90

Huxley, Laura, 64, 112

hyperkinesia, 69

I Love You, Alice B. Toklas, 150

ibogaine, 11, 17, 41; arrival in New York, 19, 36, 39; effects of, 137–8; treatment for addiction, 16, 39–40, 159, 181, 191–2, 194–5, 197, 220n18

I-Ching, 96

Illumination of the Buddha, The, 149

India, 31, 35, 51, 144, 166, 167, 199

Inner Space, 130

Island, 73, 135, 225n57

Italy, 104

Itkin, Michael, 88–9, 148, 149

Japan, 25, 38, 99, 151

Jofen, Jerry, 134–6

Johansen, David, 124

Jones, LeRoi, 33, 58, 96

Joplin, Janis, 34, 124

Josiah Macy Jr Foundation, 69

Kadis, Asya, 78

Kapralov, Yuri, 163, 165–6

Kaprow, Allan, 133

Kastor, Jacaeber, 193

Katzman, Allen, 97–8, 127, 129

Kefauver-Harris Drug Amendment, 79

Kennedy, Robert, 226n61

Kerouac, Jack, 19, 27–9, 33, 34; discovers psilocybin, 46–8

Kesey, Ken, 8, 9, 10

Kessler, Stephen, 158

King, Martin Luther, 183

INDEX | 261

Klein, George, 71
Kleps, Art, 12, 38, 170–2
Knauer, Alwyn, 63
Koota, Aaron, 155, 157–8
Kring, Walter, 148–9
Krippner, Stanley, 74, 83, 100,
110, 120, 136, 143, 147, 151, 202;
discovers psilocybin, 57–8
Kusama, Yayoi, 151–2

L.S.D. (... Just the High Points ...),
192–3
Larocca, Peter, 144
League for Spiritual Discovery,
114–15, 120–2, 133, 146, 148, 150,
173, 184
Leary, Jack, 43
Leary, Marianne, 43
Leary, Rosemary (née Woodruff),
115, 117, 141, 168–70
Leary, Susan, 43
Leary, Timothy, 5, 63, 67, 73, 78,
80, 89, 90, 160, 173, 175, 184, 185,
204, 212n57, 220n18, 244n2);
and Isaac Abrams, 139, 141; and
alcohol, 43, 117, 147, 149, 155; and
Burroughs, 57; and Cassady,
45–6; Experiential Theater
Evening, 143–4; and film, 149–50;
and Friedman, 52–3, 54–6, 58–61;
and Graboi, 111–12, 114–18, 122,
147; and Peggy Hitchcock, 90;
and Huxley, 44–5, 52–3; and jazz,
51–3, 55, 106, 144; and Kerouac,
46–8; legal issues, 5, 10, 112, 146,
168, 178; and LSD, 87, 171; and
the media, 12, 13, 15, 53, 54, 87,
91, 115, 117 ; and mescaline, 49;
and Millbrook, NY, 6, 15, 92,
122, 139; narcissism, 55, 116–17,
131, 219n9; and the prisoner
rehabilitation experiment,
52–3; and psilocybin, 14, 42–3,
44–62, 85, 170; Psychedelic

Celebrations, 17, 133, 146–9; and
The Psychedelic Experience, 92;
and the psychedelic movement,
7, 9, 15, 16, 44–62, 90, 93, 103,
106, 107, 114–18, 133, 161, 168,
170, 174, 191, 197; and sex, 43, 50,
51–2, 229n109; and spirituality,
46, 67, 92, 108–9, 110, 112, 114–15,
122, 145–6, 147–9, 171; and USCO,
144–5; and Wasson, 55–7; and
Rosemary Woodruff, 115, 141, 147
Lent, Norman, 158
Levy, Murray, 121–2
Life magazine, 9, 14, 34, 42, 57, 78,
87, 157
Limelight, 194
Lincoln Center for the Performing
Arts, 133, 156, 192, 238n83
Lindsay, John, 124, 133, 134, 183
Loeb, Eric, 36, 87
Long Island, 157, 227n84
Los Angeles, 38, 68, 108, 109, 112, 123
Lotsof, Howard, 11, 16, 181, 191–2,
194–5, 197, 199; convicted for
possession, 159; discovers
ibogaine, 39–40; meets Isaac
Abrams, 137
Lowe, Bob, 149
Lowell, Robert, 48–9
Lowinger, Paul, 80–1
Lownes, Victor, 74
LSA, 39
LSD, 16, 17, 39, 40, 54, 62, 110, 112,
131, 173, 181, 191, 196, 197, 199,
200; and alcoholism, 67; and
art, 132, 138–9, 141, 150, 151, 154,
181, 185, 187, 192–3, 201; and
autism, 64, 69, 70; in California,
5–6, 8, 113; and the CIA, 65–7,
69, 85; controversies, 10, 80–1,
82–3, 91–2, 115, 155, 157–8, 172;
counterculture, 106–7, 114, 119–
20, 174, 191; decline in quality, 10,
161–2; and depression, 73, 77–8;

262 | INDEX

distribution, 104–5, 124, 125–7, 129, 136, 158, 159–60, 162–3, 164, 172–3, 176, 181, 184–5, 186, 190, 192, 194, 195; early non–medical uses, 9, 87–97, 141; early research, 9, 63–5, 65–7, 68; effects of, 11–12, 14–15, 69–70, 72, 74, 75, 77, 82, 86, 88, 92–3, 102–4, 108, 125, 127, 150, 151, 154, 160, 161, 169–70, 174, 177–8, 184, 185–6; historical overview, 6–7; and hypochondria, 79; and labouring, 78; and the media, 13–14, 15, 86–7, 127–31, 157, 158, 172; and migraines, 69; and nature, 182–4, 201; and nightlife, 11, 100, 176, 187–8, 194; and parapsychology, 67; and the police, 120, 158–9, 181, 185, 190, 192, 195; and politics, 107, 133; and psychoanalysis, 64, 71–2, 74–5, 76–7, 82, 84, 138; and psycholinguistics, 81–2, 84, 85; and psychosis, 63–4, 73, 84; regulation, 11, 79–81, 157–8; and religion, 115, 118, 121, 122, 144–6, 147–9, 150, 153, 178, 181, 184–5, 188, 201; replaces psychedelic plants, 45, 62; and sex, 83, 119; subculture, 100–3; users, 14, 17, 68, 70, 71, 88–91, 92–7, 100–4, 106, 113, 114, 116, 117–18, 121–2, 124–7, 142–3, 150, 151, 153, 157, 159, 160–1, 164, 167, 168, 169–72, 176, 177–8, 182–5, 188, 194, 195, 203–4; and youth, 13–14, 155–6
LSD-OM, 185
Luce, Clare Boothe, 14, 87
Luce, Henry, 14, 45, 87, 157, 199
Luhan, Mabel Dodge, 9, 16, 21–3, 24, 51, 199

Madison Avenue, 17, 74, 121, 149, 173–4, 178, 179, 199
Mafia, 31, 158, 160, 162, 164

Mailer, Norman, 53–4, 169
Malitz, Sydney, 70, 82
Maloney, William, 63
Mancuso, David, 11, 92, 187–8
Manhattan Island, 184
Manhattan State Hospital, 83
Manson, Charles, 186, 193
Marihuana Tax Act, 26
Martin, Tony, 100
Marzani, Carl Aldo, 76–7
Maslow, Abraham, 111–12
Massachusetts, 52, 88
Masters, Robert E.L., 81, 82, 83, 110, 113, 142, 143, 151, 196
Max, Peter, 174–5, 185
McLean, Jackie, 135
McLuhan, Marshall, 144, 175
McLure, Michael, 145
McNeill, Don, 117–18, 123
McReynolds, David, 107–8, 160–1
MDA, 66, 159, 161, 190, 194
MDMA, 17, 193–4, 200
Mead, Margaret, 71
Menninger Foundation, 71
Merck, 194
mescaline, 6, 7, 14, 19, 32, 82, 84, 134–5, 139, 146, 203; distribution, 36, 38, 49, 74, 101, 159, 163; in the media, 54; medical use, 54, 67, 78, 82–3; research, 9, 23, 54, 63–6, 67, 69, 71, 82–3, 85, 86; users, 38–9, 45, 49–50, 54, 74, 90, 101, 135, 136, 137
methedrine, 162
Metro Transit Advertising, 174
Metronome, 39
Metropolitan Museum of Art, 184
Metropolitan Opera House, 192
Metzner, Ralph, 91, 92, 112, 113, 117, 144, 147, 149
Mexican immigrants, 26
migraines, 69, 70
Millbrook, 6, 92, 114, 115, 116, 118, 122, 139, 144, 145, 146, 148, 149,

151, 169, 170, 171, 173, 182
Mingus, Charles, 51, 97, 106, 144, 149
moiré, 138
Monk, Thelonious, 50–1, 106
morning glory seeds, 16, 19, 39
Morningside, 105
morphine, 20, 23, 25
Mount Sinai Hospital, 39
multimedia art, 8, 132–4, 144, 146–7, 152, 176
multimedia light shows, 132–3, 144–8, 152, 175, 179, 194
Museum of Modern Art, 138

N-bomb, 196
Nagrin, Daniel, 97
Naiderman, Harold, 38
Naked Lunch, 57
National Institute for Drug Abuse (NIDA), 191, 194, 195, 197
National Institute for Mental Health, 71
National Science Foundation, 80
Native American Church, 146, 148, 186
Native American Indians, 23, 118
Natural Church, 96–7, 199
Neuman, Osha, 95
New Consciousness gallery-store, 122
New Jersey, 9, 45, 55, 62, 80, 104, 138
New Orleans, 20
New Riders of the Purple Sage, 186
New School for Social Research, 110, 113
New York Academy of Science, 86–7
New York Advertising Club, 115
New York City, as capital of the arts, 132–4, 141, 154; and crime, 20, 24, 28, 122, 156, 159–60, 163; during the Depression, 25; fiscal crisis, 8, 156, 180; as "fun city", 124; as a global capital, 7–8; immigration, 7–8, 20, 21, 22–3, 26, 31, 95, 109,

157–9, 166; and mental health, 64, 69; narcotic peak, 10, 165; pharmaceutical industry, 9, 18, 23–4, 39, 49; protest and activism, 11, 30, 76, 89, 95, 112, 128, 156, 169, 178, 181, 186, 191; and religion, 25, 29, 89; upper class, 90, 173
New York City Board of Health, 39
New York Dolls, 124
New York Medical College, 74
New York Neurological Society, 63
New York Psychoanalytic Institute, 21, 25
New York State, 26, 36, 83, 96
New York State Council on Drug Addiction, 10
New York State Department of Mental Hygiene, 84
New York State Psychiatric Institute, 63, 84
New York State Psychiatric Institute Department of Experimental Psychiatry, 63, 65, 70, 199
New York University, 71, 94, 123, 138, 166, 190, 195
Newsweek, 34, 128
Newton, Massachusetts, 44, 46, 60
nitrous oxide, 45, 163

On the Road, 28, 34
op art, 138–9
opium, 20–1, 23, 28, 32, 154
Orange County, 5
Orange Sunshine, 161, 166, 184–5
Orlovsky, Lafcadio, 45
Orlovsky, Peter, 34, 45, 49, 117
Osmond, Humphry, 41, 67, 71
Oster, Gerald, 138
Owsley Stanley III, Augustus, 8, 172

Pahnke, Walter, 110
Paik, Nam June, 151
Paradise Garage, 188

264 | INDEX

paraphernalia, 99, 125, 150
parapsychology, 29–30, 67, 85, 110, 111
Parapsychology Foundation, 29–30, 67
Parker, Charlie, 19, 24, 26, 27, 28, 51, 97
Parsifal, 192
Pau, Sylvia, 55
PCP, 185
Peace Eye Bookstore, 164
Pennes, Harry, 65
Perkins, Jeff, 88, 91, 97, 119
Perls, Fritz, 64, 73
Peters, George, 110
peyote, 7, 9, 16, 39, 41, 42, 44, 51, 86; and Buddhism, 37–8, 75–6; distribution, 36; effects of, 21–2, 36–8; in Greenwich Village, 18, 19, 21–3, 33; medical use of, 75–6, 78–9; and Native American Indians, 21–3, 136, 186; replaced by LSD, 88; users, 21–3, 36, 37, 45, 90, 136
Playboy, 74, 83
Playboy Club, 149
Playhouse of the Ridiculous, 142
police, 20, 22, 36, 40, 54, 95, 97, 120, 122, 126, 141, 156, 157, 164, 167, 169, 181, 194, 195
Polish National Home, 146
poppers, 189
portable camera, 151
Preminger, Otto, 150
prison, 5, 27, 28, 52, 90, 112, 158–9, 180, 190–1, 194
prostitutes, 20, 27, 28, 88
psychedelic art, 10, 49, 54, 83, 99, 100, 142, 143, 181, 183, 187, 196, 201; coined by Isaac Abrams, 132, 138; commodification of, 174–5; context, 133, 138, 154; first exhibition, 139–41; and politics, 133

psychedelic art survey, 143
Psychedelic Celebration, 144–9
psychedelic experience: and deconditioning, 108; and individual transformation, 74, 112, 132, 139, 142, 143, 203; and language, 52; meaning of, 12, 201; and set and setting, 14–15; and spirituality, 37–8, 67, 92, 106, 114, 118, 119, 145–6, 174–5; and therapy, 68–72, 74
Psychedelic Experience, The, 92, 93
Psychedelic Information Center, 130–1
psychedelic movement, 7, 12, 14, 41, 89–90, 118, 141, 144–5, 150; end of, 168–70; initiated by Leary and Huxley, 44–5
psychedelic nightclubs, 10, 100, 152, 176–8, 192, 199, 249n129
Psychedelic Peace Fellowship, 148
psychedelic rock, 8, 15, 152, 169, 175, 186, 189
psychedelic showcase, 121–2, 131, 174
Psychedelic Solution Gallery, 193
Psychedelicatessen, 125–7, 164
psychotomimesis, 63–5, 73
psilocybin, 7, 9, 15, 16, 17, 41, 43, 44, 45, 51, 56–7, 86, 90, 134, 200; effects of, 46–9, 52–4, 55, 58–61; marketed as Indocybin, 45, 46; in the media, 54, 57; mushrooms, 195; and music, 192; replaced by LSD, 62, 87, 89; research, 70, 80, 85, 110, 220n18; as a sacrament, 153; and sex, 51–2; and the upper class, 54–5, 170; Wasson coverage of, 42
Puerto Ricans, 31, 95, 163, 165
Pure Food and Drug Act, 21

quaaludes, 187, 189, 190
Queens, 64, 69, 160, 195
Quixote Bookstore, 32

raids, 36, 97, 126, 159, 164
Ram Dass, 167–8
Rapée, George, 52
Rappaport, David, 71
Rattiner, Dan, 97–8
Rauh, Ida, 22
Rauschenberg, Robert, 134, 141, 240n9
real estate, 14, 52, 53, 60, 86, 93–4, 156, 179, 200
Reincarnation of Jesus Christ, The, 148–9
religious freedom, 96, 144, 145–6
religious revival, 89, 93
Research Center for Mental Health, 71, 82, 138
Rinkel, Max, 63–4
Riverdale, 51
Riverside Church, 122
Riverside Museum, 144
Robbins, Jerome, 147
Robbins, Trina, 127
Robinson, Carolyn, 28
Rockefeller Drug Laws, 180
Rollins, Sonny, 19
Rosenfeld, Ed, 35, 37, 40–1, 42, 88, 92, 96–7, 114, 115
Rosset, Barney, 49, 50
Rothstein, Arnold, 24
Rotolo, Suzan, 95
Rubin, Jerry, 5, 169
Rumsey, Charlie, 173
runaways, 31, 123, 156–7, 164, 165, 166, 202

S.B. Penick, 39
Sabina, María, 136
Sacred Mirrors, 187
San Francisco, 5, 8, 20, 104, 109, 123, 128, 149, 198
San Remo Café, 24, 28–9
Sand, Nick, 136, 172–3, 184, 185
Sander, Ellen, 35, 105

Sanders, Ed, 128, 164
Sandoz, 9, 11, 13, 45, 55–6, 58, 62, 65, 70, 74, 80–1, 82, 87, 92
Sandoz Foundation, 81
Sansert, 70
Saperstein, Henry, 243n73
satori, 29, 48
Scheinbaum, Stanley, 143
Science, 80–1
Scientology, 244n10
Scully, Tim, 172–3, 184
Seitz, William, 138–9
set and setting, 14, 15, 46–7
Shankar, Ravi, 150
Shelton, Gilbert, 129
Sheridan Square, 32, 53, 94, 189
Siegel, Eric, 151
Sinclair, John, 237n65
Sisko, Bob, 191–2
Skidoo, 150
Sklar-Weinstein, Arlene, 138
Smith, Jack, 135–6, 142
Smoke-ins, 253n62
Sokei-an Sasaki, 25, 29
Solomon, David, 38–9, 40, 53–4
South Bronx, 27, 185, 191
speedball, 33–4
Spiegelman, Art, 129
spiritual awakening, 29, 37, 91, 93
spiritualism, 22, 89
Spring Grove State Hospital, 65
St Marks Place, 98
St Regis Hotel, 142
Stafford, Peter, 103, 130
Stampfel, Peter, 36–7
Staten Island, 40
Steppenwolf, 146–7
Stern, Gerd, 43, 133, 151, 196; and cannabis, 28; collaborates with Leary, 144–5
Stern, Rudi, 133, 145, 175, 177, 199; collaborates with Leary, 146–8; rift with Leary, 149–50
Stevenson, Borden, 176, 178

266 | INDEX

Stickney, Chad, 185
Stoll, James, 89
Stonewall Inn, 53, 156, 188
Storyk, John, 152
STP, 10, 162
students, 13–4, 27, 36, 68, 70–1, 91, 101, 104, 110, 138, 157, 159, 190, 195
Summer of Love exhibition, 196
Sunshine Girl, 129
Susskind, David, 87
Suzuki, D.T., 29
Swallow, Steve, 144
Swing Rendezvous, 30–1
Synthetic Drug Abuse Prevention Act, 196

tabloid, 13–4, 34, 129
Tate Liverpool, 196
Tavel, Ronnie, 142
Teague, Howard, 74
Temple of the True Inner Light, 193
thalidomide, 79
theological art, 239n7
Third World, The, 149, 182
This Week, 42
Thompson, Hunter S., 198
thorazine, 102
Time magazine, 9, 14, 34, 68, 87, 110, 128, 130, 138, 157
Timothy Leary Defense Fund, 112, 168
Tocqueville, Alexis de, 203
Tomorrow, 30, 67
Tompkins Square Park, 98, 105, 125, 127, 128, 129, 137, 163, 166, 167, 186
Town Hall, 155
transcendentalism, 203
trauma, 14–5, 65, 66, 67, 76, 113
Travia, Anthony, 158
Trilling, Diana, 147
Trilling, Lionel, 147

Ukrainians, 31, 167
UML-491, 70
Underground Press Syndicate, 129

underground therapy, 7, 85
Underground Uplift Unlimited, 99
United Nations, 60, 196
United Nations Convention on Psychotropic Substances, 196
United States Public Health Service, 70
upper class, the, 9, 16, 41, 43, 45, 51, 54, 61, 89–90, 141, 142–3, 157, 169–73
Uris Brothers, 52–3, 60–1
USCO, 133, 144–5, 151

Vaccaro, John, 142
Varieties of Psychedelic Experiences, 81, 83
Veterans Administration, 80
Vietnam, 107, 133
Vigus, Larry, 152–4
Village Gate, 169–70, 175
Village Theater, 127, 147, 186
Village Vanguard, 26, 94, 144
Village Voice, 9, 12, 98, 102, 117, 127, 139; and drugs, 53, 124–5, 128, 130, 162, 189–90
Vollmer, Joan, 27
Volstead Act, 24
von Schlebrugge, Nena, 141

Walker, Peter, 147
Wallace, Mike, 55
Warhol, Andy, 141, 154, 196
Washington Square Park, 23, 25, 29, 88, 94, 105, 111, 113, 119, 124
Wasson, Gordon, 42, 44, 70, 145; rift with Leary, 55–7
Wasson, Valentina, 42
Watt, James, 77–8
Watts, Alan, 29, 58, 90, 110, 113, 144, 169
Weed, Susun, 125–6, 164, 201
Wescott, Roger, 75
Westchester County, 123
White, Joshua, 161

White Horse Tavern, 24, 116

Whitney Museum of American Art, 17, 196

Wilcock, John, 53–4, 98, 129, 166

Wilfried, Thomas, 132, 146

William Alanson White Psychoanalytical Institute, 25, 26, 76, 82, 84

Wilson, Bill, 67

Wolf, Van, 54, 90, 113, 139, 171, 173

Wolfe, Tom, 8–9

Woodstock, NY, 136, 182–3, 187

Woodstock Festival, 161, 185–6

Wooster Group, 192–3, 197

working class, 8, 20, 23, 86, 95, 157, 163, 178, 191, 197, 200, 214n34

Yablonsky, Lewis, 125, 182

Yalkut, Jud, 151–2

Youngblood, Gene, 153

Zazen, 34

Zen, 25, 29, 33